Eli Lilly: A Life, 1885-1977

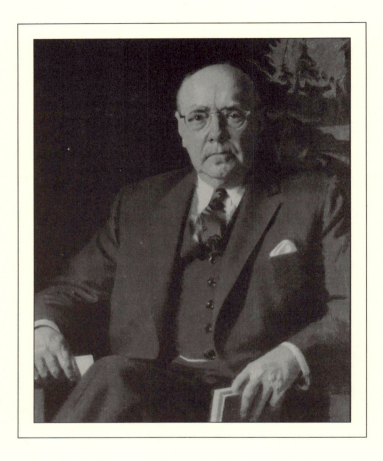

Copy of 1959 portrait by Joseph Allworthy, located at the Indiana Historical Society.
The original is owned by the Lilly Endowment, Inc.

Eli Lilly: A Life, 1885-1977

James H. Madison

Indiana Historical Society

Indianapolis

1989

The paper used in this publication meets the minimum requirements of American National Standard for Information Sciences—Permanence of Paper for Printed Library Materials, ANSI Z39.48-1984. ∞

Library of Congress Cataloging-in-Publication Data

Madison, James H.
    Eli Lilly, a life, 1885-1977 / James H. Madison.
        p.   cm.
    Bibliography: p.
    Includes index.
    ISBN 0-87195-047-2 : $29.95
    1. Lilly, Eli, 1885-1977.   2. Businessmen–United States–Biography.   3. Philanthropists–United States–Biography.   4. Eli Lilly and Company–History.   5. Pharmaceutical industry–United States–History.   I. Indiana Historical Society.   II. Title.
HD9666.5.L55M34   1989
338.7′616151′092—dc20
[B]   89-15261
                                                                                                    CIP

For Jeanne

Contents

Preface

"My whole existence has been rather humdrum," Eli Lilly wrote in his eighty-eighth year, "and I can't imagine who on earth would want to read even the best possible sketching of my life."[1] At first glance there is some temptation to accept Lilly's self-analysis. A wealthy businessman and philanthropist, he seemed conservative in his politics, traditional in his beliefs, and provincial in his attachments to Indiana and Indianapolis. He spoke in a soft voice and for decades went out of his way to avoid public notice, even of his many benefactions. By the popular standards of twentieth-century America, he was not a heroic figure. Short, plump, and bald, he appeared as an ordinary man.

Yet the image of a bland, humdrum existence disappears as understanding of the man grows and as realization develops that such an image derived from Lilly's sense of privacy and genuine modesty rather than from the life he actually led. One of the most obvious of many fascinations of his life centers on his accumulation of wealth. In his ninety-one years (1885-1977), Lilly earned many millions of dollars, nearly all in the pharmaceutical company his grandfather founded in 1876. Even more interesting than large sums of money, however, are the contributions he made to Eli Lilly and Company as it evolved from one among many small pharmaceutical businesses to one among a few giants in the industry. Eli Lilly led his company into the twentieth century, pushing it to become a big business not just in size but in manner of operation as well. Lilly energetically brought mass production, systematic management, harmonious labor relations, overseas expansion, and biochemical and pharmacological research to the Indianapolis company. These were the hallmarks of modern American business, and it was Lilly's vision in significant part that brought them to McCarty Street and thereby made the company he led one of America's most successful. While building a modern business Lilly attempted also to keep the rapidly growing firm close to the familial corporate culture his father and grandfather had nourished. In this he was largely successful, although new challenges of size and structure by the 1940s made it increasingly necessary to rely on the symbolic force of his own personal leadership, a force that would diminish but never expire as he withdrew from active management after 1948.

Lilly was certainly a very successful businessman, but the widening range of his interests contradicts images of narrow-minded pursuit of profit. In his forties he began stretching to wider horizons beyond the pill factory, seeking first in archaeology and then in history, historic preservation, and Chinese art diverse stimulation and companionship. In these and other areas he made substantial and enduring contributions as participant and patron. He was not an intellectual who engaged in abstract thought, but he became more thoughtful and intellectually disciplined than most businessmen and perhaps most academics. His active mind struck on large rather than small questions, ranging from the mysteries of a Delaware Indian narrative called the Walam Olum to the intricacies of character development and moral behavior in children. Some of his intellectual pursuits might be judged romantic, naive, and even foolish, but all showed a man passionately engaged in quests that were fundamentally important not only to him but to many others.

From his own life experience Lilly was convinced of the importance of family. His father, Josiah Kirby Lilly, Sr., was the polestar of his being, especially as a young man. His brother, J. K. Lilly, Jr., played an important role too. Eli Lilly also knew both marital happiness and unhappiness and the disappointment and frustration of loving a child whose behavior contradicted some of his strongest personal values. He knew too the experience of taking stock of his own life, of deciding in his early forties that he was not the person he wanted to be and setting out to change himself, to develop by force of will what he thought would be a proper outlook on life.

Contradicting also Lilly's profession of a humdrum existence were the many millions of dollars he gave away. Personally and through the Lilly Endowment he quietly became one of the major philanthropists of twentieth-century America, directing his wealth to religion, higher education, community services, history, archaeology, art, and other areas. He was different from many rich benefactors, however, for he stood personally at the center of his giving, actively engaged in setting agendas and passionately striving to ensure that his gifts would have consequences for others and even for the human condition.

_____

This is a narrative biography. It seeks to let Lilly's life unfold without intrusive analysis from the author. It fails, perhaps inevitably. Henry James advised, "Never say you know the last word about any human heart."[2] I certainly do not know the last word about Eli Lilly's heart. While he left thousands of letters and other documents and while it was possible to interview several dozen people who knew him, it was not possible to reconstruct accurately and fully this man's life. Like all biographers, I wish there had been even more evidence. But had there been ten times as many sources available, this complex life would not be fully revealed. Lilly's private and inner thoughts often can only be guessed. I have tried to allow the reader the freedom to think and conclude rather than force a particular meaning on the evidence. Yet this is not a perfectly objective biography, no more than any other biography. My own interpretation and occasionally my own heart shaped the selection and organization of material, sometimes subtly, sometimes more openly. I have tried neither to debunk Lilly nor memorialize him. I admire much that he did and thought but by no means all. Rather than burden the reader with my personal beliefs, however, I have tried to present a man I never met as honestly as possible, hoping that understanding and perhaps even some touching of human hearts will result for readers.

This is not an "official" or "authorized" biography. Neither the pharmaceutical company nor the Lilly family supported the project financially, nor did they seek to influence the making of the book. I am most grateful, however, to Eli Lilly and Company for allowing me free and full access to its well-organized archives. The company's enlightened policy in this regard is an essential prerequisite for serious study of twentieth-century American history and ought to be emulated by other institutions.

I am especially grateful to the Indiana Historical Society, which played a critical role in initiating and supporting this study. Former Executive Secretary Gayle Thornbrough and the Society's Board of Trustees, especially Herman B Wells, urged me to undertake this project, offering fellowship support for an academic year and research expenses. The time free from teaching and other responsibilities and the encouragement from Gayle

Thornbrough and her successor, Peter T. Harstad, have greatly assisted in my work.

During the last year of research and writing I was appointed the Fischelis Scholar of the American Institute of the History of Pharmacy, located at the University of Wisconsin. This fellowship allowed additional opportunity to devote full time to the book. I am grateful to the Institute and its head, Gregory J. Higby, not only for this financial support but also for the expression of confidence in a newcomer to the field.

One other institution played a major role in making this book possible. Indiana University provided sabbatical leave in the fall of 1984 and a summer faculty fellowship in the summer of 1988. Equally important was the university library. As I followed the many and diverse trails of Lilly's life I became ever more conscious of the significance of a first-rate research library and knowledgeable reference librarians. I am grateful also to the history department, which allowed leave time to work on this project and which provided the collegial environment that helps make scholarship so joyful.

Many people have assisted in this book. Among my largest obligations are those to the several dozen people I sought to interview. All agreed to talk with me. They are listed, with dates of interviews, in the note on sources. Without their rich memories this would be a much poorer book.

Many other friends and strangers provided assistance and advice in the writing of this book. I am particularly grateful to Susan Conner, James E. Farmer, Gregory J. Higby, Ann January, Gene E. McCormick, John Parascandola, Christopher Peebles, Glenn Sonnedecker, David Vanderstel, and J. Reid Williamson, Jr. Among the several scholars who read individual chapters and made suggestions to improve them were James B. Griffin, Barry V. Johnston, James H. Kellar, C. Ellis Nelson, L. C. Rudolph, and John Swann. I am especially grateful to the historians and friends who read the entire manuscript: John Douglas Forbes, Ralph D. Gray, George Juergens, Anita Martin, Irene D. Neu, Martin Ridge, and Gayle Thornbrough contributed substantially in the revision process. The expert advice of these readers greatly improved the book, though none bears any responsibility for its shortcomings.

At the Indiana Historical Society Peter T. Harstad, Thomas A. Mason, Paula Corpuz, Kent Calder, Megan McKee, and Kathy Breen all read the manuscript and made numerous improvements. I am most grateful that the Society maintains a tradition of careful copy editing, checking of sources, and proofreading and thereby saved me from many large and small errors.

My largest obligations are, as always, to my family: to my grandmother and parents, who taught me the first steps; to my children, Julie and John, who provided the essential diversions; and to Jeanne, for whom this book is dedicated.

Note to the Reader

Wherever in text and notes the name Lilly is used without other identifying reference, it refers to Eli Lilly (1885-1977). His grandfather, of the same name, is designated by use of his Civil War title, Colonel.

Chapter 1

The Early Years, 1885-1907

"I am a great nut on family influence," Eli Lilly wrote near the end of his long life.[1] Indeed he was. In nearly everything he did family exerted its influence, from his career in the pharmaceutical industry and his activities in philanthropy to his pursuit of avocational interests and his struggles to develop a proper outlook on life. Grandparent, parent, wife, brother, child, aunt—all were intimately part of who he was and what he did. Such family influence is not unusual, of course, except that Lilly was uncommonly aware of the importance of family and of the fact that he himself was a "great nut" on the subject.

Lilly was born in Indianapolis on 1 April 1885, "causing great joy and creating great expectations in the families," his father later wrote, "for a new Eli had come."[2] In the style of many middle-class American families, he was the male heir, bringing joyous expectations and named therefore for his grandfather and for a long line of Eli Lilly men who had preceded him. His birth announcement listed his name as Eli Lilly, Jr.[3]

The patriarch of the Lilly family in 1885 was Colonel Eli Lilly. The title was not honorary. In 1862, at the age of twenty-four, he organized the Eighteenth Indiana Light Artillery Battery. His recruiting posters called for volunteers "who will fight manfully for our just and holy cause" and promised that this would be "the crack battery of Indiana."[4] The men who joined were Hoosier farmers, clerks, craftsmen, and students from Wabash College and Indiana Asbury (later DePauw) University. In the custom of the day they elected their captain, selecting Lilly. The battery eventually joined John T. Wilder's mounted infantry, the Lightning Brigade, and saw its first bloody action at the Battle of Hoover's Gap in 1863 and then at Chickamauga. Later Lilly joined the Ninth Indiana Cavalry as a major. Captured and imprisoned by Confederates, he was released and mustered out in 1865 as a colonel.[5]

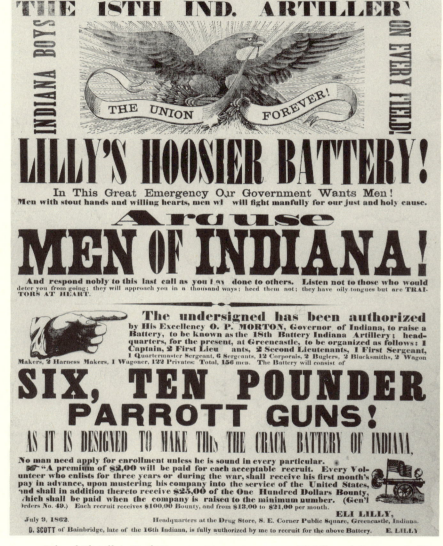

Colonel Eli Lilly's Civil War recruiting poster.   *Eli Lilly and Company Archives*

His grandfather's military career was a source of great delight for young Eli. Many Sundays he listened eagerly as the Colonel narrated stories of battles and skirmishes, following the action in a huge atlas spread on

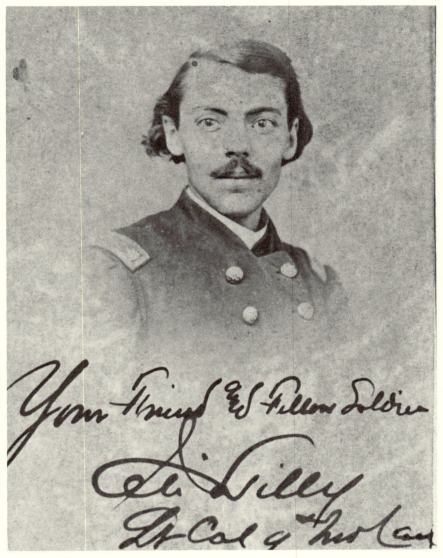

Eli Lilly, Civil War officer.   *Eli Lilly and Company Archives*

the floor. The highlight of Civil War memories came in 1893, when the Grand Army of the Republic held its annual encampment in Indianapolis. Tens of thousands of Union veterans and their families came to the city and joined in a huge parade and in smaller reunions of their regiments and companies. Colonel Lilly was chairman of the entire affair. But more impressive to the eight-year-old boy was the fact that his grandfather's home was headquarters of the Eighteenth Indiana Battery and the Ninth Indiana Cavalry. In the yard was a large tent, surrounded by red, white, and blue decorations and a great flag. Under that flag gathered the men the boy knew from his grandfather's stories. They sang Civil War songs and told their tales. One warm evening they gathered to listen to their old commander, Brigadier General John T. Wilder of the Lightning Brigade. It "was the high-water mark in the life of the wide-eyed, eight-year old," Lilly recalled.[6] The Colonel's grandson never abandoned his interest in the Civil War. Long after his grandfather was dead he corresponded with his men, some of whom addressed him as "Dear Adopted Comrade," and at least one of whom he supported financially. And he participated actively in the Indiana Commandery of Loyal Legion, a Civil War veterans group to which his father and grandfather had belonged.[7]

Lilly's grandfather and grandmother lived for a time only two doors south of his childhood home on Tennessee Street, and Eli often joined them for meals or a between-meal treat, such as a cracker heavily weighed down with butter and sugar. Great-Grandmother Eleanor Sloane also lived there, and Eli sat long hours with the elderly woman, listening to her scary stories of Indians as she recalled her childhood on the early nineteenth-century Ohio frontier.[8]

Though Eli did not fully understand it at the time, Grandfather Lilly was one of the most important men in late nineteenth-century Indianapolis. Earlier he had tried several business ventures without much success. He was an experienced chemist, working in the drug trade in Lafayette and Greencastle, Indiana, before the Civil War, and in Paris, Illinois, and Indianapolis afterward. In 1876 he decided to venture on his own. He obtained a small, two-story building on Pearl Street, a side street just off the city's main business avenue. Soon he was making sugar-coated pills, fluid extracts, elixirs, and syrups for sale in Indianapolis and surrounding communities. Although the new enterprise was one among hundreds of such concerns in Gilded Age America, it grew in size and scope. By the late 1880s sales exceeded $200,000, and the Colonel employed a hundred men and women and had moved to larger facilities on McCarty Street, in the city's expanding industrial south side. By now one of the most prominent manufacturers in Indianapolis, Colonel Lilly also became one of its most civic-minded residents. He was the driving force in organizing the

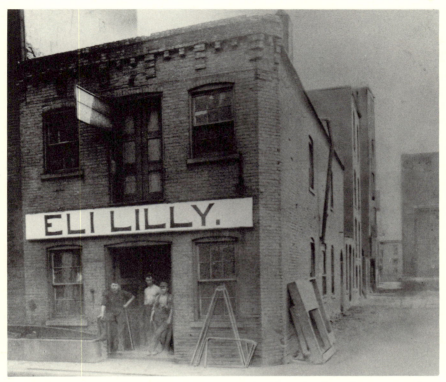

The first laboratory, opened at 15 West Pearl
Street, Indianapolis, 1876.   *Eli Lilly and Company Archives*

Commercial Club in 1890, dedicated to improving the well-being of the
city through such means as street paving, new sewer facilities, and improved
railroad crossings. And he was supportive with his time and money in
charitable and relief activities, particularly in organizing assistance to the
large number of unemployed citizens during the depression that began in
1893. A summary of his career a few years after his death in 1898 concluded
that Colonel Lilly "did not have a superior among his contemporaries either
in the practical achievements of business or in the civic pride and energy
which have made Indianapolis a great city."[9]

Colonel Lilly's heir was Josiah K. Lilly, his only son, born 18 November 1861. He had a loving but unsettled childhood. His father was away
in uniform during his first years, and his mother, Emily Lemon Lilly, died
in 1866. Josie, as the family called him, lived for a time in Greencastle,

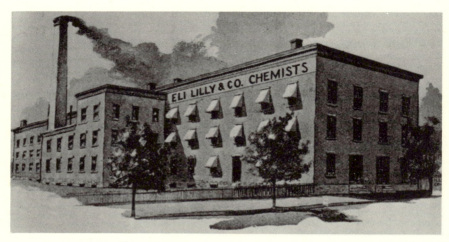

McCarty Street plant, ca. 1886.   *Eli Lilly and Company Archives*

Indiana, with his grandparents, Gustavus and Esther Lilly, staunch Methodists strongly opposed to slavery and alcohol. He was a shy and sensitive boy, frightened by hog butcherings and by the shouts of drunken farmers in the Greencastle streets on a Saturday night. When the Colonel married Maria Cynthia Sloane in 1869, Josie went to live with them in Paris, Illinois, and then in the mid-1870s to Indianapolis. In 1876, just a month after his father began his new pharmaceutical business, and not yet fifteen years old, Josie quit school and went to work full time in the Pearl Street plant. As was the custom of the time, the boy worked long and hard, ending the day so tired that he would sometimes fall asleep at the dinner table. As the business improved, the Colonel decided that his son and the new company would both benefit from more technical expertise. In 1880 he told Josie that he had decided to send him to the Philadelphia College of Pharmacy. "The Cinderella of the laboratory felt himself a prince," J. K. Lilly later recalled. He was an excellent student and greatly enjoyed the two years of pharmacy school. He received a first-class education, one that not only hardened his commitment to pharmaceutical manufacturing but also gave him tools to carry the business beyond the beginnings made by his father. Soon after he returned to Indianapolis in 1882 J. K. Lilly became superintendent of the laboratory. By 1890, when the Colonel was more interested in civic activities, the son was de facto head of the growing company.[10]

While enrolled in the Philadelphia College of Pharmacy, J. K. Lilly became engaged. He had met Lilly Ridgely on a visit with relatives in

Lexington, Kentucky. She was his second cousin, born in Lexington in 1862. He later described her as "a beautiful woman, blonde, about five feet, six inches in height: of a merry, vivacious disposition; a devout Episcopalian with a keen sense of duty which she always discharged in full." She was not well educated, but she read extensively. On Josiah's twenty-first birthday, 18 November 1882, they were married.[11]

The first memories of the son born to this couple on 1 April 1885 were of the Lilly home at 476 North Tennessee Street. The house was brick, of Greek Revival style, with two stories and a small front porch. A picket fence separated it from the brick sidewalk. The front parlor and sitting room provided ample space for magic lantern shows. In the sitting room was a coal-fired stove, next to which were the preferred seats on cold winter days. Gas fixtures provided illumination for evening games and reading. The boy slept upstairs in a small room next to his mother and father. His mother's sister, Aunt Margaret Ridgely, also had an upstairs bedroom. Upstairs too was the bathroom, equipped, unlike most homes of Indianapolis, with a flush toilet. The small boy was deathly afraid of owls, however, and believed that pulling the chain that released water from the large tank above the toilet not only caused a roar of water but might also set free a swarm of owls. "Each trip was a horrid adventure," he later recalled, and ended with a flight down the hall at full speed. There was also the alternative of visiting the small backyard structure with the customary half-moon cut in the door.[12]

Located in what was referred to as the "new north side," Tennessee Street (renamed Capitol in 1895 in honor of the new state edifice constructed eight blocks south of the Lilly home) was one of the most popular streets in Indianapolis. Many of the more prominent and prosperous residents of the city lived on the street, though it was not as grand as Meridian Street, two blocks to the east. North Tennessee Street was a genuine neighborhood where eggs and milk were borrowed and lifelong friendships were made. In his eighties Lilly could still name and remember something about nearly every family who had lived along the street in his youth. The wide street was lined with cottonwood and maple trees. On the sidewalks in summer

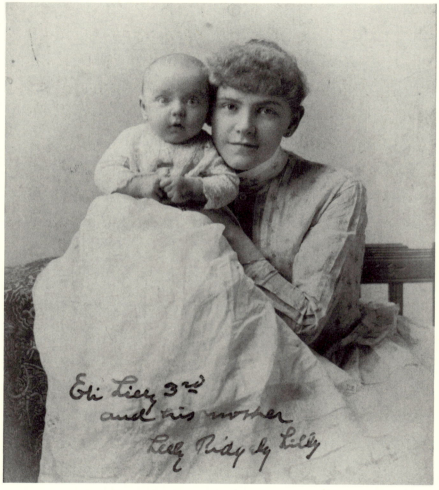

Eli Lilly and mother, Lilly Ridgely Lilly, 1885.   *Eli Lilly and Company Archives*

evenings Eli and the neighborhood children would play games and race tricycles, their shouts mixing with the sounds of two neighborhood girls practicing their piano lessons. As the sun faded, the lamplighter would light the gas lamps on the corner, the young boy would climb on the lap of his father, sitting on the front porch, and soon Papa would carry him to his bedroom. When the seasons changed, Tennessee Street became the site of sleigh races, and the boy thrilled to the whirl of the fast horses and handsome cutters flying down the street. Tennessee Street was also the route to Crown Hill Cemetery. Funeral processions often were wonderful spectacles, led by a brass band playing a slow and reverent piece to the cemetery and returning with a jaunty number, such as "A Hot Time in the Old Town Tonight." Throughout the year the boy, wearing his knee-length pants and sometimes the special red boots his Grandfather Lilly had given him, took short walks with his mother to the local bakery, sweet shop, and the family grocery. On occasion he accompanied his father to the Cathcart and Cleland bookstore on Washington Street, where J. K. Lilly was one of the best customers. Most Sundays the family attended Christ Church, the Episcopal church in the center of the city, where Eli was a choir boy.[13]

Indianapolis was the state's capital and largest city at the end of the nineteenth century. Yet in some ways it was still a small town, as its best-known writer, Booth Tarkington, so vividly portrayed it. "The members of this society live on terms of singular intimacy with one another, almost as in a village," Tarkington wrote in a 1902 essay. "When the warm weather begins one has only to stroll or drive about certain pleasant portions of the city during the early evening to see nearly all his friends, who will be lounging each on his lawn, or comfortably taking the air on the broad porches." Of course, Tarkington concluded, such intimacy "entails an amusingly large quantity of amazingly small gossip."[14] Tarkington's fellow Indianapolis author, Meredith Nicholson, conveyed a similar view of the city, describing it as "neighborly and cosy, . . . a place of industry, thrift, and comfort, and not of luxury," inhabited by people who were "home-loving and home-keeping."[15] There were some pretensions toward high society, however, most evident in the social directories that began to appear near the end of the century. In formal Victorian tones these blue books and red books set out rules for dinner parties, theater attendance, and social calling. "A formal call should not exceed a quarter of an hour," the *Red Book of Indianapolis* for 1895 admonished. In these directories men and women listed their clubs and the days women would be home to receive callers. Eli's grandmother chose Mondays as her reception day. His mother did not specify a day.[16] There was also the May Festival, the climax of the city's social season. Colonel Lilly was director of this musical extravaganza, and he and other gentlemen attended in white tie and tails, while the ladies, his grandson later wrote, "dressed within an inch of their lives."[17]

Indianapolis had been laid out on a grid pattern in the early nineteenth century, broken by four diagonal streets that extended out from the center, which was known as the Circle. On the Circle at the end of the

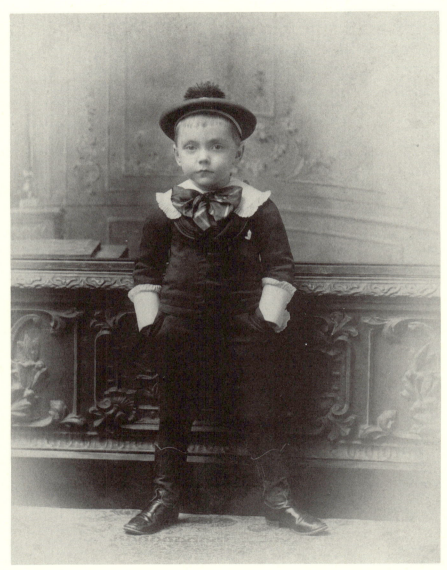

Eli Lilly, ca. 1890, wearing the red boots given   *Eli Lilly and Company Archives*
him by Grandfather Lilly.

century rose the Soldiers and Sailors Monument, which, along with the new state capitol two blocks to the west, was the best-known landmark in the city. Visitors to Indianapolis would arrive at the newly built Union Train Station and soon be shown the Circle, the statehouse, and the north-side neighborhoods in which Tarkington, Nicholson, the Lillys, and nearly all other of the more prosperous families lived. Newcomers would probably not see the poorer neighborhoods where the city's black residents lived, nor the small cottages that housed the German, Irish, Italian, and native-born workers, most of whom lived south of the Circle. Nor would they likely tour the stockyards, packinghouses, factories, and warehouses on the south side. Only very interested friends visiting the Lillys would likely travel through this commercial-industrial area to see the family pharmaceutical business, seven blocks south of the Circle.[18]

The Hoosier capital was growing rapidly at the turn of the century. Its population increased from 75,056 in 1880 to 169,164 in 1900 to 314,194 by 1920. New stores and offices lined Washington Street, new factories sprouted to the south, and new suburbs grew in all directions. And as Tarkington wrote in his best novel, *The Magnificent Ambersons,* "New faces appeared at the dances." The city was changing, Tarkington realized. It "was heaving up in the middle incredibly; it was spreading incredibly; and as it heaved and spread, it befouled itself and darkened its sky. Its boundary was mere shapelessness on the run."[19] Tarkington did not much approve of such changes—of the newcomers, the new suburbs, and the new industries, spewing black coal smoke that hung heavy over the city. In his resistance to change Tarkington reflected a judgment Nicholson made, that "Indianapolis was a town that became a city rather against its will."[20]

With urbanization and industrialization, Indianapolis experienced conflicts and challenges common to other American cities. But the edges were less jagged, the transitions more moderate, and the responses and remedies less radical. The city's population was far more rooted and far less transient than that of most other cities. Tenements and slums developed with economic and social change, but such housing conditions were not widespread compared to many other urban places. Single family home ownership remained very high, so that Indianapolis boosters who proclaimed that theirs was a "city of homes" were not exaggerating. Well into the twentieth century fundamental features of the town remained, particularly evident in a comfort in small-town ways and in a certain reluctance to change. This wariness of change Colonel Lilly and later cautious reformers discovered as they tried to address the needs of a growing city. In its moderation and caution, the capital was comfortably representative of the state's citizenry. Hoosiers generally tended to seek the middle of the road. Hoosier moderation permeated Indianapolis.[21]

Lilly's favorite spot outside Indianapolis was Lake Wawasee, located in Kosciusko County about 125 miles north of the state capital. Colonel Lilly began vacationing at the lake in the early 1880s and in 1887 built a cottage on the northern shore. His grandson first visited about 1888 and returned every summer until 1976. For an impatient boy in the 1890s it was a long train ride to the lake. Leaving early in the morning on the Big Four line from Union Station, the steam engine poured smoke and cinders as it slowly pulled the cars northward, stopping at every Indiana small town and finally at Milford Junction. There Wawasee-bound passengers changed to the Baltimore and Ohio line for the last few miles. Finally, the boy caught a first glimpse of grandfather's cottage and the lake, which was "every bit as good as Christmas morning," he later recalled.[22]

Once he arrived, there was everything to do. With Billy Kappes, Harry Hauser, and other boys, young Eli explored the three dozen miles of shore, roaming the woods and swamps and stealing apples from the Riddle orchard. But the lake itself provided the prime amusements. Swimming was usually on the day's agenda. So, too, was boating. His grandfather loved sailing and gave the ten-year-old a twelve-foot dingy with a spritsail. Fittingly named the *Alpha*, it was the first in a long line of sailboats Lilly would own. Billy Kappes had a similar vessel, and soon the boys were enacting great naval clashes from the War of 1812. On a cool, rainy day they enjoyed watching Jess Sargent in his woodworking shop as he repaired a sailboat or fashioned an object of wood. There were also books to read on such days. Eli's favorites were "The Gunboat Series" by Harry Castlemon. The set had belonged to his father, and young Lilly loved its tales of masculine adventure and Victorian virtue. He kept his favorite book in the series, *Frank, the Young Naturalist*, to the end of his life, as one of his "most treasured possessions," and could recite at will its opening lines. July Fourth was always the most special day at the lake. Grandfather Lilly made sure of an exciting celebration and provided the boys with strings of firecrackers. At dark Roman candles, pinwheels, and colored flares filled the sky over the lake. The most difficult day for the boy was Sunday. Grandfather and Grandmother Lilly strictly enforced their prohibition of sailing, fishing, and swimming and allowed no music other than hymns.[23]

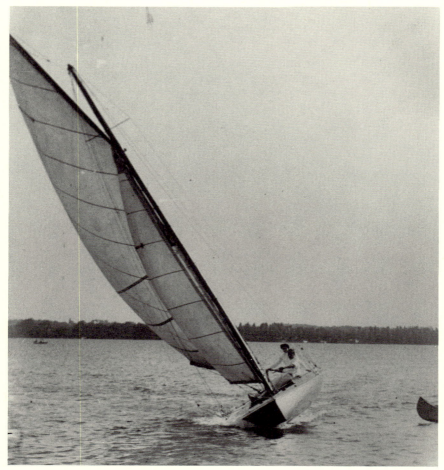

Eli Lilly and Aunt Margaret Ridgely sailing at   *Eli Lilly and Company Archives*
Lake Wawasee, ca. 1905.

There were other occasional trips for young Eli. In 1889 he traveled with his mother to Florida, where she recuperated from an attack of quinsy. Even more exciting was the trip to northern California with his father in 1895. After a long rail journey they rode the last miles in a dusty stagecoach, with Eli sitting much of the time on the high seat next to the driver. They arrived at their destination, Great-Grandmother Lemon's home, and soon joined in fishing, hiking, and social gatherings. An uncle surprised Eli with

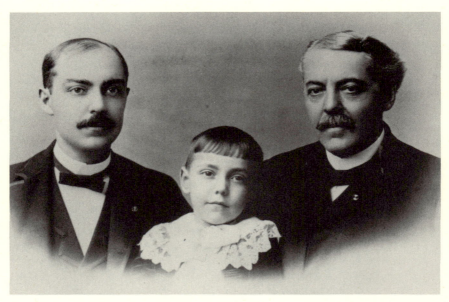

Three generations: Josiah K. Lilly, Sr., Eli Lilly,   *Eli Lilly and Company Archives*
Colonel Eli Lilly.

a gift of a pair of yellow chaps and a cowboy hat. From Modoc County father and son traveled to San Francisco, where they watched the sailing vessels in the harbor, rode the cable cars, and visited Chinatown. Later he traveled with his parents to Yellowstone and to the Adirondacks.[24]

With the exception of these trips and the summer vacations at Wawasee, Eli Lilly spent his childhood in Indianapolis. That childhood was filled with love and security, but was not without its rough spots. One came with the death of his grandfather in 1898, a strong blow to the entire family. The Colonel had been an important influence in Eli's life. Long after his death the grandson would remember him by such acts as placing in the wall of his new house a stone from the Colonel's Maryland birthplace. J. K. Lilly took full charge of the pharmaceutical company after his father's death and with the Colonel's widow, Maria Lilly, shared in the estate, which he gradually passed to his sons. Eli loved his father, too. J. K. Lilly had a kindly, sensitive disposition and a droll, whimsical sense of humor. He delighted in word play and parody, and he became one of the great admirers of fellow Indianapolis resident James Whitcomb Riley. Often J. K. Lilly walked through the house on Tennessee Street singing or whistling popular tunes from Stephen Foster and Gilbert and Sullivan or snatches of arias from *Rigoletto, Il Trovatore,* and other operas. J. K. Lilly participated in campaigns to improve the city's public schools and in local charitable ventures, but he did not have the driving civic interest of his father. His first love beyond his family was the pharmaceutical company, and he worked very hard to improve it.[25]

When his son was about eight J. K. Lilly moved his family to a larger home on North Pennsylvania Street, only three blocks east of Tennessee Street. It was a lovely residential neighborhood, home to some of Indianapolis's first families, including the Tarkingtons. Like other prosperous, north side families, the Lillys had hired help—usually young women from rural Indiana and Kentucky who did the cooking, washing, and ironing, and a man, Martin Clark, who for thirty years took care of the family horses and buggies and did other chores. Only about 5 percent of Indianapolis families at the turn of the century had such live-in help. Not far from the Lilly residence was the home of Benjamin Harrison, who had just completed his term in the White House. Eli later recalled the day he and friends accidently threw a ball through a window in the former president's carriage house.[26] But the event he remembered most vividly from the Pennsylvania Street home was the birth of a brother.

On 25 September 1893 a baby boy was born to J. K. and Lilly Ridgely Lilly. They named him Josiah K. Lilly, Jr. Eli was sent to his grandmother's house for lunch that day. In the afternoon he came home from school to deposit his books, eager to run outside again, for the boys of the neighborhood were in turmoil over the news that Court Van Camp's rabbits had escaped. As they organized scouting and recovery parties, their excited shouts penetrated inside the Lilly house, where Eli's father informed the boy that he had a new baby brother. After a quick visit upstairs to see the baby, Eli bolted to run outside, but his father grabbed him and forcefully sat him in a chair. By the time he was released the great rabbit hunt was over. "This was," Eli Lilly later recalled, "an inauspicious beginning of our relationship and was not strengthened by my parents always taking Joe's part in our childhood altercations. It was simply armed neutrality until we grew to appreciate each other properly."[27] Lilly remembered, on another occasion, that "my brother and I hated each other like poison until we were grown. He was 8 years younger and no matter what happened, being the younger, he always got our parents' ear."[28]

Eli and J. K. Lilly, Jr., did eventually develop a fraternal respect and affection for each other, though they grew up to be very different kinds of men who shared few interests beyond the pharmaceutical business. Their relationship as adults tended to be formal rather than casual and spontaneous. And there were hints even in adulthood of sibling rivalry. Eli, for example, made certain to inform the corporate historian in 1969 that a contribution he had made to improving human relations at the company in the 1930s "was absolutely independent from the brilliant work of Mr. J. K. Lilly Jr."[29] Eli did come to love his brother, but he never forgot or forgave the parental partiality he detected toward him in childhood. He did not blame his father. Indeed, among his personal papers are numerous references to his father, all in terms of respect and admiration. Even more revealing is the life Eli Lilly lived: it leaves no doubt that he loved his father and that his desire to please him was a guiding force of his life—a desire perhaps intensified by the presence of a brother named after their father.

In the thousands of pieces of paper Eli Lilly left as record of his life there is not a single, revealingly significant mention of his mother. Always his references to her in correspondence and memoirs were short and formal. A chapter about his life written in the early 1970s for the internally produced history of the pharmaceutical company, which Lilly read and approved, makes no significant mention of Lilly Ridgely Lilly. He seldom talked about his mother, even to close friends and associates. When he did, on only a few occasions, he indicated that not only did she shower her attention and love on her younger son but that her discipline of the older boy was strict, erratic, and unpredictable. Sometimes she hit him with a hairbrush, he remembered. It stung all his life. He felt unloved by his mother.[30]

Some of the affection that might have gone to his mother young Eli directed toward his Aunt Margaret. Orphaned at the age of fourteen, Margaret Ann Ridgely moved in with her sister's family on Tennessee Street. She never married. Eli grew to adore her as a source of comfort and counsel. She mediated fights with his brother without always taking Joe's side. She listened sympathetically to his pangs of adolescent love. As late as 1927 she addressed a letter to him as "Dearest Bub Eli," a family childhood nickname. In his "Reminiscences" he referred to her often as "Dear Aunt Margaret Ridgely." On her death he established a memorial library for her at Christ Church. And in the history of that church, which he wrote in the 1950s, he called her "a real saint" and wrote that "doubtless God could have made a better aunt, but doubtless he never did."[31]

School joined with family and neighborhood to form the great triad of Eli Lilly's childhood. His school days were generally happy and successful, leaving many warm memories. They began in 1890 in Nora Farquhar's kindergarten, located on North Pennsylvania Street. Eli and the other children learned spelling with lettercards, wove strips of colored paper, molded clay, and sang such songs as "Good Morning Merry Sunshine." Many of these children remained Lilly's lifelong friends. In 1951 he organized a sixtieth reunion for the class. Nineteen attended and received a booklet Lilly had printed with their names and the songs they had sung in 1890-91. Included also was a class photograph, which the 1951 gathering imitated, with Lilly sitting again in the shy, downward looking pose of sixty years earlier.[32]

From kindergarten Lilly moved to School Number 2, later named the Benjamin Harrison School, located eight blocks from his North Pennsylvania Street home. Among his fondest memories of his first eight years of public school was reading about the Trojan Wars, which sparked all manner of debate as he and his friends walked home. Lilly regretted that he did not learn how to spell in these years. Throughout his life, he thought, his spelling remained "hilarious." He was especially fond of Jane Graydon, a teacher who "had an unusual element of freshness, and electricity of the spirit" and who "inspired me out of my arithmetic slump to make a perfect grade on my final test."[33]

In 1900 Lilly entered Shortridge High School, one of two in the city at the time. He got off to a slow start, with four Cs at the end of his first term. His father decided to send Eli to Culver Military Academy in northern Indiana. He returned to Shortridge after an unhappy term at Culver and received in this Indianapolis public school an excellent education. Lilly was not a brilliant student but did above average work, especially in his last two years. He found Latin very difficult but liked geometry and history. He also took classes in English, government, biology, chemistry, physics, and art. Lilly thought the faculty outstanding, and indeed they were, for Shortridge was well on its way to acquiring a wide reputation as one of the finest public high schools in the nation. Decades later he still remembered most of his teachers. There was English teacher Charity Dye: "I can just see her reciting with closed eyes one of her favorite quotations from Henry Van Dyke, 'A little that is pure is worth more than much that is mixed.'" And there was Laura Donnan who taught government—"a host in herself who could and would crack her bull-whip at the first suggestion of injustice or unfair dealing." "Surely if there was any good material in our

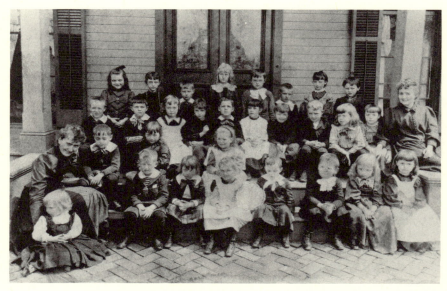

Farquhar kindergarten class of 1891. Eli Lilly is in second row, far left.   *Eli Lilly and Company Archives*

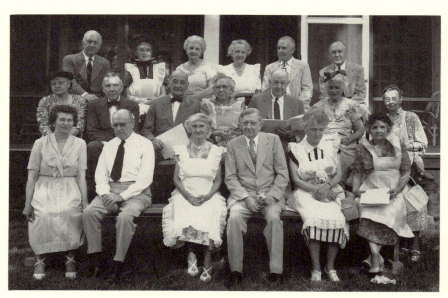

Sixtieth reunion of Farquhar kindergarten class, with members taking position and pose of 1891 photograph.   *Eli Lilly and Company Archives*

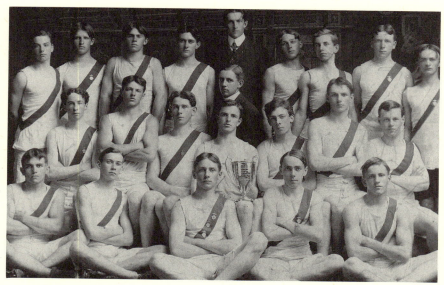

Shortridge High School track team, 1903. Eli   *Eli Lilly and Company Archives*
Lilly is in front row, second from right.

high school companions," Lilly recalled, "these fine teachers could bring it out."[34]

At Shortridge Lilly participated in the wide range of activities the school offered. There were dances and plays and social fraternities, one of which he joined. For Lilly and many of his peers the greatest enthusiasm was for athletics. He attended most events and participated in some. He was not much of an athlete, but he did make the football team as a substitute halfback, standing 5 feet, 9 inches and weighing 135 pounds. His athletic career peaked when he won a school letter in track for his performance in the hurdles. Lilly was well liked by his peers; they elected him president of the 1903 junior class.[35]

At about the age of fifteen Lilly developed two strong interests—astronomy and girls. He began to study the constellations with an energy and care that would reappear later in other avocational pursuits. In several scrapbooks he made in 1900 and 1901 he carefully pasted newspaper and magazine articles, using as one of his general sources a book titled *Popular Astronomy*.[36] But interest in stars began to fade in the brighter light of female beauty. In his second year at Shortridge he was smitten with Isabel Gates, who gave him a lucky dime to put in his shoe for the track meet in which he won his letter. Such a good omen did lead to romance, but not with Isabel Gates.[37]

When Isabel invited Eli to watch her play in a basketball game against the girls of Knickerbacker Hall, a private school, he readily accepted. But at the game it was the forward on the Knickerbacker team who took Lilly's fancy. She was beautiful, and he already knew her. Evelyn Fortune was the older daughter of William Fortune, who had worked closely with his grandfather in organizing the Commercial Club, in planning the GAR encampment of 1893, and in other civic projects. Eli soon learned that Evelyn would be spending the summer at Lake Wawasee. Her father and Wawasee carpenter Jess Sargent had built a large, two-story houseboat for the Fortune family's vacation there. Soon after the Fortunes arrived at the lake, Eli came to visit, bringing a dinner invitation from the Lillys. That summer and the next several summers Eli and Evelyn sailed, swam, and went for walks. Sometimes they attended dances at the Wawasee Inn. One summer she sewed a pennant for his favorite sailboat. They saw each other in Indianapolis, too. The Fortunes lived in Woodruff Place, a beautiful suburb northeast of the Circle. Eli would pick her up to go riding in his horse and trap. Sometimes they just sat in front of the fireplace or went for long walks among the ornamental statuary and fountains that adorned Woodruff Place. It was a quiet, happy courtship. Neither had had such a close relationship before.[38]

In addition to courting Evelyn Fortune and attending Shortridge High School, Eli directed his adolescent energy to the pharmaceutical company his grandfather had begun in 1876. As long as he could remember, the company was a part of his life. As a small boy he eagerly accompanied his mother in the family's fringe-topped surrey to McCarty Street to pick up his father. "Those were the days when we boiled a good deal of asafetida and other odoriferous things," he once recalled in a story told by his parents, "so when approaching the plant from downwind, my face would light up and I would say to Mother, 'Oh, Mama, I smell the business!'"[39] At the age of ten he began working in the plant during school vacations. He started washing bottles and eventually worked in nearly every department. One employee at the time later recalled that "from the beginning he endeared himself to the old employees because he did the dirty work of the department where he was employed just as cheerfully as the choice tasks."[40] Lilly himself later remembered that "it was my chief delight to go home to dinner thoroughly saturated with some evil odor that would cause my banishment from the table."[41]

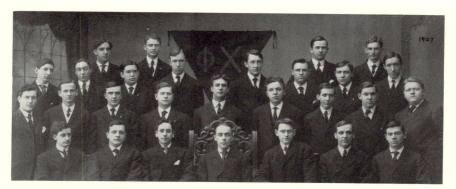

Eli Lilly, front row, center, president of his frater-   *Eli Lilly and Company Archives*
nity at Philadelphia College of Pharmacy, 1907.

Eli Lilly "was born into the business," he once said, and "never thought of doing anything else."[42] In the fall of 1904 he began a three-year course of study at the Philadelphia College of Pharmacy (PCP), the alma mater of his father. It was the oldest and perhaps most distinguished pharmacy school in the nation, founded in 1821. At the head of PCP was Joseph P. Remington, author of the first modern American pharmaceutical textbook and the leading figure in American pharmacy. Remington had been J. K. Lilly's teacher and invited his son to Sunday dinner. He showed the wide-eyed Lilly the room in which he was revising the *United States Pharma-copoeia,* the standard compilation designed to insure uniformity in the quality and therapeutic strength of medicinals. Lilly soon decided that his approach to learning at PCP had to be far more serious than it had been at Shortridge. He began to study hard and formed a habit he would follow the rest of his life of underlining his books in red ink. The effort brought rewards, for he finished his first year at the top of his class and repeated the honor his second year.[43]

Lilly worked hard at PCP, but there were some amusements, too. He joined several clubs and a fraternity and in his third year was elected its president. He visited the historic and cultural sights in Philadelphia and went for long walks in Fairmount Park and along Wissahickon Creek. His favorite recreation was the theater. At least weekly he and his friends rushed to get a first-row seat in the gallery, where they saw the great stars of American and English theater. Lilly especially enjoyed the light musicals. To the end of his life he could sing songs from the turn-of-the-century American stage. PCP also provided many personal and business friends, most notably Ralph Reahard, who joined his classmate in a long career at Eli Lilly and Company.[44]

Lilly was not entirely happy at PCP because Evelyn Fortune was hundreds of miles away. He sent her flowers, sometimes every week. Just before coming home for Christmas in 1904 his father wrote to promise that a hack would meet him at the train station "so you can drive over to Woodruff Place on the way home." In a letter to Aunt Margaret, Eli confessed that she had been replaced in his affections by Evelyn, though he assured Aunt Margaret that she, too, was "mighty sweet." At Wawasee he proposed marriage, and in 1906 they announced their engagement, with plans to marry soon after his graduation.[45]

Lilly graduated from the Philadelphia College of Pharmacy in 1907 with a degree as a pharmaceutical chemist. He had achieved a goal and was now prepared for a career, for marriage, and for adulthood. Though he had a youthful face, his hair was already beginning to thin on an inexorable march toward baldness. Reaching his twenty-first birthday a year before, he received a letter from his father, a letter of congratulations and of love of the kind J. K. Lilly, Sr., usually wrote to mark each 1 April. The senior Lilly sent with the letter a check for $2,712.07, which represented payment of Eli's $1,000 reward for not smoking before his twenty-first birthday and $1,712.07 as his share of income from his grandfather's trust fund. J. K. Lilly, Sr., also told his son that he would be elected to the board of directors of Eli Lilly and Company at the next election and that "if you want some stock in the Red Lilly I think it can be arranged."[46] But these monetary and business rewards came at the end of the letter. At the beginning, and doubtless more important to Eli, was the father's praise "that you have always been a *good boy*. You have never given us any concern as to your morals." And, J. K. Lilly continued, "I love you dearly and we must be the closest kind of partners as long as I remain with you."[47] The son honored his father's wish to the end of their lives.

Chapter 2

Into the Business, 1907-1919

In 1907 Eli Lilly entered the adult world. He graduated from the Philadelphia College of Pharmacy, joined the pharmaceutical company his
grandfather had founded and his father now managed, and married his
high school sweetheart. Happiness, achievement, and affection lay ahead,
as such a felicitous start in life might indicate, but the way was not always
easy or clear for young Lilly. There were shadows mixed with the sunlight.

Marriage to Evelyn Fortune brought large bursts of sun to his life.
The small, family wedding took place at noon on 29 August 1907 in the
library of the Fortune home in Woodruff Place. Afterward, the couple took
the train to the family cottage on Lake Wawasee, "the very best place" for
their honeymoon, Lilly's father told him.[1] J. K. Lilly, Sr., and William
Fortune were much pleased by the marriage of their children, for it united
families that had long been close. In the years to come the families often
exchanged visits and gifts, with Evelyn's father giving Eli such books as
The Federalist Papers and James Bryce's *American Commonwealth*.[2] The
young couple usually had a Sunday noon meal at the home of J. K. and
Lilly Ridgely Lilly and a Sunday supper with "Father Fortune."[3]

Eli and Evelyn lived the life expected of a young couple of their time
and circumstance. They settled first at 12 East Eleventh Street, in a house
with little charm, though it was near enough to novelist Booth Tarkington's
North Pennsylvania Street home to hear the noise of his parties. About
1912 they moved to the corner of St. Joseph and Meridian streets and then
in the early 1920s to Delaware and Thirteenth Street, where they lived in
a Victorian-style house next door to Evelyn's sister Madeline and her husband
Bowman Elder. All three homes were in the north side neighborhood of
Eli's boyhood and only a few blocks from his father and mother's home on
North Meridian Street. The young couple lived modestly, with Evelyn sewing
many of her own dresses, though like many middle-class Indianapolis

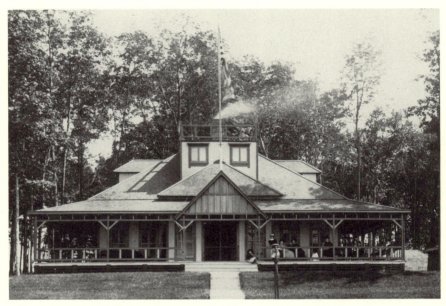

Lilly family cottage, Lake Wawasee.   *Eli Lilly and Company Archives*

families they had a hired girl to help during the day. They seldom traveled, except occasionally to meetings of the drug trade and once with William Fortune to visit Colonel Eli Lilly's Civil War battle sites in Tennessee. Their social life was restrained. They entertained a few close Indianapolis friends and only occasionally went out dancing. Eli did not care much for dancing, although he knew the steps of the day. His passion was sailing, a sport he indulged during their summer vacations at Lake Wawasee.[4]

Evelyn and Eli usually spent the month of August at Wawasee. They took the train to the lake, walking the last distance from the station to the cottage. Later, when Eli had a Ford motor car, they drove, meeting the challenges of flat tires and dusty roads. The cottage had hot water only on Saturday, when a fire was built under an outside water tank. There was no kitchen or dining room in the first years, so they ate all meals at the inn nearby. Later they converted a boathouse to a dining room. Nearly every day they would sail, often to Buttermilk Point, stopping at the spring house for a glass of cool buttermilk. In the afternoons they swam, though neither was an expert swimmer. Evenings they sat on the spacious front porch of the cottage, reading, sewing, talking, sometimes with friends from Indi-

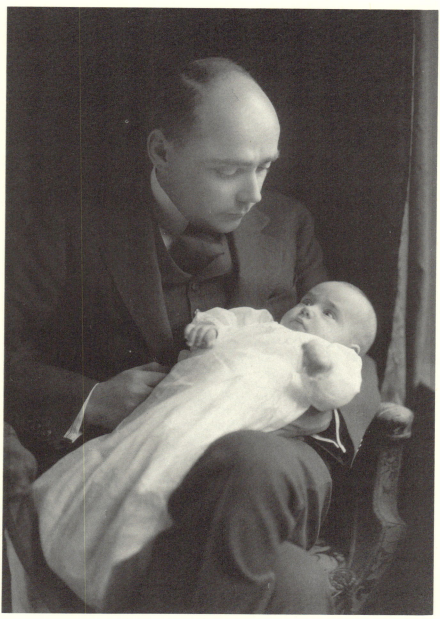

Eli Lilly, holding one of his two sons, both of whom were named Eli and both of whom died in infancy.

Eli Lilly and Company Archives

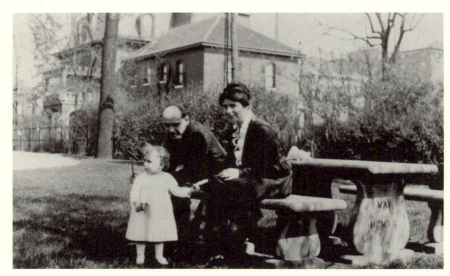

Evie, Eli, and Evelyn Lilly, ca. 1919.   *Eli Lilly and Company Archives*

anapolis, especially Bob and Mary Failey, who came to visit. On clear nights Eli would point out the stars and identify constellations by name.[5]

The only early shadow of sorrow fell soon after the birth of their first son. Born on 7 June 1908 and named Eli, the baby died a month later. A second son, also christened Eli, was born 25 March 1910 and lived only seven months. There were now two small stones near Colonel Lilly's monument in Crown Hill Cemetery, markers of two tragedies the father and mother never forgot. Despite their sorrow, the couple remained eager to have children. Evelyn had several miscarriages in the 1910s, and, after visiting a specialist in Boston, underwent an operation to correct a prolapsed uterus. To their great joy a child was born on 25 September 1918. They named her Evelyn but always called her Evie. Fearful for the survival of the prematurely born baby, they hired a full-time nurse to care for her. There would be no son to follow, however, no Lilly male to constitute their contribution to the fourth generation of the pharmaceutical family.[6]

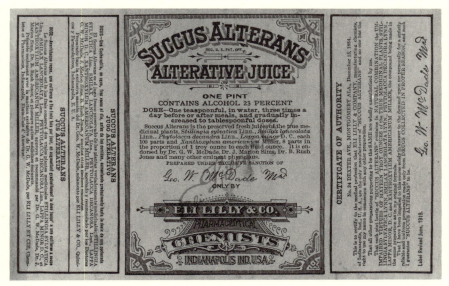

One of Eli Lilly and Company's best sellers at beginning of twentieth century.

Eli Lilly and Company Archives

In addition to his family and the pleasures of Wawasee, the great passion for Eli Lilly was the pill factory. The company and the industry he entered in 1907 were still very much like that his grandfather knew in the two decades after 1876. Plants provided much of the raw material for American pharmaceutical manufacturers; handwork constituted the primary method of production; research was limited largely to insuring uniformity and quality of the drugs; and unproved claims for efficacy provided the means of enticing consumers to buy the product. Eli Lilly and Company was a respected manufacturer, more careful in making and selling drugs than the patent medicine men of the era, but there was little sophisticated research on McCarty Street or anywhere else in the industry at the beginning of the twentieth century. Indeed, although the Indianapolis firm attempted to distance itself from the less reputable patent medicine makers, it remained ambivalent about scientific research. One of its best sellers at the turn of the century was Succus Alterans. Produced from a secret formula, purportedly derived from Creek Indians, Succus Alterans was sold primarily as a "blood purifier" and treatment for "syphilitic affections" but also recommended for "certain types of rheumatism and especially skin diseases like eczema, psoriasis, etc."[7]

The Indianapolis company in 1907 manufactured hundreds of drugs with a work force of approximately four hundred people. The business was small enough and simple enough for J. K. Lilly, Sr., to manage it largely unassisted. Supervision of employees, as one of them later recalled, "was a personal thing performed by word of mouth."[8] That task was easier because J. K. knew most of his employees by name and had close contact with every phase of the business. He was determined that the company would grow and prosper and that it would remain a family-run organization.

Father and son planned wisely for Eli's introduction to the business. There was no need to prove he could do the dirty work of washing bottles, cleaning out hogs' stomachs, or grinding foul-smelling pokeroot. That Eli had already demonstrated during summer work while still in school.[9] And rather than taking a job belonging to an employee or carving out a narrow corner of the operation, father and son agreed that he would become head of the newly created Economic Department.

The Economic Department consisted of a single desk manned by Eli Lilly. On 1 June 1907 he entered the job, fired with ambition to succeed. His task was to find ways to save money and introduce efficiency into the company. Roving through the plant, carrying his black notebook, the head of the Economic Department sought ways to cut costs as he learned the business of making drugs. His interest in mechanical devices often led him to the company machine shop, where he worked on new production equipment and soon became a "'spark plug' for mechanical gadgets."[10] One of his first gadgets was a bottle-filling machine. It filled bottles of varying sizes to an exact height, avoiding the spillover and waste of prior methods. Lilly designed the machine and oversaw its construction and installation. His father proudly noted in his annual report for 1907 that Eli's new bottling machine would save the company more than $7,500 a year.[11]

Other gadgets and production improvements sprang from the Economic Department. Lilly's precise quantitative studies in the Fluid Extract Department demonstrated that wooden barrels caused a loss through absorption of several pounds of alcohol. He installed copper-lined barrels, effecting a savings of $15,000 a year. He assisted also in installation of new pill-counting machines, which increased the speed of production and gave exact counts of pills. He investigated the merits of bottle labeling machines and the possibilities of making vaginal tampons. And for the company's powdered extracts Lilly designed a sloping shoulder bottle, which allowed an ordinary spatula to reach any part of the interior.[12]

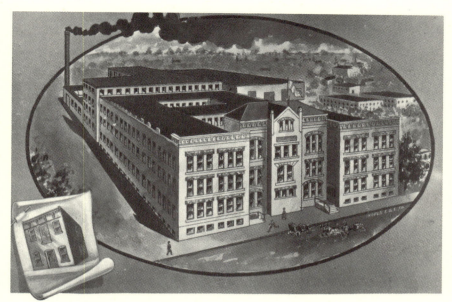

Eli Lilly and Company, 1905, with the Pearl
Street laboratory of 1876 in lower corner.

Eli Lilly and Company Archives

Lilly did not spend all his time on new products or gadgets to be
made in the machine shop. He also studied flows of production, attempting
to devise the most efficient methods of moving products through the plant.
As a result of his calculations he announced in early 1909 that the company
was purchasing chemicals in too large lots, bearing inventory costs that
were wasteful and unnecessary. His study of shipping proved that it was
less costly for the company to own its own drays than to hire this service.
Even more important was his plan to blueprint manufacturing tickets.
Drug manufacturing necessitated gathering, processing, and packaging large
numbers of items in great variety. To carry on production quickly and
accurately became a more challenging task as the company grew and as
the size of output increased. Lilly's blueprinted manufacturing tickets were
a major step in ensuring rapid and precise movement of a large volume
through production. Under his system the formula for a drug was type-
written on transparent paper, and multiple copies were made by blueprint-
ing process, each an exact duplicate of the original. These blueprint copies
were distributed to all departments and used to check each drug as it

moved through the department. Verbal instructions, handwritten notes, and individually typed orders gave way to this new system of blueprinted manufacturing tickets.[13]

The young head of the Economic Department spread his message of efficiency by word as well as deed. Six months after beginning work, he brought out the first issue of *Laboratory Notes*, a company publication designed "to establish good fellowship and the spirit of economy around the Lab."[14] In the first issue he suggested closer attention to turning off unnecessary electric lights and was soon gratified to see the savings effected. Again and again he emphasized that "business is made up of little things." Competition was so keen, he admonished, that "in many lines the margin of profit is so small that little savings or little wastes make all the difference between success and failure." He urged each employee also to take "pride in keeping the things in his charge as clean and neat as possible." [15]

For two years Eli Lilly's one-man Economic Department pushed out ideas and gadgets to cut costs and speed production. The pride of accomplishment for young Lilly was equaled only by that of his father. While vacationing at Wawasee in late summer 1909, Eli received a letter from his father, telling him that he had not written much "about business for I wanted you to be free as a deer and grow fat." But, the senior Lilly added, it was soon time to return, for on 1 September "you will be given charge of the manufacturing division."[16] The new responsibility was not only a promotion but also a commendation unsurpassed for a son eager to please the father he so loved.

───────────────────

Lilly's promotion to a full and responsible management position in 1909 came just as the company was entering a period of rapid growth and change. The new superintendent of the laboratory, as the manufacturing division was called, was at the center of this change and often out in front leading the enterprise in new directions. Well might his father write him from his Florida winter home in early 1911, "Dog on it boy where is the Old Biz going to."[17]

The period of expansion began in 1909. It was a year of record sales and profits. The board of directors approved four new buildings for the

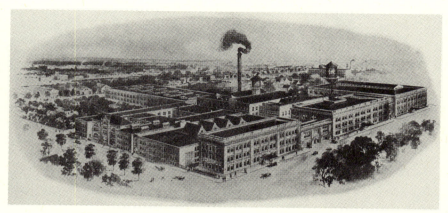

Eli Lilly and Company, ca. 1920.   *Eli Lilly and Company Archives*

McCarty Street plant. The first major addition was the Science Building (Building 14), completed in 1911. Laboratories occupied the second and third floors, and animal and sample rooms were located in the attic. Eli Lilly and other managers of the company had new offices on the first floor of the building.[18]

The other major addition was a new capsule plant (Building 15), opened in 1913. The manufacture of gelatin capsules had become an increasingly important part of the business, but it was a tedious and difficult process of hand labor and often produced capsules that stuck together or shattered. Eli Lilly effected some improvements in production by installing instruments to determine the temperature and specific gravity of the gelatin solution, rather than relying on the worker's guess, but demand continued to exceed the company's ability to produce quality capsules. A major change came in 1909 with installation of ten Colton automatic capsule making machines. Others were soon added. Completion of the new capsule plant allowed systematic layout of a battery of fifty machines and the introduction of air conditioning so that the humid Indiana summers would no longer cause a halt in production. In 1917 *Scientific American* devoted a full article to the wonders of "the largest capsule factory in the world," capable of producing 2,500,000 capsules a day. Capsule production soon exceeded the company's own requirements and provided sales to others in the trade, including abortive arrangements to sell capsules to Russia and Germany just prior to the opening guns of August 1914.[19]

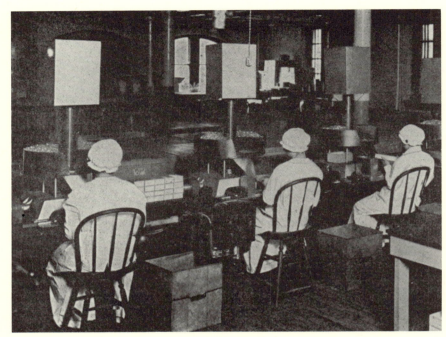

Gelatin capsule work at Eli Lilly and Company.   *Reproduced from* Scientific American, *117 (15 Sept. 1917): 194*

The automatic capsule machines and the new plant to house them were among the most visible signs of change at Eli Lilly and Company during the second decade of the century. Continued growth in output required relentless attention to the details of the business and to the overall system that organized those details. Such a system, Lilly came to believe, must move the materials quickly through the production process. "Our principal concern," he later wrote, "was with the time required for a given factory or laboratory operation. We wanted to perform the individual operation in less time."[20] To do this Lilly drew from his experience in the Economic Department and from his unusually large attention to the writings of management experts.

Exactly when Lilly began to read the books and articles written by scientific management experts is uncertain, but by the beginning of the second decade of the century he was well versed in their views of labor, production, and management. He read Henry L. Gantt, Frank B. Gilbreth, and, above all, Frederick W. Taylor, the founding father of scientific management. Taylor's major publication, *The Principles of Scientific Management*, Lilly later wrote, "had more vital influence on the history of Eli Lilly and Company than any other."[21] These experts had differing notions of the proper form for scientific management, but all stressed the need for rational, systematic analysis of the processes of production and of the means of managerial supervision and control. Responding to disorderly growth in size and complexity of American factories, management experts urged the substitution of what they described as scientific methods for the intuitive, rule-of-thumb methods that predominated in shops and factories. They advocated introduction of improved tools and machines to be placed and used in the most productive manner. Their prescriptions included also large attention to selection and training of workers. And they carefully studied each worker's task to determine the most efficient way to perform it and to ascertain precisely the amount of time required. To provide incentives for labor productivity, workers received, instead of hourly or piece-rate wages, bonuses based on their efficiency in meeting and exceeding standards. The tools of the scientific manager were many, but most ubiquitous was the stopwatch, symbolizing the orderly, scientific precision of the doctrine. Some workers and managers resisted the introduction of scientific management, fearing its dehumanizing tendencies and its potential to exact more work from them. Older employees were more likely to prefer doing their jobs in the old way, trusting to intuition and time-proven, seat-of-the-pants procedures. Younger workers and managers more often eagerly embraced the new doctrine.[22]

In early 1911 Eli Lilly formally introduced scientific management to McCarty Street. His work at the Economic Department was a prelude to the symphony of change he hoped to orchestrate. "Eli's stop watch scheme will surely wake things up," J. K. Lilly, Sr., wrote from Florida.[23] Armed with his stopwatch Lilly and his assistant, Ralph Reahard, began the search for the most efficient way to perform the innumerable tasks in the manufacture of pharmaceuticals. By systematic study they set methods and standards of output so as to reward efficient workers with bonuses rather than the piecework rates Taylor and his disciples so despised. Lilly and Reahard made one of their initial time studies in the Capsule Filling Department. Most of the workers were young women (always referred to as "girls"). The work was dirty and foul smelling, and tapping the capsules produced calluses on their fingers and often cracked the skin. Lilly and Reahard studied the task, agreed on the most efficient ways to fill the largest number of capsules, and concluded that following their method would enable an efficient worker to fill 8,568 capsules a day. Women meeting this standard would receive $1.16 for their day's labor. Lilly soon discovered, however, that his stopwatch had not allowed for human nature. In late 1912 he complained to the head of the Capsule Filling Department that when the time experiments were made we "thought the girls were working as hard as they could comfortably, but that was not the case as evidenced by the 2:30 and 3:00 sewing parties which go on." Change was necessary; henceforth, "no girl will be allowed to leave the department until 5:30 and must work up to that time steadily." Extra bonuses for capsules filled above the standard requirement encouraged women to continue working until quitting time.[24]

The new bonus system did not solve all the problems in the Capsule Filling Department. Many new workers were not immediately proficient enough to meet the daily standard and were likely to become discouraged and quit. Nevertheless, in the Capsule Filling Department and elsewhere Lilly saw welcome progress derived from the introduction of scientific management. His special pride was the Gelatin Coating Department, where time studies and a bonus system resulted in increasing workers' pay by 40 percent and their output by 90 percent. The new ways were not yet fully developed or implemented throughout the company, however.[25]

Two years into his campaign to introduce scientific management Lilly called on outside help. Seeking to find additional sanction and guidance for his program, he hired the Emerson Company to undertake an intensive study of the McCarty Street operation. Harrington Emerson was one of the nation's most popular exponents of scientific management. Less doctrinaire than Taylor and tending toward expedient promotional techniques, Emerson laced his gospel of efficiency with moral appeals to discipline, common sense, initiative, character, and fair play. His consulting company was based in Chicago but had offices in six cities and claimed a hundred employees. Often Emerson could claim success for his clients in improving plant output and raising wages for workers.[26]

The Emerson experts first visited McCarty Street in the fall of 1913 and after a month of study produced a 369-page report. The consultants praised the system of blueprinted manufacturing tickets and the bonus system already in place in the Gelatin Department. They strongly suggested elimination of piece rates still existing in some departments, to be replaced by a guaranteed wage for the worker and "a bonus incentive to constantly draw him on to better work in which he will use his head as well as his hands." The experts commended the new capsule plant as the best operation in the company and condemned the Elixir Department as the worst— "the general loafing place for the porters." They urged "more rigid discipline" of workers but also suggested increase in the average pay. And they noted that the company policy of allowing workers with five years experience a week of annual vacation with pay was unusually generous, since most American factories allowed no paid vacation to employees. Finally, they included many pages of stopwatch data from their time studies, arranged by specific drug and operation.[27]

Lilly was pleased with this preliminary report. As part of his campaign to convert his brother, J. K. Lilly, Jr., to the cause of scientific management, Eli sent a copy to Joe, then completing his last year of pharmacy studies at the University of Michigan.[28] And he immediately recalled the Emerson consultants to Indianapolis to undertake a more detailed six-month study, beginning in mid-December 1913. The emphasis now was on expanding scientific management, particularly on further implementation of the bonus system. Lilly continued to be the main company contact with the Emerson experts, but he assigned several young men in the company to work with them. Among them was Earl Beck, for whom "time study work came as second nature." Beck would soon rise high in the company. Beck and others conducted hundreds of time studies, detailed down to the point of constructing efficiency curves for each employee in several departments. As they expanded the incentive bonus system Lilly reported proudly that production costs decreased and wages increased. The Emerson experts had certified his initial forays into the realm of scientific management and aided in carrying that cause further along.[29]

While the Emerson Company's work in 1913-14 focused on time studies and implementation of the bonus system, Lilly began to introduce more systematic management in other ways. One nagging problem was high labor turnover, which led to a large proportion of new, inexperienced employees. Much of the cause for this turnover was the seasonal demand for pharmaceuticals, which was largest in March and October. The company hired new employees in the month or two prior to this high demand and then released them when peak sales passed. Lilly and Reahard attacked the inefficiency of this procedure by planning to produce ahead of demand. To do this they determined those drugs that were low in material cost and therefore less burdensome in inventory costs. Production of these items during slow seasons filled the valley of labor demand and enabled the company gradually to move toward a more stable and experienced labor force.[30]

Related to the problem of seasonality was that of determining the most economical lot size for each product. High inventory costs argued for small lot sizes, while the lower unit costs of large lots urged manufacture of great quantities of each item. Lilly and Reahard laboriously devised for each class of product a formula that balanced these variables and enabled a rapid and accurate determination of the most economically sized lots. These formulae guided production decisions for decades afterward.[31]

Lilly's dedication to systematic management extended to all the details of manufacturing, details he closely monitored and supervised. The task of producing a large variety of products at high volume, consistent quality, and low cost demanded careful planning, intense supervision, and meticulous record keeping. Lilly insisted on standard, uniform procedures. A typically short memorandum he sent to all supervisors in early 1914 indicates his thinking: "No changes in details of manufacture or packaging shall be made except by written memoranda. No written memoranda seeking to effect changes in details of manufacture or packaging shall be authority for such changes unless it bears the following stamp." Here and in many other ways Lilly replaced older, more informal means of communication and control with formal, routinized methods of manufacturing.[32]

Though less interested in nonmanufacturing areas of the company, he participated also in decisions to implement a new accounting and inventory system. This step toward more systematic management was aided by a study done in 1916 by the accounting firm of Ernst and Ernst. Soon thereafter the company installed Hollerith sorting and tabulating machines to meet the demands of the more detailed record keeping.[33]

By the time of World War I, Eli Lilly and Company was well on the way to becoming a modern big business. System gradually replaced hit-or-miss methods of production. Speed of flow through the plant increased, and unit manufacturing costs decreased. Control became more formal and structured. Eli Lilly was not alone responsible for these changes, but he was actively involved in all and led in most. In his struggle to bring more modern, systematic management to the company, he acquired in 1914 a most useful ally, J. K. Lilly, Jr.

The younger Lilly brother graduated from the Hill School in Potts-town, Pennsylvania, in 1912 and then completed the two-year course at the University of Michigan School of Pharmacy. After graduation in 1914 he married Ruth Brinkmeyer, an Indianapolis woman, and in November of that year began work at McCarty Street. He soon showed the kind of approach to business that appealed greatly to his older brother. In 1916 he prepared a 154-page report on employment, a very detailed, analytical document with a strong scientific management cast, based on readings of the experts his brother found so appealing and on visits to employment officers at Sears, Roebuck, Montgomery Ward, and Marshall Field. In late 1916 Joe became head of a newly formed division, the Efficiency Division, which included the Employment and Service Department, the Payroll and Bonus Department, and the Methods and Standards Department. He thus took immediate charge of time studies, bonuses, and other functions his brother had inaugurated earlier. This responsibility was soon interrupted, for with the United States entry into the World War Joe enlisted in the army and soon was in France organizing a medical supply unit.[34]

The Lilly brothers were two points of a family triangle. At the apex was J. K. Lilly, Sr., a man of unusual talent and character. His influence on the company that his father had founded in 1876 was profound, not only in a direct way, but also through his two sons. There is no doubt that Eli and his father were as close as sons and fathers can be, exchanging confidences, sharing the details of their daily lives, mutually encouraging and lifting each other through the crises and disappointments, and providing a haven of familial love safe from the larger world.[35]

Family members do not always make good business partners, however, even in families of constant love. Nor do family-managed businesses always succeed, even in families with large business talent and dedication. J. K. Lilly, Sr., was talented, and he was dedicated to the business. Even from his Florida winter home or on his many travels he frequently wrote his sons with requests for information about a particular product or about the latest set of sales figures.[36] The success of the company was exceedingly important to him, even as he spent more time away from Indianapolis. But the company was always second to the family. Eli Lilly and Company would always be a family business, he insisted. Often he expressed his pride in the family-run enterprise. When considering the prospects of a merger with Parke-Davis in about 1918, J. K. Lilly, Sr., carefully listed the advantages and disadvantages. At the top of his list of disadvantages was his conviction that "the Lilly family would completely lose control of its destinies, reducing them to subserviency to a board of directors, consisting partly of strangers." And he added, "No 3 men in the U.S. have the interest in a Pharmaceutical house as J. K., Eli & Joe. All others are minor stockholders, absentee landlords having no family pride in family achievement, looking only to *dividends* no matter how acquired." Although he listed many advantages to merger, he would have no part in such a corporation. If forced to merge, "my personal interest would be sold only for cash and I would take my doll rags and go home."[37]

J. K. Lilly, Sr., believed that a family business was the best kind, that the success of Eli Lilly and Company derived in large measure from the fact of its family ownership and management. But there were challenges peculiar to family businesses. Two were of fundamental importance to Eli Lilly and Company by the second decade of the century. One was the problem of succession, of bringing new family members into management. Younger family members could be incompetent, lazy, or unsuited to the business. Older members could be rigidly set in their ways, holding on tightly until only death relaxed their grip. At the Du Pont Company, for example, young Pierre S. Du Pont quit the family firm in anger, embittered because older members would not listen to him. And at the Ford Motor Company, Edsel Ford, even as president, remained intimidated and cowed by his imperious father, Henry. Another common problem in family businesses was bringing nonfamily managers into positions of authority. As a company grew in size and complexity, it became increasingly difficult for family members to manage it alone. Yet sharing power with professsional, nonfamily managers sometimes proved difficult for the family and the outsiders.[38]

These two challenges the Lilly triumvirate met and largely conquered in the 1910s. There were no spoiled playboys in the third generation of the pharmaceutical family. Eli and Joe prepared themselves first through relevant technical training and then eased into the company by beginning with general-purpose assignments and moving gradually to positions of increasing authority. Both young men showed a capacity for hard work that immensely pleased their father. At the same time father and sons knew that the three alone could not manage the rapidly growing company no matter how hard they worked. Unlike many of his contemporaries, J. K. Lilly, Sr., knew that "A Ten Million business cannot be comfortably handled by a force and organization that easily conducted a One Million Affair."[39] His first major step in sharing power with nonfamily members was to appoint Charles J. Lynn general manager in 1907. Lynn had joined the company as a salesman in 1895 and remained close to J. K. Lilly, Sr., throughout his life. When Eli moved into management in 1909 he joined the two older men, Lynn and his father, as the three top managers in the company. But it was not enough, J. K. Lilly, Sr., thought, especially in preparing for the future, to have only "one young, active partner for this business." As the company expanded rapidly, he wrote in his 1910 annual report that "unless active, brainy partners are gradually acquired to share the responsibilities with our one youngest partner, the inevitable growth of this business in the next ten years will be a genuine calamity."[40]

Such partners were soon acquired. And they were allowed to purchase shares in the family-held enterprise. Lynn was the first nonfamily associate to purchase stock, two hundred shares in 1909. A year later John S. Wright, with responsibilities in sales, and Woods A. Caperton, in charge of advertising, were allowed to buy fifty shares. One of the most important additions to management came in 1910, when Nicholas H. Noyes joined the company. A graduate of Cornell University, Noyes in 1908 married Marguerite Lilly, a cousin of J. K. Lilly, Sr. Noyes's expertise in finance led in 1914 to his appointment as treasurer and his joining Lynn on the board of directors. In his thirty-eight years in the company Noyes acquired a reputation for fiscal stringency that spread throughout the organization.[41]

The movement of these men into positions of responsibility reflected the Lilly family's accurate understanding of the growing demands of managing a large corporation. The Lilly brothers alone were not going to have to bear the managerial burdens as the company grew and as their father began to remove himself from day-to-day involvement. Equally important, however, the addition of new men to the ranks of stockholders, directors, and managers did not disguise the locus of fundamental decision making or the source of basic strategy. The Lilly family remained fully in control. In 1916, in the midst of working out new inventory and accounting systems, J. K. Lilly, Sr., wrote from Florida to his sons that on his return he wished "to get you two in a closet and lay my plans before you, then when we have them all thoroughly digested (*we three*) we can let the others in and then go to it along systematic and thorough lines."[42] Three winters later he wrote in a similar vein about a four-year plan under consideration: "I will want to go over it with you before we release it to a meeting."[43]

The human business environment for Eli Lilly in the 1910s thus included his father, his brother, just entering the business, and Lynn, Noyes, and other new managers. It was natural to expect that as Lilly grew in experience his responsibility would increase. It was natural also to expect

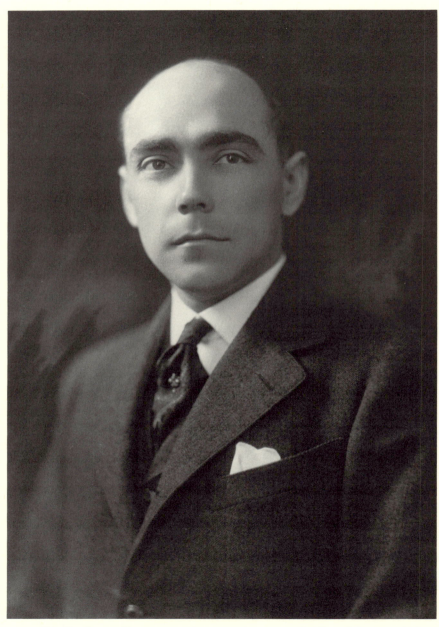

Eli Lilly, driving force in systematic management.   *Eli Lilly and Company Archives*

that young Lilly wanted that process of maturity to proceed more rapidly than it in fact did. He had ideas and goals of his own for the company. They did not always match those of his fellow managers.

In particular, not all his colleagues shared Lilly's zeal for scientific management or rapid change. Using his Wawasee sailing imagery, Lilly complained that some dragged anchor and did not pick up on changes in the wind, particularly time and efficiency studies.[44] He later recalled: "I brought the first stop watch into Eli Lilly and Company, and you would have thought that I had brought a barrel full of virulent plague for the stir it made, not among the workers but among some of the officers who feared that I intended to work our people to death or cut the quality of their work."[45] On another occasion Lilly noted that "Joe and I both had our troubles in the early days in getting ideas accepted. New ways were suspect, and many were long and loud arguments—resulting in an occasional broken window."[46] One such new idea was a machine to paste labels on bottles. Others were convinced that it would not work, that only hand application could accurately place labels.[47]

The center of resistance to labeling machines, stopwatches, and other new ideas was Charles J. Lynn, general manager and right-hand man for J. K. Lilly, Sr. Lynn was as blunt and strong as the cigars he smoked. He was also a perfectionist who feared the imperfections that might accompany innovation. Lynn began his career in sales and remained ever after more concerned about that part of the business than production. Eli Lilly kept pushing for changes and after more than a decade of resistance from Lynn decided to clear the air.[48]

In October 1919 he drafted a memorandum for circulation to his fellow officers—the two other Lillys, Noyes, and Lynn. The memorandum was titled "Too Much Conservatism." Lilly began by asserting, "The writer is so profoundly convinced that we are afflicted with too much conservatism that he wishes to put into writing his ideas on this subject." The major issue he chose to illustrate his general contention was the fear of his fellow officers of a sudden decrease in prices, a fear that had hampered company growth for several years. The result of this fear was purchase of raw materials in too small quantities, manufacture in uneconomical size lots, and maintenance of inventories inadequate to meet demand. Consequently "we have lost thousands of dollars worth of business." Lilly also pointed to the ultraconservative policy on the purchase of coal, which produced an excessive, three-month supply. A six-week stock of coal was adequate, he argued, and far less costly. And he challenged his colleagues who had adopted the position that "because the Government takes away a lot of our excess profits that it does not justify us in making these additional profits." This foolish idea must be abandoned; "the sooner we regard Government Taxes simply as an incidental expense of doing business the better for all concerned. . . . I do not advise throwing conservatism to the winds," Lilly concluded, "but too much of it is as bad as too little of it."[49]

Lynn was furious. He took the memorandum, Lilly later explained, "as a severe personal criticism of his management" and suggested that Lilly "be removed from the head of the manufacturing division and banished to the provinces of the sales division and placed under his direction."[50] Lilly refused that offer. Both men appealed to a higher authority, J. K. Lilly, Sr.

Eli had shown the memorandum to his father before distributing it. The senior Lilly had approved its circulation, but, he soon made clear, he did not agree with his son's analysis of the business. He wrote Eli, "Of course I take your observations good naturedly, otherwise I might take great umbrage at what might appear on the surface of it to be a wholesale condemnation of the management of this business." J. K. Lilly, Sr., proceeded to answer each one of the specific criticisms his son had made, explaining the reasons for decisions and policies, indicating no regrets, and suggesting the possibility of change only in the matter of coal inventories. "I laid awake last night for hours thinking of this," he concluded, and "as long as I am connected with the business we shall not depart from a proper policy of conservatism, at the same time being progressive but safely so. . . . It is infinitely better to lose some profit occasionally than to jeopardize the solidity of the business."[51]

But while he rebuffed Eli's general argument of too much conservatism, J. K. Lilly, Sr., did not reject his son. On the contrary, in response to Lynn's suggestion that Eli be banished from McCarty Street, J. K. Lilly, Sr., shifted his two colleagues' responsibilities, giving Eli full charge of the manufacturing and scientific divisions and making Lynn, who had been general manager, responsible for sales and other divisions, each to report directly to President Lilly.[52]

The episode of 1919 was never forgotten, but it soon receded in significance as new challenges burst forth at McCarty Street. Indeed, the next five years would be the most important in the history of the company. Eli Lilly would have further chance to show the merits of his progressive ideas, and his eager desire for change would be more than fulfilled. These early years, beginning with his introduction of scientific management ideas in the 1910s and continuing into the mid-1920s, he later wrote, were for him and his brother, "the most satisfying and creative periods in our lives."[53] Despite all the achievements and recognitions that came in later years he remained immensely proud of his work with stopwatches, economical size lots, labor force variation, and other details of production and management. It was through these achievements in the hard details of drug manufacturing that he proved he could make his own contribution to the company his father and grandfather had built.

Chapter 3

The Revolutions on McCarty Street, 1919-1932

The years between 1919 and 1932 were years of great changes for Eli Lilly. The company he joined in 1907 became a gigantic modern manufacturing enterprise, due in significant part to the application of his driving interest in mass production and due also to the development of new ventures in scientific research.

The American pharmaceutical industry changed rapidly in the late 1910s and 1920s. World War I increased the demand for pharmaceuticals and cut off supplies of German drugs and chemicals, forcing American companies to speed up development of their own capabilities in production and in scientific research and development. Two months before American entry into the war, J. K. Lilly, Sr., wrote his sons urging preparation to help defeat "Damnable Barbaric Germany." Regretting that the pharmaceutical company could not produce guns, he instructed Eli and Joe to increase production of typhoid vaccine.[1] With entry into the war in April 1917 the company turned full energy to production of necessary medicines and the execution of large war contracts. As male employees went off to war, women in khaki bloomer suits took their places. From McCarty Street and the personal resources of the Lilly family came also financial support for a Red Cross base hospital in France and energetic participation in several Liberty Bond drives. And while Eli and his father managed the company Joe enlisted in the army and served as an officer in the medical supply service in France.[2]

The difficulties of meeting the large wartime demands and the profits made during and immediately after the war encouraged Lilly management to increase productive capacity once the international crisis was ended. So, too, did longer term, general trends in the pharmaceutical industry. It was evident by 1920 that some firms were growing larger, evolving into the gigantic corporations that were the hallmark of early twentieth-century

American industry. Those firms that did not grow were likely to fall by the wayside in this intensely competitive industry.[3] The Lillys were determined to grow, and in 1919 and 1920 they began systematically to prepare the way.

J. K. Lilly, Sr., sounded the trumpet in a lengthy memorandum of October 1919. Titled "A Plan for Promoting the Affairs of Eli Lilly & Company during the Years 1920-21-22-23," the document was forty-six pages long and was filled with statistical data and reasoned arguments. The senior Lilly urged the need for energetic sales work; the development of a personnel department to reduce labor turnover and avoid labor unrest; the formulation of plans "for additional land, buildings, warehouses, power house, rebuilding and trackage on a scale to provide for growth of the business for many years"; and, finally, the establishment of a "department of Experimental Medicine" to function "on 'result getting' lines."[4]

The four-year plan announced in the fall of 1919 was the kind of marching order an ambitious Eli Lilly needed. His conflict with the conservative Charles Lynn was still brewing. With his father's four-year plan and with his promotion to full control of the manufacturing and scientific divisions that year, he now had at last the authority to expand the company in directions he had so long wished.

Since joining the company in 1907 his first love had been production. Now in the early 1920s he was able to bring to fruition the wisdom that had come from years of reading the literature of scientific management and from his experience on the production floor. His objective simply was high-volume production at the lowest possible cost, and he set immediately to work. In early 1920 he reported to his father that he had prepared a general building plan. At the next board of directors meeting he was made chairman of the committee to carry out expansion of the Indianapolis plant.[5]

The expansion program of the early 1920s included many components, but the crowning achievement was Building 22. Located on the northeast corner of Delaware and McCarty streets, Building 22 represented Eli Lilly's long-nourished ideas about pharmaceutical production. Completed in 1926, the new plant enabled raw materials to enter one end and exit the other as finished drugs, moving through the production process in a near straight line by means of an elaborate system of conveyors, lifts, pipes, and chutes. Lilly worked very hard to design the layout for this straight-line production system so as to meet his dictum that "the less time required in applying motion to material, all other things being equal, the more profitable the business."[6] Increasing the speed of movement and reducing human

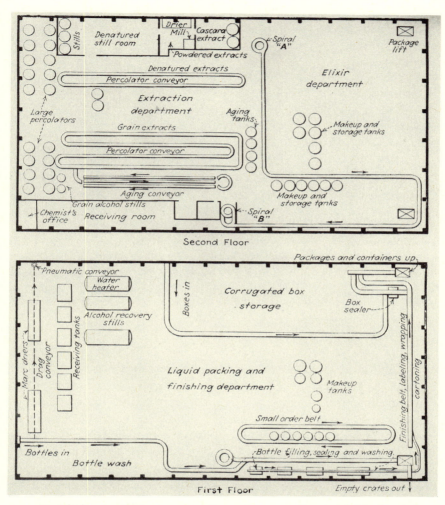

Straight-line production system on first and
second floors of Building 22.

Chemical & Metallurgical
Engineering 35 (1928): 82

handling by means of conveyor transfer of materials had long fascinated
Lilly. He had begun to investigate the possibility of using mechanical conveyors
as early as 1907, after only two weeks on the job. His reading of Frederick
W. Taylor and his work with the Emerson Company extended this interest,
as did a tour of the Ford Motor Company's famous River Rouge plant just
after World War I.[7]

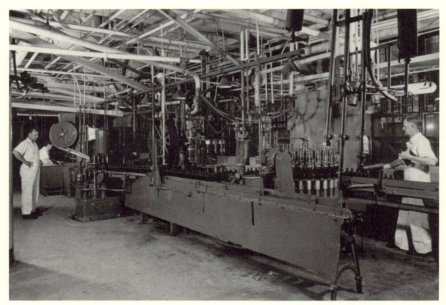

Wet Finishing Department, filling and finishing   *Eli Lilly and Company Archives*
belt, Building 22.

The introduction of conveyor systems was only the most obvious illustration of the new straight-line production at Building 22. More important and difficult to achieve were the detailed planning and coordination necessary to make the system work efficiently. This had to be done by applying the techniques of scientific management, including time and motion studies, not simply to one operation but to the entire plant. The challenge was particularly difficult because, unlike the builders of the automobile assembly lines, Lilly had to plan for the production of approximately 2,800 different products in Building 22. A myriad of pills, tablets, ointments, elixirs, and syrups, derived from all manner of raw materials, had to be produced, bottled, and packaged in many forms and quantities requiring careful attention to detail. Through the early 1920s Lilly labored over the details of setting up the complex new system so as "to permit the logical flow of work from operation to operation with the minimum of handling."[8]

By the time he finished Lilly had meticulously laid out five floors of production in such a manner that Building 22 received the highest praise from a visiting editor of *Chemical & Metallurgical Engineering*. Even more important was the pride of Eli's father and the impressive improvements

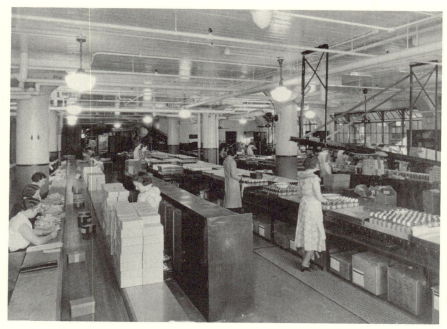

Dry Finishing Department, Building 22.   *Eli Lilly and Company Archives*

in productive capacity and efficiency that came with the opening of Building 22 in February 1926, just in time for the celebration of the company's fiftieth anniversary. Few if any achievements in Lilly's long career in business were more important to him than straight-line production and Building 22.[9]

While he concentrated his attention on setting up the straight-line production system Eli Lilly also worked with his father and especially brother Joe on continuing and expanding other efficiency measures. With Joe he established a Planning Department to centralize production planning, "so that a continuous stream of materials is flowing into the points of the system, as needed."[10] And he and his brother improved personnel measures to reduce labor turnover and avoid the kind of strike that a major competitor, Parke-Davis, suffered in 1920. Eli and Joe developed more careful hiring procedures and provided employees with improved working conditions, including a new cafeteria and a new emphasis on job safety. And they expanded the bonus system begun in 1911 and began to award efficiency or "E" buttons to employees who exceeded their standards. Often the button arrived with a personal note to the employee from Eli Lilly.[11]

The Lilly brothers continued their interest in time and motion studies, applying them even to the porters' chore of polishing the brass on entry doors. They also expanded earlier efforts to eliminate seasonality in production, moving to a system of larger inventories of finished goods. And they developed methods of insuring the quality of the finished product, including the deliberate introduction of errors into the system to test employees and inspectors.[12] By 1928 their company was one in which a zealous employee would use the word "efficiency" four times in one sentence, and a Methods and Standards Department Manual would advise workers that "both hands should be busy; if they are not, surely some change can be made to keep them busy all the time."[13]

Eli Lilly's hard-driving presence was apparent not only in the general efficiency campaign but in the oversight of production details. A mix-up of heroin hydrochloride and calomel tablets, for example, was a matter for his attention, as was a monthly report of broken tablets.[14] He made frequent personal inspection tours through the factory, accompanied by his secretary, Ruth Allison, who took notes of all irregularities. His monthly housekeeping inspections were exceedingly thorough in attention to cleanliness and order, particularly in Building 22. In the unfortunate department that he judged most distant from his high standards he placed a sign proclaiming "This is the Dirtiest Place in the Plant." His reputation among employees in the 1920s came to be that of a fair but very strict, no-nonsense manager.[15]

Indeed, in his drive to produce more pharmaceuticals at lower cost Lilly sometimes encountered opposition from associates who grumbled that he was "Fordizing" the plant. High-speed mass production, they feared, would lead to drugs of inferior quality. Lilly's old nemesis, Charles Lynn, sent him all customer complaints as a way, Lilly thought, of showing opposition to the whole concept of straight-line production. But Lilly kept a careful record of complaints and eventually could demonstrate to Lynn that the number actually declined as the new methods were introduced.[16]

There were difficulties also on the shop floor in integrating the centralized planning system into the straight-line production of Building 22. Lilly worked closely and intently with only a few associates, unwisely ignoring the heads of the operating departments. Consequently, when problems developed there was a tendency for these foremen to take the position, as one later recalled, "I had nothing to do with it—you make it work—you made the layout." Eventually one of the braver men developed the courage to discuss the problem with Lilly, which caused him to organize a foremen's group to provide closer consultation between shop floor heads and management. The experience was a lesson that Lilly would apply well in later years.[17]

The 1920s brought record-setting profits to Eli Lilly and Company. The business had a particularly good year in 1923. In his annual summary J. K. Lilly, Sr., reported profits of over 17 percent of sales, "the most profitable year in the history of the business." These record profits, he noted, were about evenly divided between a very large increase in general sales and the sale of one new product, known to the Indianapolis company as Iletin and to the world as insulin.[18]

Insulin brought more change to McCarty Street than did any other drug in the company's history. Its consequences were revolutionary, but, like most revolutions, the production of insulin had a deep and broad historical context. Insulin production developed from the changing nature of pharmaceutical research in early twentieth-century America generally and specifically from fundamental changes at Eli Lilly and Company.

American pharmaceutical companies as late as World War I were still not far removed from their nineteenth-century origins as apothecaries and patent medicine manufacturers. Consequently, their research activities and products were still held in very low regard by many physicians and university scientists. In 1915 the Council on Pharmacy of the American Medical Association concluded that drug company research was of little scientific merit and asserted that "it is only from laboratories free from any relation with manufacturers that real [pharmaceutical] advances can be expected."[19]

Most of the work done in pharmaceutical company laboratories was of a routine nature, concentrating on testing of raw materials and finished products in order to manufacture standardized, reliable drugs. In analytical laboratories technicians adjusted preparations to the standards of the *Pharmacopoeia* and, after its passage in 1906, of the Pure Food and Drug Act. These quality control measures were important and sometimes difficult steps in drug manufacture, especially with the rise of mass production techniques, but this growing attention to testing and standardization did not lead directly to significant basic research or efficacious new drugs. The 1905 revision of the *United States Pharmacopoeia* contained, by a modern estimate, only a handful of worthwhile drugs.[20]

The initial impetus for fundamental change in pharmaceutical research came from outside the American drug companies, particularly from the university and industrial laboratories of Germany. There, beginning in the 1880s, scientists applied organic chemistry to the production of synthetic drugs, leading by the turn of the century to aspirin, barbiturates, and other new products. This research culminated in the discovery of arsphenamine (a treatment for syphilis), the first in a long line of chemotherapeutics. In German laboratories also scientists developed around the turn of the century a variety of biological serums, vaccines, and antitoxins. German science so dominated new medicines in the United States that 228 of the 592 drugs listed in the 1916 edition of *New and Nonofficial Remedies* were imported from Germany.[21]

World War I cut off this supply of drugs and the scientific expertise behind it and led as well to the American government's abrogation of German patents. The resultant opportunities for American scientists and companies to produce their own established products and develop new medicines sparked a surge of research activity and the beginnings of substantial cooperation between university and industrial scientists. The search for new drugs derived also from the increasing respect for science generally and from the professionalization of medical care specifically, with better medical schools educating physicians who demanded efficacious medicines. And with growing material prosperity and education in the early twentieth century there were more Americans willing and able to pay for these new drugs.[22]

These industry-wide developments were directly important to Eli Lilly and Company. By World War I many of its old standby sales leaders were declining in popularity. Succus Alterans was perhaps the best example. By the second decade of the new century Lilly managers were very much aware that the days were numbered for the old Creek Indian remedy and for similar concoctions, as medical schools were warning their students against use of such dubious products.[23]

In the four-year plan announced in October 1919 J. K. Lilly, Sr., urged the creation of a new "department of Experimental Medicine . . . on 'result getting' lines."[24] Four months later he reported to the company directors that "the development of new specialities of large possibilities by this house is extremely unsatisfactory." While the Scientific Department had performed well in the "insurance of routine quality, we are forced to confess that as a speciality producer it is a complete failure."[25] The senior Lilly could afford to be so critical of the company he headed because he and his elder son had already begun a major initiative to bring change. Eli Lilly reported to his father in early 1920 that he had begun the revival of the Scientific Division with a shift to experimental research "on broad lines." The critical step had come with the hiring of George Henry Alexander Clowes.[26]

Clowes was born in Ipswich, England, in 1877. He studied chemistry at the Royal College of Science in London and then earned a Ph.D. in chemistry at the University of Göttingen in Germany. In 1901 he emigrated to America, where he worked at the New York State Institute for the Study of Malignant Disease in Buffalo until the United States entered the World War. Then Clowes went to Washington, investigating mustard gas for the Chemical Warfare Service. His research publications and growing reputation brought him to the attention of the Indianapolis company. In 1918 Eli and his father invited Clowes to the Hoosier capital for lunch and an interview.[27] In the summer of 1919 Clowes joined the firm as director of biochemical research. He described his new situation in a letter that same year in which he refused an offer to become head of the Division of Chemistry in the United States Hygienic Laboratory in Washington. Eli Lilly and Company, he wrote, "have created a purely research position for me, in which, for the first time in my life, I am free to devote my attention to those fundamental problems on the border line field of physics, chemistry, biology and medicine. . . . They have provided me with ample laboratory facilities and assistants and have arranged to let me carry on the biological side of my work at Woods Hole [Massachusetts] during the summer months."[28]

In providing such opportunities, Eli and J. K. Lilly, Sr., had large hopes of expanding the company's research operation. Announcing Clowes's appointment in the *Budget,* they indicated that "for some time we have realized the inadequacy of the conventional methods of studying pharmacological problems, and believed that an attempt should be made to apply physico-chemical principles to the study of such problems as the penetration and mode of action of drugs on living tissues."[29] Clowes was an expert in biochemical research, with particular interest in cell division and cancer. But the Lillys brought Clowes to McCarty Street for more than his technical research expertise. He had, first, an unusually sophisticated

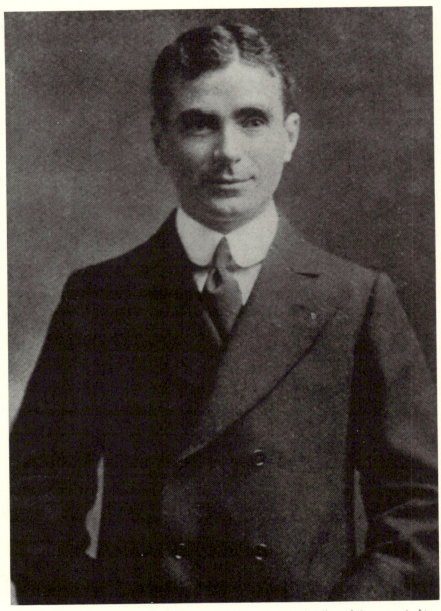

George Henry Alexander Clowes, 1919.   *Eli Lilly and Company Archives*

and practical vision of the purpose and nature of scientific research in an industrial setting. In his annual report for 1921, he indicated his goal to substitute "systematically planned small scale, wide range laboratory experiments for hit-and-miss large scale, narrow range laboratory experiments, thus diminishing the time required for an experiment and increasing its chance of success." And to this sensible research strategy he added the urgent need for the company and its scientists to secure "the recognition, respect and confidence of scientific and medical organizations and individuals all over the world."[30]

Clowes brought also to Indianapolis a determined, energetic drive and a forceful, optimistic personality. "He lived," Eli Lilly later recalled, "more hours per day than any man I ever knew."[31] Nor was he a modest man. Despite strict company rules on employee parking, Clowes, as an associate recalled, "parked his derned automobile anywhere he wanted to."[32] Many employees thought him arrogant. There were often conflicts and even raised voices. He had an impatience for detail, abhorred committees, and was never happy as a bench worker in the laboratory. Rather, his skills were in seeing research problems in their large dimensions and in inspiring and convincing others of their importance. To this end he deluged Eli Lilly, who had responsibility for the Scientific Division, with memoranda and reports, even while Lilly was on vacation. And he corresponded with university scientists and traveled to laboratories wherever there was a possibility of research relevant to the company's interests.[33] It was this man, J. K. Lilly, Sr., predicted to his sons in early 1920, who "will some day hit some great thing that will make him famous and rich."[34]

Clowes began the journey that would hit some great thing on Christmas Day, 1921. Leaving his disappointed family in Indianapolis he set off for the American Physiological Society meetings in New Haven, Connecticut. There he heard a paper by J. J. R. Macleod, Frederick G. Banting, and Charles H. Best on "The Beneficial Influences of Certain Pancreatic Extracts on Pancreatic Diabetes." The three scientists reported on their research at the University of Toronto, where they had induced diabetes in laboratory dogs and then administered a pancreatic extract to work against the diabetes. They reported that their extract, which they called insulin, reduced blood sugar and kept alive two diabetic dogs. Most listeners in the New Haven audience were wary. Clowes was the exception. He spoke with the Toronto researchers immediately after their presentation and suggested the possibility of collaboration in commercial preparation of insulin. The Toronto men politely refused.[35]

The disease that Macleod, Banting, and Best were fighting was one for which there was no effective treatment in 1921. Diabetes meant that the body could not burn nutrients in food. Carbohydrates especially were not fully metabolized and turned into energy, but rather were passed from the body as sugar in the urine. The result was weight loss, weakness, and many other serious symptoms. A child diagnosed as having diabetes could expect to live about one year. The primary therapy was a "starvation" diet, in which the diabetic's food was severely limited on the assumption that giving the body only the fuel it could metabolize would slow the destructive march of the disease. This treatment ultimately led to a choice of death by starvation or death from diabetes. Prior to death it meant the agony of patients, many of them children, slowly starving, their bodies reduced to skin and bone.[36]

It was this dreadful disease and its relationship to the regulation of metabolism by the pancreas that was the subject of the New Haven meeting. Returning to Indianapolis, Clowes did not forget about the work of Macleod, Banting, and Best. Encouraged by Eli Lilly to pursue the possibility, Clowes wrote Macleod, again suggesting collaboration, and in early May he met with him in Washington. By the spring of 1922 the Toronto researchers had made great strides. They had begun experimental injections of insulin into human diabetes patients with near miraculous results, but they were experiencing great difficulty in producing the hormone, which required carefully controlled alcoholic extraction from pancreas glands. Clowes's offers to help became increasingly attractive as the Canadians contemplated also the inevitable difficulties in moving from small-scale laboratory preparation to large-quantity manufacture of insulin. They invited him to Toronto.[37]

Clowes and Eli Lilly traveled to Toronto to meet the insulin discoverers on 22 May 1922. Following several days of discussion in the King Edward Hotel, Lilly, Clowes, and the Canadians reached an agreement for the commercial development of insulin. The Indianapolis company would have an exclusive license to produce and sell insulin in the United States for a one-year experimental period. The Canadians and Americans promised to share techniques and knowledge throughout the experimental period. Although the university scientists were wary of commercializing their work through collaboration with a profit-oriented pharmaceutical manufacturer, they were attracted by Clowes's high standing in the scientific community and by the company's generous support of his work. They knew also of the company's broadening interest in research and its specific interest and growing expertise in gland products such as insulin. And they knew that the business had at its command a large supply of equipment, capital, and skilled chemists and workers able to produce a complex drug in high volume.[38]

The agreement signed on 30 May 1922 between the Indianapolis pharmaceutical company and the University of Toronto signaled the beginning of hard work for Lilly, Clowes, and their associates as they struggled to produce insulin in large quantities at consistent standards. Charles Best, a young graduate student at the University of Toronto who had worked closely with Banting, was in Indianapolis by 2 June to help with the first production effort. He and Eli Lilly became good friends; they continued to visit and correspond into the 1970s. Best made nine trips to Indianapolis in 1922, carrying information to and from Toronto.[39] In mid-June Lilly reported to Macleod that the company was producing insulin but only on a small scale. Difficulties continued for the next several weeks as Lilly and Harley W. Rhodehamel, chemist and jack-of-all-trades, concentrated their energies on the challenge of production.[40] By the end of July they had made considerable progress, enough to allow Lilly to join his wife and daughter for a few weeks of vacation in New England. He stayed in close touch, however, writing his father for details on insulin. J. K. Lilly, Sr., informed his son that production was improving significantly, up to 1,500 units a week by August, and assured him that "Rhodie is right on his toes" and "sailing in for a finish."[41]

There were setbacks in production, however, particularly a problem with deterioration of insulin potency that occurred in the fall of 1922, but even that setback led to progress. It stimulated the company's chief chemist, George Walden, to develop a process of isoelectric precipitation that greatly enhanced the stability and purity of insulin and constituted a major advance in insulin manufacture. By the spring of 1923 the basic production problems were solved, and Clowes was able to boast that the company had the capability now to supply the entire world with Iletin, the trade name of its insulin product.[42] Eli Lilly and his associates had worked long, hard hours to reach this point. His special recognition came in May when his father, from on board the *Samaria* on which he was sailing around the world, wrote him: "A glow of pride pervades my being as I contemplate the splendid manner in which you steered the good ship Iletin to the Harbor of success."[43]

Eli Lilly's hand was not the only one on the ship's tiller, of course. Clowes, Rhodehamel, Walden, and J. K. Lilly, Sr., played major roles, too, in this cooperative effort. And there was the absolutely essential work and cooperation of the University of Toronto scientists. Much later, in 1962, when thoughts of a new company history were in the air, Lilly critiqued the earlier history written by Roscoe Collins Clark and published in 1946. Commenting on Clark's chapter on insulin, Lilly urged that Clowes should receive more credit and that Eli Lilly and Company "is given too much credit on the development of Insulin and Toronto not enough."[44]

Lilly was always careful in later years to praise the Toronto scientists and commend the "perfect cooperation" between the company and Toronto.[45] But in fact there was considerable friction between the university scientists and the Indianapolis businessmen. In the resulting controversies Lilly became the company's guardian of business profit, usually quietly and tactfully, but sometimes firmly. He and his father knew the advantages that could result from insulin and were determined to obtain them. The scientists at Toronto had little interest in, or sympathy for, the bottom line of an Indianapolis pharmaceutical company.[46]

From the first meeting in Toronto in May 1922, Lilly insisted that the company be permitted to distribute its insulin under the trade name of "Iletin." This insistence on a trade name was supplemented with exclusive and, until January 1923, free distribution of insulin to selected physicians, all in the hopes of bonding their loyalties to Iletin. Once the year of monopoly production and sale concluded, other pharmaceutical companies would be able to enter the insulin market, but none could call their product Iletin. The Lillys hoped that because of their head start doctors and diabetics would always ask for Iletin rather than insulin. The scientists at the University of Toronto initially paid little attention to this side of the matter. As they became more knowledgeable about the pharmaceutical business and as they organized their Insulin Committee to oversee the new product, they began to object, fearing that use of the trade name would give the Indianapolis company an unfair advantage over competitors. Toronto's Insulin Committee pushed hard to make the company drop "Iletin" and market its product simply as "Insulin (Lilly)." At one point Clowes agreed to this concession, doubtless in the interests of scientific harmony, but Eli

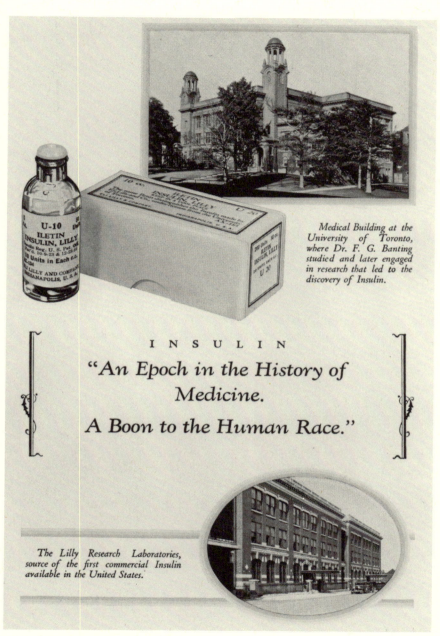

Medical Building at the University of Toronto, where Dr. F. G. Banting studied and later engaged in research that led to the discovery of Insulin.

INSULIN

"An Epoch in the History of Medicine.

A Boon to the Human Race."

The Lilly Research Laboratories, source of the first commercial Insulin available in the United States.

Advertising insulin, ca. 1930.   *Eli Lilly and Company Archives* and J. K. Lilly, Sr., overruled him. They did eventually agree that although labels on their bottles would include the words "Insulin, Lilly" the word "Iletin" would precede in letters of the same size.[47]

Eli Lilly forcefully expressed his views on the trade-name controversy though Clowes, who, with his usual verbosity, reported to Macleod in April 1923 that "Mr. Eli Lilly has asked me to remind you that on the occasion on which he and I paid a visit to Toronto at the time at which the preliminary contract was drawn up and signed, that this question of a trade name was brought up by him and that he himself particularly stressed its great importance for our corporation. He stated that in his opinion it was the most important factor from the business standpoint and that without the authorization to use such a trade name Eli Lilly and Company would not have considered making a provisional agreement without being granted a subsequent monopoly." Mr. Lilly, Clowes concluded, was "not prepared to make any further concessions on the matter."[48]

While the controversy over the trade name brewed in the spring of 1923 another business issue began to heat up. The company applied for a patent on George Walden's isoelectric precipitation method, a patent, the Insulin Committee feared, that might give the company a virtual monopoly on insulin beyond the one-year experimental period. The Toronto scientists counterattacked by initiating arrangements to patent a similar process developed independently at Washington University in St. Louis. They also began steps to stall the American Medical Association's approval of "Iletin" as a trade name. Through letters and at least two trips to Toronto, in May and June 1923, Eli Lilly helped arrange a compromise: the Insulin Committee agreed not to block AMA approval of "Iletin," and Lilly agreed to give Toronto the patent on Walden's isoelectric precipitation process, which would thus eventually be available to other licensed insulin manufacturers.[49]

After another flare-up over the use of the word "Iletin" in April 1924, Lilly wrote the prickly executive secretary of the Toronto Insulin Committee: "It is unfortunate that these little instances seem to happen right along, but they are only natural I suppose in the pioneering of a new project. Our competitors will probably give less trouble along this line than we have, on account of the fact that the policies which have been worked out on us can be given them in perfect form." And Lilly added, doubtless recalling his own boyhood, "You know that the first child in a family catches all the discipline!"[50]

Lilly's effort to smooth over the differences between Toronto and Indianapolis pointed to the fundamental problem and the larger issue. It

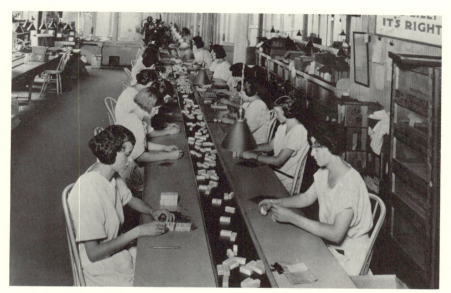

Insulin finishing line, 1923.   *Eli Lilly and Company Archives*

was not that the Toronto researchers were interested only in pure science and the Indianapolis businessmen only in profit. The differences were more subtle than that. They derived from the challenges of what Lilly described as "the pioneering of a new project." Not only did the pioneers have to work out the technical details of insulin production, they had also to develop the patterns and modes of cooperation between two different institutions on such matters as trade names, patents, licenses, and prices. There were few precedents or models, for as one scholar has written, this was "the first long-term, large-scale case of biomedical collaborative research between a North American university and a pharmaceutical firm."[51] In this context the controversies are less significant than the successes, the flare-ups less meaningful than the long-term cooperation that for decades benefited both the University of Toronto and its scientists and the Lilly family and company.

The business savvy of Eli Lilly and his father produced immediate returns from insulin. Company profits soared in 1923, with about half deriving from Iletin even though commercial distribution did not begin until October of that year.[52] To the company's benefit, competition was slow to develop. The Insulin Committee agreed in September 1923 to license other United States firms to produce insulin, but they were slow to get their products on the market. Not until mid-1924 did Eli Lilly and Company face competition. The company's two-year head start and its unique right to its trade name helped maintain the early dominance.[53]

More than financial profit resulted from insulin. Most important were the suffering averted and the lives saved by the new drug. By the fall of 1923 nearly twenty-five thousand Americans were receiving insulin. Newspaper stories told of diabetics revived from their deathbeds by the wonder drug. Elizabeth Hughes was fifteen years old, weighed forty-five pounds, and was barely alive when she received her first insulin in August 1922. In the next five weeks she gained ten pounds. By Thanksgiving she was home. Elizabeth Hughes later went to college, married, and had three children. She lived until 1981. Such a drug could only bring prestige and recognition to all associated with it. To the Toronto scientists, Banting and Macleod, insulin brought the Nobel Prize in 1923. They and their colleagues enjoyed worldwide acclaim. Clowes's role as an essential intermediary was specially recognized in 1947, when the American Diabetes Association gave him its Banting Medal.[54]

For Eli Lilly and Company the development of insulin certified a position as a first-rank, research-based pharmaceutical manufacturer. "We are now flooded by propositions from scientists both in this country and abroad to cooperate with them to develop their new item," J. K. Lilly, Sr., proudly wrote in 1924.[55] The days of Creek Indian remedies were gone. As the senior Lilly wrote a competitor, "If every house can get a few good Specialities we won't be so keen about cutting one another's throats on Fluid Extract of Spunkwater or Tincture of Chickweed."[56]

Insulin was the most important drug in this transition and in the history of the company, doing more than any other drug or process to make the Indianapolis firm one of the major pharmaceutical manufacturers in the world. It brought prestige and profit. And it also gave company managers and scientists the experience and the confidence that encouraged them to seek aggressively new drugs and new ways of manufacturing them. It was, as one employee later recalled, as though "we got our first pair of long pants in 1922."[57]

But insulin alone did not bring the change. Behind the success of this single drug were years of company growth and development. Specifically important was the research initiative begun in 1919 and marked by the hiring of Clowes. And generally important was the gradual improvement in production capability that flowed from Eli Lilly's long, hard push toward

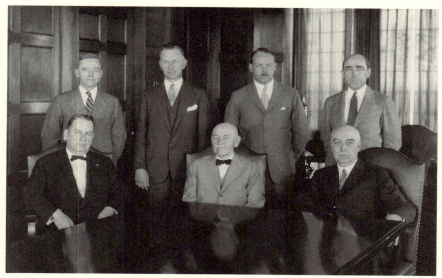

Eli Lilly and Company Board of Directors, 1927.   *Eli Lilly and Company Archives*
Left to right (seated): C. J. Lynn, James E. Lilly,
J. K. Lilly; left to right (standing): J. S. Wright,
N. H. Noyes, J. K. Lilly, Jr., Eli Lilly.

systematic management. Without these preparations the Indianapolis company would not have been ready for the long trip to Toronto. "It was," Lilly later recalled, "as if we had rushed ourselves to a point of readiness just to participate in this momentous event."[58]

The success of insulin helped spark the rapid evolution of a more sophisticated and systematic research effort at Eli Lilly and Company. Eli and J. K. Lilly, Sr., were determined to develop new specialities. They hired more scientists, who devoted more effort to research. And they paid more attention to developing ties with university scientists. These trends toward more emphasis on research were under way also at a few other American pharmaceutical companies, but the Indianapolis firm was in the very front rank of this shift.[59]

Although not an active scientist himself, Eli Lilly became increasingly involved in research administration during the 1920s, often building on his experience with insulin and generally bringing to bear his enthusiasm for more systematic procedures. One of his major initiatives was establishing formal ties to university scientists. Building on the German model, several American research-oriented companies began closer cooperation with universities in the 1920s, and university scientists, in turn, became more receptive to industrial research, though there remained some academic reluctance and even stigma associated with commercially supported science.[60] Lilly's major reach into the ivory tower came with a program of research fellowships, which he began in 1928. Within a year he had set up fourteen fellowships, extending from Yale University to the University of California. By 1930 the number had expanded to eighteen, including a fellowship at the University of Munich, "to keep in touch with the important work going on in Europe."[61]

In planning the university fellowship program Lilly evidenced his customary attention to system. Rather than depend solely on Clowes's personal ties to the scientific community, as had been the case before insulin, Lilly developed a program that relied on other members of the research staff and depended on the growing prestige of the company rather than on one individual. These fellowships, Lilly wrote in 1929, "have increased the friendliness of the faculties of the various Universities for our house. Various members of our staff are now very welcome in most of the medical centers." As part of the fellowship program, Lilly established procedures to identify productive university laboratories and to prepare a "cream list" of "the men most important in research." He encouraged company researchers always to travel with this cream list, especially as they made their periodic visits to fellowship holders.[62]

As the research program expanded in size and importance, there was the inevitable growth of confusion and uncertainty about objectives and responsibilities. As director of research, Clowes had the vision to see the need for generously supported fundamental research. Clowes worked hard and deluged Lilly with proposals and questions.[63] But Clowes had an impatience for detail and for the day-to-day administration of a growing research laboratory. He became, some thought, more stubborn and aloof, and there was often friction with other scientists. His long absences in the summers, when he worked in the company-financed laboratory at Woods Hole, Massachusetts, left the Indianapolis staff to their own devices, often happily so.[64] One particular conflict developed over a proposal to set up a company-sponsored research clinic at Indianapolis City Hospital. Clowes and Leon G. Zerfas, the physician in charge of the clinic, had many quarrels over details of the project. In such instances Lilly often became the arbiter, though on one occasion, at least, he, too, lost patience. Writing Clowes at Woods Hole in September 1924, Lilly exploded: "I suppose our whole clinical effort will have to wallow along like a dismasted frigate until you return. In the meantime I wash my hands of all responsibility, and will have nothing to do with it."[65]

The combination of company expansion and Clowes's particular interests doubtless prompted Lilly's reorganization of the Scientific Division in 1926, giving more responsibility to others, particularly Harley W. Rhodehamel, who served as director of research development. Even more important, in the late 1920s Lilly took the responsibility to call and chair regular research committee meetings. In contrast to Clowes's informal and eclectic methods, Lilly sent a formal agenda in advance of the meeting and encouraged those attending to discuss issues and proposals openly, with the result, Zerfas later remembered, of "an oftentimes verbal knock-down, shake-out on some subjects."[66] Each scientist had his say directly to Vice-President Lilly, who often made the necessary decision. "It was a marvelous feeling," one scientist recalled, to have Lilly chair these sessions.[67] These regular research meetings replaced the "time-consuming, irregular jumble" of conversations with Clowes and brought more systematic communication and decision making to the growing Scientific Division.[68]

The stepped-up attention to research in the 1920s produced results. The most important products introduced by the company, in addition to Iletin, were Amytal, Merthiolate, ephedrine, and liver extract.[69] Amytal was a barbituric acid derivative, the first American sedative of this kind and an indicator of the growing sophistication of the Indianapolis company's work in organic chemistry. Merthiolate was the antiseptic and germicide introduced in 1930 after it had been formulated at the University of Maryland with suppport of a company research fellowship. Ephedrine was more exotic. It derived from the work of Ko Kuei Chen. Born in China, Chen was educated at the University of Wisconsin, where as a pharmacy student he had visited Eli Lilly and Company. On his return to China, Chen isolated ephedrine from the Ma Huang plant and demonstrated its effectiveness as a vasoconstrictor, useful in treatment of asthma, hay fever, and allergies. Following his return to the United States in 1925, he met with Eli Lilly and convinced him of the value of ephedrine. By 1926 the company was receiving more orders for the versatile drug than it could fill. Three years later Chen joined the company as director of pharmacological research, the position he held until his retirement in 1963. Highly impressed earlier

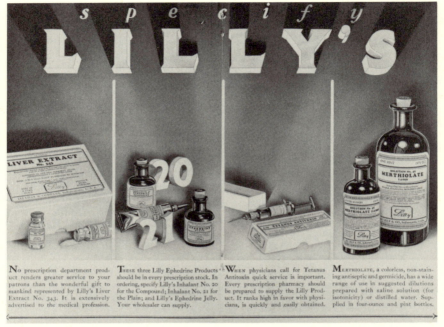

Advertisement, early 1930s.   *Eli Lilly and Company Archives*

by the company's role in insulin, Chen soon became a great admirer of the Lillys and the independence they permitted researchers. His highly productive research career later won him the Remington Medal of the American Pharmaceutical Association. Chen was a man of broad tastes. He had an interest in Chinese art and later advised Eli Lilly on collecting it. Chen also loved playing the tuba and watching the spectacle of college football marching bands.[70]

The development of liver extract came close to home for the pharmaceutical family. Eli's mother, Lilly Ridgely Lilly, began to suffer from pernicious anemia, an abnormality in blood production that was once nearly as deadly as diabetes had been. By early 1927 she had reached the stage where she could not tolerate the blandest foods. Through Zerfas, who had been studying the condition before Mrs. Lilly developed it, the family was able to bring to Indianapolis George R. Minot, a Harvard physician who was then making important breakthroughs on pernicious anemia. Minot prescribed a treatment for Mrs. Lilly of a calf's liver extract that had, in the short term, near miraculous results. This incident intensified the company's earlier interest in pernicious anemia and contributed to formal collaboration with Minot and his Harvard colleague, William P. Murphy. The Harvard scientists agreed to the joint venture because they were impressed with the Indianapolis firm's expertise in preparing liver extracts and with its earlier success in the collaboration with the University of Toronto. Together they developed the processes for mass production of a potent and uniform liver extract (Liver Extract 343), which the company began to sell in 1928. This project with Harvard also helped set up a collaboration with George Whipple of the University of Rochester, in 1929, which produced a treatment for secondary anemia that was put on the market in 1930 as Liver Extract No. 55.[71]

All parties to the two anemia projects benefited in profits and prestige. Minot, Murphy, and Whipple shared the Nobel Prize for medicine in 1934. The Indianapolis company basked in the reflected glory of its second Nobel Prize collaboration in ten years, proudly and liberally using as its slogan "Progress Through Research."[72] And anemia patients lived.

The work on anemia and the collaboration with Harvard and Rochester built on the model of the insulin project. As Lilly had predicted, the lessons learned from that first university-pharmaceutical company collaboration contributed to smoothing the bumps of later joint ventures. Businessmen and scientists had a fuller appreciation of each other's interests, and such matters as drawing up agreements and assigning patents and royalties, which Lilly oversaw, proved much easier in the late 1920s than they had in 1922-23. By then Lilly was developing his "contract paragraph book," which contained several versions of standard agreements, from among which he would select appropriate paragraphs in drawing up contracts with outside researchers. What had been so difficult in 1923 had been subjected to Lilly's drive for efficiency and system.[73]

That drive was unrelenting during the 1920s and brought success upon success. By the standards of the American business culture that so pervaded the decade, Eli Lilly had reached the top rung of the ladder. Nurtured by his father, he combined hard work with a wide vision of the dictates of modern business to build one of the most successful companies in America. He was not, however, a happy man.

Chapter 4

The Middle Years, 1907-1948

Eli Lilly was a hard-working, intense young man in the early 1920s. He spent long, pressure-filled days setting up the straight-line production system, laying out Building 22, establishing the insulin project, and administering the new initiatives in research. His active and forceful drive for efficiency and productivity was apparent to all. So was his temper. He had a "reputation of being a stickler for perfection," one employee later recalled, and was "a little hard to get along with on a day to day basis out in the plant."[1] Production workers saw his attention to detail and his passion for order and cleanliness occasionally burst forth in an outraged kick at an example of carelessness or disorder. He once fired a worker on the spot for using a chemical from an unlabeled container. Those employees tempted to sneak off for a coffee break (in the days when such a distraction was uncommon in American industry) knew they risked his periodic raids to flush out slackers and get them back to their production lines or desks. Lilly later admitted that "I was sometimes so intent on my job that I would look serious and people would take that for anger and they would worry about it and wonder 'who's going to get hell now.'"[2]

His father knew well this side of Eli. Although not often inclined to include negative criticism in letters to his son, on one occasion at least he made clear the problem. Quoting an epigram he had come across—"The test of mastery is restraint"—J. K. Lilly, Sr., wrote: "You have mastery and you have more restraint than I have. Yet you could use a little more."[3] Since the senior Lilly was in fact a most restrained man, the force of this tactfully understated criticism was all the stronger. In his twenties and thirties Eli Lilly had the unrestrained intensity of a very ambitious young man. Impatiently he pushed ahead, determined to prove that though born to the business he was fully capable of making his own contribution to its success.

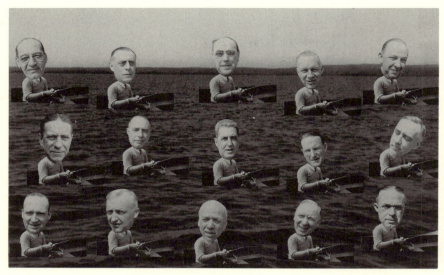

Rowdy Revelers, 1930s. Top row, left to right,
Anton Vonnegut, William H. Stafford, Eli Lilly,
Nicholas H. Noyes, Robert B. Failey; middle row,
left to right, Garvin M. Brown, Charles Latham,
Fred Appel, George L. Denny, Sylvester Johnson;
bottom row, left to right, Roger Wolcott, Robert
Parrott, G. Barret Moxley, Robert Scott, W.
Hathaway Simmons.

Charles Latham, Jr.

There was consequently little time for diversion or frivolity in the
1910s and 1920s. He traveled often for the company but seldom for pleasure. He enjoyed Lake Wawasee the most, especially on one of his sailboats.
And there was the fishing club known as the Rowdy Revelers. His father
began the annual gathering in about 1898, inviting male friends to spend
a week at the family cottage on the lake. After he discontinued it in 1916
Eli began his own Rowdy Revelers, with about a dozen men gathering at
Wawasee the last week in April to fish, play cards, sail, indulge in practical
jokes, and talk. Lilly kept careful records of the number of fish caught; he
was among the leaders, with a total of 106 fish for the years between 1916
and 1931.[4] He had very few other diversions or interests. He took little
pleasure in his house or garden and did not enjoy hosting dinner parties
or other formal entertainments.[5]

   Part of the intensity and much of the eventual unhappiness of the
1920s came from a marriage that was failing. Eli and Evelyn Lilly had once

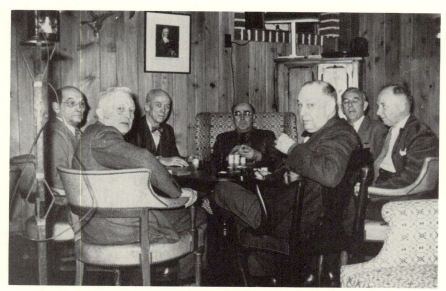

Rowdy Revelers in basement (the "hilarium") of Wawasee Cottage, 1950s. Left to right: Anton Vonnegut, Robert Parrott, G. Barret Moxley, Eli Lilly, Robert B. Failey, Sylvester Johnson, Robert Scott.

Eli Lilly and Company Archives

fully loved each other. By the mid-1920s that was no more. Evelyn grew to desire a more outgoing, active life, and she became more strong-willed and independent. She tried to encourage other interests for Eli, such as collecting antiques. She wanted to give more dinners and parties. She wanted to travel. Eli had neither the time nor the interest for such diversions.[6] He later admitted that "I . . . was probably selfish and remiss in not doing and being what she wished, and I do not blame her a lot more than myself in the eventual outcome." He did blame her for a "lack of maternal instinct," however, which along with his own inexperience he believed contributed to the death of their two infant sons. And he accused her of being affectionless, cold, and uncompromising.[7]

Evelyn began to make her own life. In 1913, when, in an unusual break from the routine of work, Eli joined his father on a two-week Caribbean cruise, Evelyn traveled to Washington, D.C., to visit Catherine Beveridge, wife of Indiana's former Senator Albert Beveridge. The two women became close friends. Beginning about 1920 Evelyn began to spend summers in a small house on the Beveridge property at Beverly Farms, Massachu-

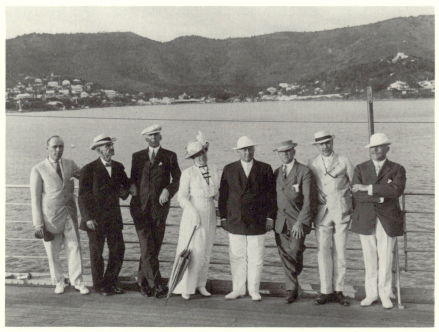

A Caribbean cruise, 1913. Left to right: Eli Lilly,   *Eli Lilly and Company Archives*
Thomas Spann, William Wheelock, Mr. and Mrs.
Smith, W. J. Brown, J. K. Lilly, Sr., and George R.
Sullivan.

setts. In the first years Eli joined her and his infant daughter for a few weeks each summer. There were no children other than Evie, born in 1918, although to the family's sadness Evelyn suffered another miscarriage in February 1922.[8]

In the late summer of 1922, while the work on insulin was still intense, Eli made an effort at marital reconciliation. Leaving Evie at Beverly Farms with a nurse, he took Evelyn on a auto trip through the White Mountains, "stopping at the most famous hotels and resorts, while I made every effort to be the devoted bridegroom." His romantic campaign to "snatch victory from defeat" failed, and the couple drifted further apart.[9] The following spring Evelyn indulged her wish to travel and joined an Indianapolis friend, Mrs. Hugh Hanna, on a trip to Paris.[10]

Eli shared his unhappiness with his father. When he mentioned divorce, however, the elder Lilly exploded and threatened to disinherit him. Eli told him that he could no longer live with Evelyn and was going to leave her,

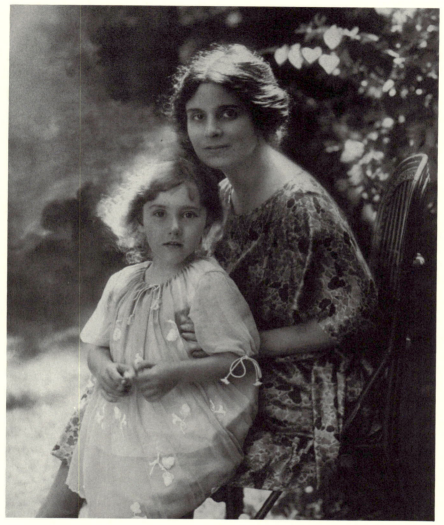

Evelyn Fortune Lilly and daughter Evie.   *Madeline Fortune Elder*

with or without his approval. Divorce came in 1926. In the settlement Evelyn received $300,000 in cash, their Lafayette touring car, their house at 1239 North Delaware Street, and most of its contents. Eli reserved for himself some family furniture, a Wayman Adams portrait of Evie and some other portraits, and his grandfather's Civil War recruiting poster.[11]

The tragedy extended beyond Eli and Evelyn. All of Indianapolis knew. It was a small town, the Lilly and Fortune families were among its most prominent citizens, and divorce was as close to scandal as many gossips could hope to come in those days. One of the last people to learn was Eli's mother. He had not confided in her. She had once warned Evelyn that the Lilly men were hard to live with and perhaps was not surprised.[12] Suffering from pernicious anemia and doubtless distraught by the deterioration of the marriage, "she asks no questions," her husband wrote Eli in March 1926, "and appears desirous of avoiding the subject."[13]

But the subject could not be avoided. There was Evie. Eli hoped that Evelyn would allow him custody of the seven-year-old child. She did not, leaving town so quickly in early March that J.K. Lilly, Sr., referred to the "abduction" of his granddaughter.[14] The court concurred in awarding Evelyn custody of the child. Eli agreed to pay $250 a month in child support and was granted rights of having his daughter with him for one month in early summer and another month in late summer plus a week in late December and a week at Easter.[15] Evelyn and Evie settled on the Beveridge property in Beverly Farms, and Eli began writing warm, affectionate letters to his daughter, telling how much he missed her: "What a lonely old house this has gotten to be without your bursting in on us every little while to rattle our old bones into some semblance of a good time!"[16] In July he reported that he and his beloved Aunt Margaret Ridgely "have just bought a house—an old victorian brick house over on Broadway near 13th street. Aunt Margaret and I have picked out a nice room for you and Dante."[17] Evie came to visit in October that first year and in later years at Christmas and during the summer, often joining her father at Wawasee. He made other efforts to stay close, taking her on a trip to Washington, D.C., in March 1928, or attempting to spark her interest in prehistoric Indians.[18] Eli never got over the sadness. He never talked of his marriage to Evelyn or his divorce, even to close friends. Neither in his personal reminiscences nor in the official published history of the company is Evelyn or his first marriage mentioned.[19]

The divorce also touched the family's pharmaceutical business. Evelyn's father was very upset. William Fortune's decades of friendship with J. K. Lilly, Sr., had included a 30,000-mile trip around the world aboard the Cunard ship *Samaria*, lasting from 24 January to 31 May 1923.[20] Earlier, their friendship and the marriage of their children had led J. K. Lilly, Sr., to offer Fortune the opportunity to buy stock in the company. He became one of the first stockholders not an officer or blood member of the family

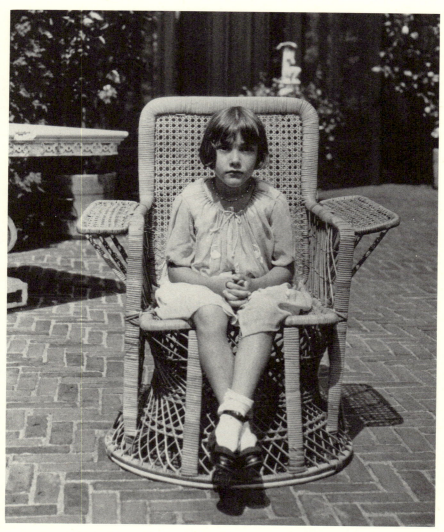

Evie Lilly, ca. 1926.   *Eli Lilly and Company Archives*

when he purchased $100,000 worth of stock in 1913. Fortune's bitterness over the divorce caused him to strike at the Lillys through the family's business. He charged that salaries paid to top managers were too high and stock dividends too low. He brought a stenographer to one board meeting, attempting to annoy the family. J. K. Lilly, Sr., advised his son that "the important thing for all of us is to keep our mouths shut on this chap's doings."[21] The bitterness persisted, with the Lillys resentful that Fortune continued to complain about high executive salaries even though his company stock by the end of the decade was worth one and a half million dollars— "An increased value to which he in no way contributed," the senior Lilly fumed.[22]

For Evelyn Fortune Lilly an unhappy marriage was followed in 1930 by marriage to Frederic C. Bartlett, a distinguished collector of Postimpressionist paintings, who at one time owned Georges Seurat's *Sunday Afternoon on the Island of La Grande Jatte*, and who was himself an accomplished painter. Evelyn Bartlett began to paint, too, and in the mid-1930s enjoyed the achievement of showings of her work in New York City and at the John Herron Art Institute in Indianapolis. She and Frederic traveled widely, entertained brilliantly, and lived happily together in Beverly, Massachusetts, and Fort Lauderdale, Florida. "Eli never brought me out the way Frederic did," she recalled sixty years after her divorce.[23]

Eli Lilly married again, too. Sharing his house with his Aunt Margaret, he "gradually determined not to let the venom and poison distilled from my marital experience . . . ruin my whole life and turn me into a complete misanthrope."[24] On 7 November 1927 he and Ruth Helen Allison wed. She had been his secretary, working in the same office for seven years. For their wedding trip they booked passage on the *Conte Biancamano,* leaving New York on 23 November for Italy. They spent their honeymoon traveling in Italy and Sicily, marred only by the news from Indianapolis of the death of Aunt Margaret.[25]

With Ruth he found finally the enduring love and affection neither Evelyn nor his mother had provided. Eli and Ruth Allison Lilly enjoyed nearly a half century of marriage, a marriage, he wrote in 1968, of "unbelieveable happiness and satisfaction." To close friends theirs was simply "a great love match."[26] Eli was devoted to her. He usually called her "Ruthie" and wrote and spoke of her always with warm affection. She was an unpretentious, kind, and friendly woman, who came to share his interests. Though she later collected expensive European watches, she also shopped for dresses on sale in the basement of the L. S. Ayres department store in Indianapolis. Every morning she read her daily Bible lesson. Often while talking her hands were busy doing needlepoint. In the evenings she and Eli would share a book by reading aloud to each other. She especially enjoyed traveling, and in the first ten years of their marriage they took trips to Florida, New Orleans, California, Toronto, Hawaii, and Bermuda. Later they would

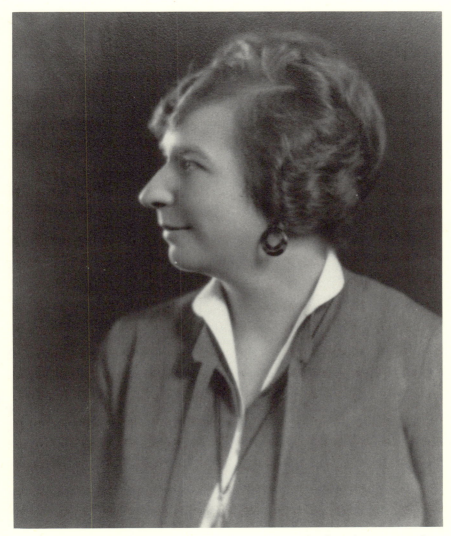

Ruth Allison Lilly, ca. 1930.   *Eli Lilly and Company Archives*

travel to Mexico and Europe. Ruth liked to collect antiques, and Eli joined her, especially in furnishing the William Conner house north of Indianapolis, which they bought in 1934.[27]

Ruth shared Eli's love for the cottage at Lake Wawasee, too. They spent several weeks there every summer and sometimes went also for a weekend in winter iceboating. Ruth worked in her flower garden and joined her husband to sail, swim, and sit on the large front porch to read and talk. One warm, moonlit evening in August 1936 the couple sailed until past midnight. At Wawasee, too, they escaped the heat of the city. Eli enjoyed checking the Indianapolis temperatures, noting as much as ten to fifteen degrees difference at the lake. They also escaped the business and social commitments of Indianapolis. Sometimes there were guests at Wawasee, but only the closest friends or most important business associates were ever invited. Eli tried hard to protect his privacy there and to keep the cares of Indianapolis at a distance. His rule of answering only life and death letters was well known to his friends and to Eva Rice Goble, his secretary at the company.[28] Wawasee was the constant delight of his life, expressed in one of the little poems he began to write after marriage to Ruth:

> I must go to Wawasee again to give my
>   heart delight
> In the ancestral cot in the woodsy lot
>   beside a garden bright
> And what I ask are kin and friends, and
>   vital to all of this
> Is Ruthie, more fair than the crystal
>   air, to fill my cup with bliss.[29]

Among Eli's occasional trips to Wawasee without Ruth were the annual spring fishing excursions with the Rowdy Revelers, which he continued until 1959. He looked forward with eager anticipation and careful planning to this chance "to clean the bats out of my belfry," as he wrote in 1937.[30] By this time his invitations to the dozen or so friends were elaborately prepared, sometimes written in humorous poetry. His poetic invitation one year he titled "An Allergy: Wrote on a Hoosier Lakeside," which concluded:

> In short, a week of friendly jubilation,
> To purge, reject, expel, by quick catharsis
> A winter's ill-digested accumulation
> Of discords, doubts, fatigue, and business farces [31]

World War II tested the commitment of the Rowdy Revelers, but they restricted their driving in order to save enough gasoline coupons to make

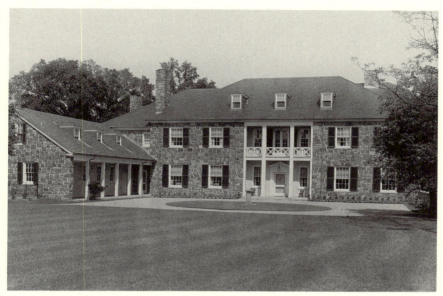

Home of Eli and Ruth Lilly, Sunset Lane, built   *Eli Lilly and Company Archives*
1930–31.

the trip. "To many of us," Lilly wrote, "it was the shining event of the season."[32]

Marriage to Ruth also led to a new home in Indianapolis. J. K. Lilly, Sr., contributed substantially to Joe's costly restoration of a home on Washington Boulevard. In order to be fair to Eli his father offered him equal amounts of money. He also offered his older son the choice of building on the twenty acres to which he had moved in 1928, located on the northern edge of the city in the town of Crows Nest. Eli accepted the offer, and in 1930 he began construction, using as a model for the house's exterior the Maryland birthplace of Colonel Eli Lilly. Situated on six acres extending from Sunset Lane to the west bank of the White River, the three-story home had four bedrooms with three baths and an additional four servants rooms with two baths.[33] Attached to the house was a four-car garage, which his father, now also his neighbor, told Eli "is the envy of all the neighborhood showfers and I am certain you can have the 'pick' of the whole bunch."[34]

In 1931, 5807 Sunset Lane became home for Eli and Ruth. It was a warm and inviting house, not at all forbidding. A survey of Indianapolis realtors forty years after the house was built ranked it among the top five houses they would choose for themselves. One of Eli's special projects in the house was a plan to paint murals in the third-floor ballroom. He very much admired the work of Grant Wood, but Wood could not accept his offer and sent instead his student, John Pusey. In the fall of 1936 Pusey painted an elaborate series of murals, depicting education, music, sports, work, and politics, and including in one panel Eli, Ruth, and Evie in front of the William Conner house. As other houses were built in Crows Nest it soon became among the most prestigious neighborhoods in Indianapolis, so attractive to top executives of Eli Lilly and Company that it came to be known as "Pill Hill."[35]

A new marriage and a new house were only part of the new life for Eli Lilly in the 1930s. He began to seek intensively to know himself and to improve himself. In 1934 he prepared a five-page guide which he titled "Plan for Developing Proper Outlook on Life." His plan began with the assumption that in life "the supreme object is the growth of personality." This growth could be stimulated "by the exercise of the proper amount of will power," because each person "can so develop his habits of indulging in expansive tendencies so as to broaden and brighten his life and surroundings." Thus he recommended development of "the constant habit of reading books and working out plans that have to be thought over and struggled over." And he urged cultivation of appreciation for music, poetry, and art. He urged getting rid of the poisons of gossip and rumor and recommended cultivating a sense of humor to recognize that "unexpected incongruities and playful exaggerations are the salt of life." He warned against "tantrums, whining, self-indulgence, boasting, irresponsibility." These and other imperfections could be diminished because "personal characteristics are largely matters of habit, and with sufficient will-power and determination we can change our modes of life."[36]

Lilly sent his "Plan for Developing Proper Outlook on Life" to his good friend Glenn Black, who responded that it was easy to "understand how you could formulate such an outline for it is you to a T." Lilly replied that in fact much of it was "a boiled-down version of Mr. Overstreet's book, 'About Ourselves.'"[37] Lilly had used his own words and choice of emphases, but the core of his plan did indeed come from his reading of H. A. Overstreet's *About Ourselves: Psychology for Normal People,* published in 1927. Overstreet was a philosophy professor at the College of the City of New York. His book addressed the ills of civilization in the jazz age of post-World War I America. He was particularly critical of the materialism, hedonism, and philistinism that he found so dominant. Above all, Overstreet used the newly popular discipline of psychology "to reveal ourselves to ourselves."[38] *About Ourselves,* the *New York Times Book Review* asserted, was a "book that ought to be profoundly helpful to any ordinary person who wants to try the experiment of remolding himself a little nearer to his heart's desire."[39]

The other major source for Lilly's 1934 plan was Benjamin Franklin. Franklin's autobiography is the classic masterpiece of self-help literature, revealing a man who rationally and skillfully disciplined himself to expand and broaden his mind and character. Lilly was a close reader of Franklin, adopting the Philadelphian's plan of making a chart on which to mark each evening the virtues that had been practiced that day. Lilly decided, like Franklin, to give particular attention each week to one specific virtue "in order to avoid the danger of too great a diffusion of effort."[40]

Whether or not Lilly kept a daily chart of his virtues, there is no doubt that he experienced a "growth of personality" in the 1930s. His horizons widened far beyond McCarty Street and the business of pharmaceuticals. He bought a farm and became knowledgeable about horses, hogs, and corn. He developed an even more passionate interest in prehistoric archaeology, where he did indeed follow his dictum to read books and work out "plans that have to be thought over and struggled over." His struggles with archaeology were among the most enjoyable of his life. He began to attend church regularly and developed a strong attachment to Christ Church, the Episcopal church on the Circle in Indianapolis.[41] He began to read about religious philosophy and psychology, about ancient Greece and Rome, and about China. He also read biography, ranging from Winston Churchill to Beatrice Webb, and history, especially Indiana history. Unlike his brother, who became a collector of rare books, Eli bought books to read and also to mark with red underlinings and scribble with marginal notes.[42] He became especially fascinated with the development of personality and character in children and near the end of the 1930s began a correspondence with college professors that led to research projects lasting for several decades.

In these and other ways, as later chapters elaborate, Lilly in the 1930s and after was no longer the narrow, intense, hard-driving businessman he had been. He became president of the pharmaceutical company in 1932 and for the next decade and a half worked hard to ensure growth and prosperity. But the pill factory was no longer the sole reason for his existence. "I need all the help I can get," he wrote a friend on assuming the presidency, "but do not propose to worry myself to death about it."[43] He retained his temper, but his outbursts were less frequent and no longer led to shouting or kicking. Sometimes only his face turned white in a way that close associates alone recognized as a sign of his anger.[44] He came to be less feared and more admired by employees as he energetically introduced new and more liberal personnel policies at McCarty Street. Most important, he made time for cultivation of his own interests away from the business. Ruth was central to this development of a proper outlook on life, as he noted in 1958 when he told an audience that "best friends say that Mrs. Lilly made a different man of me. That was a very desirable accomplishment."[45] But the changes that followed their marriage in 1927 came also because he willed them and sought them as intensely as earlier he had sought efficient, mass production of pills and elixirs.

Lilly's wider horizons of the 1930s did not lead him to abandon his attachments to his hometown and home state. Rather, his sense of place matured and deepened, reflected particularly in his expanding study of the prehistory and history of Indiana. His interest in the Indiana Historical Society developed quickly in the early 1930s into a major commitment of his time and money. And as his personal wealth grew, his philanthropy focused on Indiana and Indianapolis. This love of place would become even stronger as he grew older.

The love that remained strongest was that for Ruth and for his father. For his father the love was clear, bright, and enduring, the bond as close as it could be, the influence continuing even after J. K. Lilly, Sr., died in 1948. The senior Lilly continued to send Eli letters expressing love and approbation on his birthday and at Christmas. On Eli's birthday soon after his divorce and remarriage, his father wrote him: "I love you with my whole heart Eli, my dear son, my partner, my considerate and genial critic. . . . We have stood together through every joy and trial." In 1933 the birthday greeting began: "Forty-Eight years of sunshine and shadows finds you a fine and upstanding character, filling your place in the world cheerfully and well; a source of pride and deep satisfaction to your parents." And on 1 April 1940 he wrote that "the hopes and ambitions of those earlier days, for the little Eli, have been fullfilled. . . . You have builded a great world industry upon foundations laid by your progenitors. Best of all, you have accomplished all this while winning the love and confidence of the family and immediate associates."[46]

J. K. Lilly, Sr., remained closely interested in the pharmaceutical business even after he turned over the presidency to his elder son in 1932. Until the last year of his life, whether in California, Florida, or elsewhere, he would write Eli and Joe with specific questions about such matters as insulin production or the previous month's sales figures.[47] But J. K. Lilly, Sr., developed other interests also in later years. In the 1930s he began to grow orchids and to collect Stephen Foster sheet music and other Foster memorabilia. The Foster collection became a near-obsession, carried on in a specially built cottage, located at his apple orchard north of the city and first called Melodeon Hall and then renamed Foster Hall. By the mid-1930s he had eight full-time employees working at Foster Hall to catalog the huge collection, which he eventually donated to the University of Pittsburgh. J. K. Lilly, Sr., also constructed a family genealogy, wrote a family history, and began to collect and preserve family letters and memorabilia.[48] He provided financial assistance in the form of a monthly check to a large list of close and distant relatives. On his deathbed he gave his sons the list of "certain impecunious friends and relatives . . . to dispose of them as you see best." Eli soon began to send the monthly checks.[49]

J. K. Lilly, Sr., had a droll sense of humor, particularly delighting in using words in unconventional ways. He wrote poetry, both serious and amusing. He read books, especially history and economics. He was especially taken by Albert Beveridge's biography of Lincoln.[50] But there was a dark side, too. "Life is not all happy," he wrote in his reminiscences in 1940. "The favorite time for haunting is at night." Then "incidents of unkindness to members of my family, exhibitions of hasty and ungoverned temper, . . . and thousands of silly doings seem to be registered by white-hot irons on that part of the brain devoted to such records. . . . Many and many a night," he wrote, only a sleeping pill from McCarty Street "can close the eyes in restful sleep."[51]

One of the great sadnesses for the family was the long illness of Lilly Ridgely Lilly. Her battle with pernicious anemia continued, and by the late 1920s she was an invalid. George R. Minot's liver extract treatment brought only temporary relief. Devotedly caring for her, J. K. Lilly, Sr., spent less and less time at the office and more time at home sitting by her bed. She died on 19 April 1934.[52]

Fourteen months later J. K. Lilly, Sr., married Lila Allison Humes, a widow and the sister of Ruth Allison Lilly. He was seventy-three; she was fifty-one. Now married to sisters, father and son had additional opportunities to spend time together. The two couples traveled to Hawaii in 1936 and elsewhere. In 1938 J. K. Lilly, Sr., built a home next to the old cottage at Wawasee. He had seldom visited there in the 1920s, but now he and Lila spent their summers at the lake. Only in his early eighties did his health begin to decline seriously. He died at the age of eighty-six on 8 February 1948, leaving an estate valued at $6.5 million, most of which, after provision for his wife, went to the Lilly Endowment.[53]

In 1957, on the fiftieth anniversary of Eli Lilly's entry into the company, his photograph appeared on the cover of the Lilly Review. Several old friends remarked how closely he resembled his father.[54] The resemblance between J. K. Lilly, Sr., and Eli Lilly was more than physical, as the son well knew. Sometime in the 1950s, Eli began to jot down aphorisms and quotations in a notebook he called his "Shining Phrase Book." One entry read: "Dr. Holmes observed that every man is an omnibus in which his ancestors ride." In modestly accepting the Remington Medal in 1958, the most important formal honor of his pharmaceutical career, Lilly used Oliver Wendell Holmes's dictum as the main theme of his address. His father's example, character, and love were with him always, the omnibus in which he rode.[55]

With J. K. Lilly, Sr., and Ruth Allison Lilly as his twin sources of affection and support, Eli Lilly's familial anguish focused on his daughter. Evie was seven years old when her parents divorced. She remembered all her life that she first learned of their separation from other children on the school playground. They taunted and mocked her, and it hurt deeply. Evie also grew up feeling that she should have been a boy, the male heir in the Lilly family. Evie's troubles were those of many children of divorced parents. She felt, she once told her aunt, that no one loved her. Her father tried hard to prevent this tragedy. He made certain she visited him in Indianapolis or Wawasee as often as possible, and he went to visit her, too, in Massachusetts or in Virginia, when she began to attend Foxcroft School there. To make Indiana visits more attractive, he encouraged her adolescent interest in horses. She loved to ride and began in 1933 to show horses at the Indiana State Fair. Eli built stables at Sunset Lane, and he used the Conner farm for a large investment in horses to please Evie.[56]

Eli Lilly's most lavish display of interest in Evie was the debut he gave for her in June 1937. Evelyn Bartlett marked her daughter's formal entry into society that year with a debut at Boston's Ritz Carlton Hotel. In a very uncharacteristic display of ostentation, Lilly more than matched the

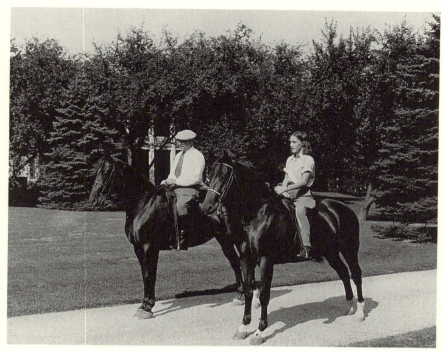

Eli Lilly and Evie Lilly, ca. 1933.   *Eli Lilly and Company Archives*

Boston crowd. The Indianapolis festivities began with a Saturday afternoon
tea at the Lilly home on Sunset Lane. In the house and in a large marquee
set on the lawn the family received five hundred guests, amidst a profusion
of flowers, fountains, and statuettes. The crowning event of the week of
parties was a dance on Wednesday evening, also held at the Lilly home.
Indianapolis society had known nothing like it. Decades later those who
were at 5807 Sunset Lane that balmy night in June remembered in detail
the festive occasion. Large tents and plants were placed on the lawn. So,
too, for dancing, was the portable wooden basketball floor of Butler University. A mind reader and other entertainment provided diversion, but the
unparalleled attraction for the hundreds of young guests was Benny Goodman and his orchestra. The King of Swing was the most popular musician
among American teenagers of the late 1930s. Lilly, whose taste in music
certainly did not include jazz, wondered "how those kids can get such a
kick out of such caterwauling . . . but somehow they do!" He was pleased,
however, when Goodman put down his clarinet and came over to sit with

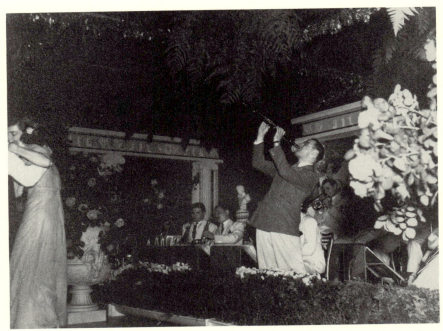

Benny Goodman and band at Evie Lilly's debut   *Eli Lilly and Company Archives*
dance, Sunset Lane, 1937.

him and was even mildly surprised that he seemed to be such a sensible
and nice young man, even if his music was not.[57]

Lilly provided Evie also with all the money she needed, and more.
He contributed $400 a month for her support in the 1930s. On her twenty-
first birthday he increased the amount to $600 and sent it directly to her
rather than to her mother, advising Evie to give some of it to charity and
also to "start a little savings fund."[58] And in 1940 and 1947 he set up large
trust funds for her, which gave her an income by 1948 of about $68,000 a
year.[59]

The shower of money brought few rainbows for Evie. She was very
independent, and many thought her a stuck-up, spoiled, rich kid. She did
not like school, and her enthusiasms in the larger world seldom led to a
completed task. Her father was very pleased when in 1939 she began
working in one of the research departments at the pharmaceutical company
and the two of them rode to work together.[60] But she soon gave up this
interest for another. In 1940 she married Francis Burrage Chalifoux. Evie's

mother strongly opposed the marriage, thinking Chalifoux something of a playboy. Evie never forgave her mother. Whether her father approved or not, he attended the ceremony at the Bartletts' grand home in Beverly, but cautiously wrote a friend afterwards: "The groom showed up and every-thing, and apparently it was a great success. Time will tell."[61] Time did tell: the marriage ended in a wartime divorce. Evie married a second time, in 1944, to Alfred M. Roberts, a dashing Navy flier. Again the ceremony was held at her mother's Beverly home, and again her father attended. Again the marriage ended in divorce. By the late 1940s Evie was drinking heavily. Her behavior deeply disappointed her mother and father, and they discussed treatment. Lilly refused, however, to sign the papers that would commit her to a sanitarium. Her mother took responsibility and had Evie commit-ted, another act the daughter held against her mother.[62]

Evie's troubles deeply distressed her father. Her visit to Indianapolis in the spring of 1948 left him saddened that her alcoholism was worsening and her sense of responsibility declining. He continued his expressions of love, but, without telling her, decided that he could not in good conscience allow Evie to inherit his fortune. In late 1948 he instructed his attorney to exclude her as a beneficiary from his will, giving the money instead to the Lilly Endowment.[63] He told no one else of this change, but with the new will he placed a handwritten letter for Ruth and another for his brother, explaining to each his decision and asking them to explain his actions to Evie. To Ruth he wrote:

> I have always appreciated deeply your sympathetic understanding of Evie's shortcomings and of my problems in dealing with them. I have done the best I could to help her make a useful, happy life. If I have erred at all it is perhaps in already giving her too much of this world's goods without having been able to inculcate in her an equal sense of responsibility.[64]

In his letter to Joe, Eli admitted that his relationship with Evie "has been an exceedingly painful one to me and I can not bring myself to discuss it freely with you even though our personal relations have always been close and affectionate." He explained his remorse: "I have deeply regretted the impact upon her of the divorce of her mother and me which probably deprived her of the family security and affectionate environment which should be every child's natural birthright." His efforts to help Evie had failed. She refused an education, so that "her life is poor in intellectual interests," which "causes her to seek happiness in physical satisfaction, in material indulgences, and in stupid idleness." And, he added, "she has become an alcoholic." In sum, Eli wrote his brother, "Her life now seems to be without purpose and she does not appear to have character, intellect, or sense of responsibility necessary to administer a large fortune wisely."[65] Evie's failure to develop what her father regarded as a proper outlook on life was a constant disappointment and sadness for him. It provided also, as later chapters indicate, stimulus for his own efforts to discourage others from the kind of life Evie lived.

———————————

As his interests matured and enlarged, Eli Lilly remained a man of simple but carefully developed tastes and habits. His outward appearance was unremarkable. A newspaper writer described him in 1939: "He always stands very erect and he walks with a springy step. He has beetling black brows and what best can be referred to as an ultra bald head. His face is genial."[66] Ostentation he abhorred, with few exceptions. He dressed conservatively, though always neatly and appropriate to the occasion. In summers he wore white linen suits, staying carefully immaculate on even the hottest of Hoosier days. He seldom attended a dinner or reception, especially out of town, without inquiring the manner of dress: "How stylish are you fellows at that meeting? Is it dinner coats or plain business clothing?" he wrote in 1942.[67] His taste in food was the simple fare of middle-class midwesterners. A nice lunch was a tongue sandwich and a piece of apple pie. His favorite drink was Coca-Cola. He seldom drank alcoholic beverages. He liked the realistic paintings of Grant Wood and later Maxfield Parrish. He found modern art without redeeming value. In music he enjoyed some opera, particularly *Rigoletto,* with Giuseppe Verdi's wonderful melodies and its story of a father's love for his daughter. But he preferred above all the theatrical tunes and folk songs of late nineteenth-century America. He and his father would sometimes get together to sing them, and late in life he still remembered the words to many.[68]

He traveled through America and Europe, but Indianapolis and Wawasee remained his favorite places. The Hoosier state's capital was still very much a small midwestern town, even though its population had reached 386,972 by 1940. "The visitor's first impression," the 1941 WPA state guide noted, "is one of spacious friendliness—broad streets, an almost Southern leisureliness, and fewer tall buildings than are seen in most cities of comparable size," adding that the town "offers little of the brilliant or the bizarre."[69] The south side of town, where the pharmaceutical company and other factories and warehouses were located, was the home in the 1930s for most working-class residents, including a small foreign-born and Jewish population, though middle-class Jews were beginning to move to the north side. Blacks were clustered along Indiana Avenue, in the near northwest area. Further north of downtown and the Circle were the middle- and upper-class neighborhoods, moving ever northward, especially on Delaware, Pennsylvania, and Meridian streets. Lilly's friends and acquaintances came from these north side neighborhoods, men and women he had known since childhood, whose parents and grandparents had been friends and neighbors, and who belonged to the same clubs and attended the same churches and schools. When Booth Tarkington published a new novel in 1945, Lilly and his friends were astir as they easily identified the Indianapolis woman on whom the novel centered and the upper-class society in which she moved. In the town of Indianapolis Lilly's roots held deep and firm.[70]

Lilly's opinions in politics were conservative but seldom passionately expressed. In his youth he had been an active supporter of Theodore Roosevelt and the Bull Moose Progressive party of 1912, working as a precinct committeeman. And he took some part in the political career of Indiana's favorite Progressive, Albert Beveridge. By the 1930s he was staunchly Republican in politics, largely because of his strong animosity for Franklin Roosevelt and the New Deal. The New Deal, he believed, was leading America to "the brink of destruction and slavery" by limiting individual freedom and restricting free enterprise. Lilly's typical business conservatism was strongly held, but he took no active part in political life beyond small contributions of money.[71]

In his middle years Eli Lilly also became a man of wealth, a multi-millionaire. As the pharmaceutical company prospered so did he. His annual income rose from $22,606 in 1920 to just over $1 million in the mid-1930s, most of it in Eli Lilly and Company stock dividends. His personal fortune by the late 1950s included Lilly stock worth nearly $31.5 million and $3.5 million in cash and tax-free bonds.[72] Wealth brought new responsibilities and problems. Like his father, he provided financial support for friends, relatives, and even strangers. With the accumulation

of wealth he gradually became more sensitive to the need to develop systematic and accountable means of philanthropy, leading to the formation in
1937 of the Lilly Endowment. Wealth also threatened his sense of privacy
and challenged his determined modesty. Unlike many of America's richest
citizens, Lilly often insisted that his gifts not be made public and that his
name not be attached to the fellowships, buildings, or programs he financed.

Wealth brought threats to safety as well as to privacy and modesty.
Most dramatic for a brief moment was an attempted extortion in 1934. At
the end of April Lilly received an unsigned letter, stating that unless he
paid $25,000 Evie would be kidnapped. With reports of actual kidnappings
and the exploits of Indiana bank robber John Dillinger filling the newspapers, this threat was not taken lightly. Lilly called the police. He also
hired Pinkerton investigators. The extortion letter instructed Lilly to take
the train from Indianapolis to Vincennes and to sit on the south side of
the coach. When he saw a white flag waving from a tree he was to throw
out the window a package containing $25,000 in small denomination bills.
Lilly followed the instructions except that he put bogus bills in the package
and brought along the police, who jumped off the train soon after the flag
was spotted near Paragon. Making investigations locally, they learned that
the flag had been used for a recent Sunday School celebration. With this
clue they soon found the two young men behind the plot and arrested
them. Their youth and the pleas of their families convinced Lilly not to
press charges. He later hired one of them to work at the company.[73]

Wealth brought new challenges, but it did not change significantly
Lilly's fundamental values. He remained attached firmly to family and
hometown, modest in his material needs, dependent on old personal
friendships. His life was as far from that of the stereotypical wealthy playboy as can be imagined. He did change in the 1930s, but this expansion
of his interests came not from growing wealth but derived instead from
his own inner assessment of who he was and who he wanted to be. In
striving to achieve something closer to a proper outlook on life he found
his largest rewards.

Chapter 5

President of the Pill Factory, 1932-1948

On 26 January 1932 Eli Lilly became president of the family pharmaceutical company he had joined a quarter century earlier. Two new buildings, both opened in 1934, symbolized his leadership. One was a full-scale replica of his grandfather's 1876 laboratory. The idea for the replica was Eli's, and he planned its construction in near perfect detail by use of an old photograph and the clear memory of his father.[1] The other new building was a research laboratory, one of the most fully equipped facilities in the world. The replica looked to the past, to the days of grinding pokeroot and mixing Succus Alterans. The laboratory looked to the future, to the continued growth of a large, modern, research-based pharmaceutical corporation. It was characteristic of Eli Lilly that in these two buildings he planned for growth and change yet remembered the past.

In the years of his presidency, from 1932 to 1948, the pharmaceutical company remained fully controlled by the family. Chairman of the Board J. K. Lilly, Sr., and his two sons owned most of the company stock. In 1934 the senior Lilly transferred to his sons 40,000 shares of stock, raising the total each son held to about 100,000 shares so as "to bring holdings of each of you more nearly to my own."[2] The Lilly triumvirate were the actual managers as well as owners. They made all important decisions and continued to work closely together, though Eli had the largest and the final responsibility. J. K. Lilly, Jr., maintained his primary interest in sales, and Eli remained more closely involved in production and research activities. On all major questions the two brothers acted only after consultation. Joe and Eli always made sure that one was in Indianapolis to watch over day-to-day business, arranging their travel and vacations with that prerequisite in mind.[3]

The enterprise grew significantly in the years from 1932 to 1948; sales increased from $13 million to $115 million, and the number of

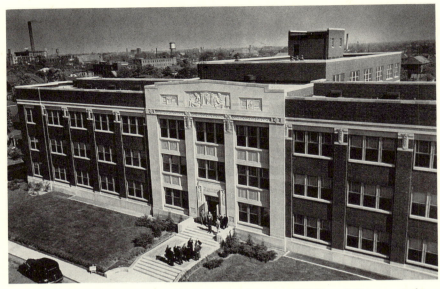

Lilly Research Laboratories, 1934.   *Eli Lilly and Company Archives*

employees grew from 1,675 to 6,912.[4] With growth came more complexity and new challenges in management, production, and sales, extended even further by expansion overseas. Growth and changing attitudes brought new expectations and new initiatives in relations between employees, managers, and owners. The business environment in these years included also the challenges brought by the economic disaster of the Great Depression, the strengthening of federal government regulation, and the multiple demands of World War II and postwar expansion. And as twentieth-century science matured, new products and methods challenged the Indianapolis company to devote even greater resources to research.

Eli Lilly was enough of a historian to know that change was the order of every day and enough of a businessman to know that he needed always to plan for change. In the pharmaceutical business by the 1930s change meant research. All his life Lilly remained proud of his company's sophisticated and pioneering initiatives in research, begun in the 1920s with the development of insulin, liver extract, and other new products. In the early 1930s he pushed hard to maintain the company's lead, focusing his energies on planning for construction of a new research laboratory. His old cigar-puffing nemesis, Charles J. Lynn, and the tight-fisted treasurer, Nicholas

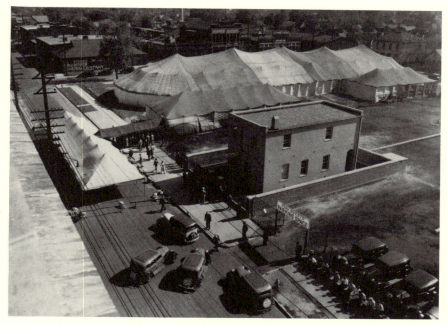

Dedication ceremonies for Lilly Research Labora-   *Eli Lilly and Company Archives*
tories, with the 1876 replica in center.

H. Noyes, argued against such a lavish building project in the depths of
the Great Depression. Lilly stood his ground, responding that research was
more important than large dividends to stockholders. Excavation began in
the summer of 1933.[5]

Dedication of the new Lilly Research Laboratories occurred on a
bright autumn day in 1934. Four hundred scientists came from major
universities in America and Europe. More than a thousand visitors gathered
for lunch under a huge tent set up outside the new building. President Lilly
presided over the ceremonies. He introduced each of the four main speakers: his father; Irving Langmuir, associate director of the Research Laboratories of General Electric Company and recipient of the Nobel Prize in
chemistry in 1932; Sir Frederick Banting, the University of Toronto scientist who had received the Nobel Prize in 1923 for his insulin work; and
Sir Henry Dale, director of the National Institute for Medical Research,
London, and one of the most distinguished scientists in Britain. A dinner
in the evening provided the occasion for remarks from seven eminent
scientists. The next day included research seminars and tours of the new

laboratories. Visitors saw a most impressive three-story building, with an entrance hall of Italian marble and with laboratories fitted out with the latest scientific equipment.[6]

The dedication ceremony was a bright showcase for the Indianapolis company's achievements in research. Nearly all the distinguished speakers commented on the company's successes, particularly the work on insulin. They could not but be impressed by the new laboratories and by the research staff, which was one of the largest in the industry. No one proposed, however, that the enterprise could rest on the laurels of insulin, liver extract, or Merthiolate. The competitive environment of the pharmaceutical industry made that clear, for at least three other companies, Merck, Squibb, and Abbott, were also building special research laboratories in the 1930s.[7]

Although the building dedicated in 1934 enabled an expansion of research activity on McCarty Street, the firm continued to rely also on cooperation with university scientists. Most important, Eli Lilly expanded the fellowship program he had begun in 1928. Through the 1930s he oversaw an increasingly elaborate system of contacts with university scientists in which company fellowships were the key ingredient. He urged careful screening of university scientists to be sure that the company was "dealing with a man or men of exceptional ability and trustworthiness." By 1942 forty-five scientists in twenty-seven universities and medical schools received fellowship support from the company. In negotiating with university researchers, Lilly pointed to the company's production and sales expertise and to its record of respect for serious research, suggesting that cooperation with Indianapolis had led to successes as grand as the Nobel Prize.[8]

Lilly continued also to chair meetings of the research committee, held in the library of the new laboratory building. Part of his challenge in these meetings was to ease the tension between those workers devoted primarily to fundamental research and those more interested in products with immediate and practical medical applications. The general problem was omnipresent in most sophisticated American companies engaged in research. One position at McCarty Street was represented most vigorously by George Henry Alexander Clowes. In a thirty-two-page confidential memorandum to Lilly, a "sort of Last Will and Testament," written in late 1944, Clowes summarized the case he had long argued. He expressed his disdain for practical-minded medical doctors and profit-oriented business executives who failed to appreciate the importance of fundamental research: "the more we build up desk executives who are not greatly interested in the fine points of research but are tremendously interested in the financial returns to the company and particularly to themselves the greater is the danger of ultimate deterioration." It was necessary, therefore, Clowes advised Lilly, to separate research into two functional divisions: a fundamental research group, headed by a Ph.D. scientist and working in a university-like atmosphere (but with higher pay than professors); and a separate industrial development group, with a staff composed largely of M.D.s who focused their energies on finding immediate medical applications for new drugs.[9]

Clowes's antagonists included Leon Zerfas, a medical doctor who headed the Lilly Clinic and urged more attention to medical application of drugs through systematic clinical studies. Also disagreeing with Clowes, and doubtless the man Clowes most had in mind in criticizing profit-oriented executives, was Adam H. Fiske, a hard-driving administrator whose increasing responsibilities in research annoyed some company scientists. Lilly tried to please both factions. He remained loyal to the egotistical and irrepressible Clowes, even when J. K. Lilly, Jr., strongly condemned "the bull-in-the-china shop tactics of our friend Clowes." Joe was furious that Clowes hastily assigned theoretical work without regard for projects already underway and then rushed off to his laboratory in Woods Hole, Massachusetts, leaving a state of "virtual chaos" in Indianapolis. Joe also condemned Clowes because, he wrote in 1940, "for five years . . . our research men have developed virtually nothing in the way of an important addition to our catalogue."[10] It was indeed the case that relatively few new products emerged in the 1930s. When in 1938 J. P. Scott, the assistant director of research development, identified the five most important drugs introduced by the company, he listed Iletin, Amytal, ephedrine, liver extract, and Merthiolate, all products of the 1920s.[11]

Eli Lilly allowed Clowes his freedom to pursue his own basic research in cancer, but he did not agree to Clowes's request that fundamental research be separated from applied research, arguing instead that the two must go hand in hand. Moreover, to Clowes's dismay, Lilly supported increased attention to medical research along practical lines. And in 1945 he appointed Clowes's nemesis, Adam Fiske, to the new position of vice-president for research, a move doubtless designed to bring more administrative order to the laboratories.[12]

Lilly's struggle to keep his scientists contented and productive was only part of his attention to the human environment on McCarty Street. Indeed, one of his most important innovations of the 1930s was his heightened level of concern for the physical and emotional well-being of employees throughout the company. Interested primarily in the techniques of mass production and the efficiencies of systematic management in the 1910s and 1920s, Lilly in the 1930s and 1940s expanded his horizons to include personnel matters generally and employee morale specifically. Doubtless this new interest was partly defensive as he saw American industries across the country melt before the hot breath of union organizing, particularly after passage of the Wagner Act of 1935. But this interest in employee welfare perhaps came no more from the threat of unionization, which was always slight at McCarty Street, than from the same inner sense of purpose that motivated Lilly's own self-analysis in the early 1930s. In creating his plan for developing a proper outlook on his own life he began to think also about the lives of his employees.

One company policy Lilly proudly instituted was a humane response to the Great Depression. He ensured that not a single employee was laid off in the 1930s even though there were many more workers than there was demand for pharmaceuticals. To avoid idle hands he instructed workers to produce surpluses of items that required the least cost in materials and the largest amount of labor. Other employees he set to work painting fences and buildings. In mid-1933 Lilly instituted a reduction in operations to a forty-hour, five-day week but increased hourly wages so that no worker would have a smaller pay envelope. These generous policies were possible in part because the company enjoyed large sales and profits even in the depression years. Aggregate sales for the years 1920-29 were $89,977,000; for the depression years 1930-39 they totaled $171,684,000. Lilly could have increased dividends to shareholders by cutting back on employee wages and benefits. There was certainly a surplus of labor in the 1930s that would have allowed such a market-oriented retrenchment policy. Because he refused to adopt such a hardheaded policy, Lilly and the company became even more attractive to employees. The people of central Indiana came to know that "Lillys" (as the company was commonly known) was an unusually good place to work. Two hundred new workers were hired at McCarty Street in 1939—from 13,231 job applicants.[13]

Lilly's interest in employee welfare went beyond bread and butter issues. Comparable in novelty to his introduction of stopwatches and time-motion studies two decades earlier, Lilly brought industrial psychology to

McCarty Street. Earlier, in the mid-1920s, Elton Mayo, an expert in industrial relations from the Harvard Business School, had visited the company and recommended employee rest periods. Lilly eventually became a strong partisan of Mayo, reading his books on industrial psychology and quoting with approval Mayo's admonitions to pay attention to the human as well as the technical side of business.[14] In 1932 Lilly hired a consulting psychologist, J. L. Rosenstein, a member of the Butler University faculty. Rosenstein devised tests to select production workers who were adept at simple repetitive operations. More important, he developed psychology courses for supervisors, in order, Lilly wrote in 1934, "to further perfect the esprit de corps of the organization."[15] These courses became the basis for Rosenstein's book, *Psychology of Human Relations for Executives*, published in 1936 and dedicated to Eli Lilly.[16]

Rosenstein also provided psychological counseling for individual employees at all levels, at first in an office downtown and later in an office set up in the plant. He worked initially with those employees likely to be fired, the ones Lilly called "our problem children." Lilly's instructions were to find "what kind of people they are" and "whether or not we can do them any good."[17] The results, Lilly later recalled, were about "20% brilliant successes, 20% flat failures, and 60% scattered between."[18]

Lilly was pleased with the new program in industrial psychology and determined to expand it. A "Personality Inventory Rating" was made for each employee, and those thought in need of counseling were referred to a psychologist. In 1936 the psychological work on McCarty Street included 131 personal counseling sessions and 83 group discussions. That same year company supervisors began meeting with employees near retirement age to discuss financial resources and to urge "the need for some activity to keep them busy upon retiring."[19] Broad attention to employee well-being also led in 1936 to the first company hobby show "to encourage the development of pleasurable and educational leisure-time activities."[20] A year later, in a move that a hard-driving Lilly would have found unthinkable two decades earlier, the company installed Coca-Cola vending machines in thirteen different locations in the plant.[21]

Eli Lilly was at the center of all these changes, consciously working to ensure high morale, a feeling of self-worth, and a sense of belonging on McCarty Street. Less and less was he the intense, austere boss, and more and more was he the firm but warm and supportive head of the family company. He began personally to meet with all new employees when they made their inspection trip through the plant. During the flood of 1936,

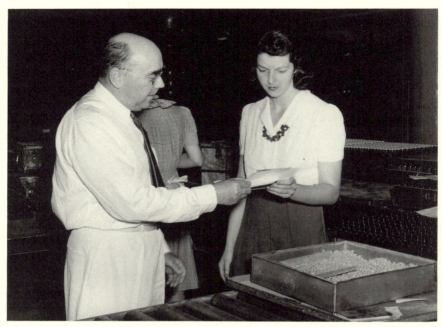

President Eli Lilly honors employee Grace Lamar,   *Eli Lilly and Company Archives*
ca. 1940.

when demand for medicines necessitated that some employees work round-the-clock for a few days, Lilly stopped in the plant after midnight with an armload of sandwiches he had bought from nearby Shapiro's Delicatessen. He even began to take a morning and afternoon Coca-Cola break, often sitting with production employees and talking about subjects such as his farm at Conner Prairie.[22] He came to know and believe, as he asserted in his presidential address to the Indiana Academy of Science in 1938, that "the one most important duty of the head of any organization is to develop and to stimulate the human material within it, for if the personnel is able and enthusiastic and of high morale, the work of the institution takes care of itself."[23]

This careful attention to morale and interpersonal relations was unusually intense but not unique to Eli Lilly and Company. During the 1930s and 1940s America's management experts produced shelves full of books and articles about industrial relations, arguing especially that workers were not motivated toward productivity solely by a paycheck or even a bonus but by the personal relations and the social environment of the workplace. The most influential analyses of the worker as "social man" were conducted by Elton Mayo and his Harvard Business School colleague, Fritz J. Roethlisberger, beginning with their famous Hawthorne studies of the 1920s.[24] Mayo's writings and his visit to the company were influential in sparking Lilly's initial interest; Roethlisberger played a role in spurring it onward.

Just as earlier he had invited the Emerson Company to assess his introduction of systematic management, Lilly decided to call in an outside expert in industrial relations. In early 1941 he invited Roethlisberger to spend a week at the company to observe human interactions. Roethlisberger's report praised the high morale within the organization and the "friendly and informal personal relations that now prevail between management and employees." Indeed, Lilly employees seemed to relate to each other "more as members of a family than as members of a highly 'rationalized' business organization," displaying "an intuitive understanding of where they stood, of what their duties, responsibilities, and obligations to each other were." After studying the "beliefs and codes of behavior" at the Indianapolis company, Roethlisberger concluded that "it is against the code of management to maintain authority by any mechanism which would tend to emphasize the social distance between management and the employees." He found that "management and employees eat lunch together; they drink 'cokes' together; they bowl together; they share the same hours of work and the same toilet facilities."[25]

Lilly was doubtless pleased by the Harvard professor's impressions of the company. An organization with a "familial orientation" was exactly what he had set out to achieve a decade earlier by means of industrial psychology and by the force of his own personality and leadership. To his father such an orientation came almost naturally. For Eli it came in the 1930s only as he assumed the larger responsibilities of the presidency and as he directed a reorientation of his own personal life.

Not all employees on McCarty Street in the 1930s were equal members of the family, however. Throughout American industry black workers were treated as second-class employees. In Indianapolis, as in most of America, blacks were also second-class citizens. Neighborhood lines between black and white in the city were tightly drawn. Nearly all black high school students attended Crispus Attucks, a segregated school constructed for that purpose in the 1920s. Public parks were segregated also, with two of them specially designated for use by blacks. Downtown movie theaters, restaurants, and hotels turned away black patrons.[26]

Eli Lilly and Company reflected the prevalent mores of its time and place. In 1934 planners of the dedication of the Research Laboratories carefully identified all local drugstores owned by blacks and all black physicians so as to be certain that they were not invited to the celebration.[27] Blacks were employed at McCarty Street, but segregation prevailed in use of company cafeterias and rest rooms. Most important, job assignments for black workers were almost exclusively as porters. Even this opportunity diminished when Lilly instructed a personnel manager in 1935 that he should "not employ another colored porter without my official O.K."[28]

Restrictive policies toward blacks eased considerably during the 1940s. Demand for labor as a consequence of World War II caused some change, but the loosening of segregation and discrimination continued after the war. Indeed, in the late 1940s Eli and Joe Lilly pushed to increase the number of black employees and to upgrade their job opportunities. As a result of the brothers' deliberate policy the number and percentage of black workers did increase, from 3.7 percent in 1942 to 5.2 percent in 1946 to 6.4 percent in 1948. Joe urged that the goal should be the same percentage of workers as there were black residents in Marion County, about 10 to 12 percent. And Eli ordered that the plant expansion of the postwar era should provide opportunities to hire black carpenters, pipe fitters, and other skilled workers. By 1948, 40 percent of black employees had jobs with higher ratings than maid or janitor. The Lilly brothers also moved gradually to eliminate segregated facilities within the plant, culminating in a general policy announced in early 1951 that all cafeterias, recreational rooms, washrooms, and locker rooms would be open to all employees regardless of race.[29]

In 1958 the *Indianapolis Recorder,* the city's black newspaper, announced its "Human Relations Honor Roll," listing those "Hoosiers who had acted to bring brotherhood nearer to reality." Eli Lilly's name was on the roll because, the newspaper asserted, his company "has set a high standard of merit employment and civilized personnel relations."[30]

Employment practices at Eli Lilly and Company in the 1930s reflected time and place in other ways as well. It was believed, in the Indianapolis Jewish community especially, that the company did not hire Jews. Some residents thought also that Catholics suffered discrimination in seeking a job on McCarty Street. White Protestant women who were not married were employed in large numbers, but primarily for jobs such as filling capsules or vials of Iletin. These conditions, too, changed in the 1940s and after.[31]

The sources of gradual change in policies and practices regarding race, religion, and gender came largely from within the company and not from government intervention. During Lilly's presidency federal and state government had little effective involvement in such matters. The presence of government in other areas, however, was powerful and becoming more so, much to the distress of the Lilly family.

As early as the 1920s J. K. Lilly, Sr., was lamenting that "we are getting too much government," necessitating, he wrote, the appointment of "a young man to keep in touch with the Washington end of our business."[32] With the depression and the New Deal the federal government became a much larger presence on McCarty Street. Eli Lilly in his 1935 annual review noted with regret "the loss of many hours of time devoted to the requirements of the ever-mounting burden of governmental regulation."[33] That year the company created a legal department and the following year hired its first full-time lawyer. Lilly noted that the Social Security Act, new tax laws, and the Robinson-Patman Act had increased the costs of business and added new confusion and uncertainty in planning. He especially deplored the ambiguity of the Robinson-Patman Act of 1936, which attempted to prevent price discrimination in retailing, but concluded that it was "fundamentally a legislative expression of the Lilly Policy which assures the fair and equal treatment of all customers."[34]

The piece of New Deal legislation designed specifically to regulate the pharmaceutical industry was the Food, Drug, and Cosmetic Act of 1938. During the 1930s popular demands grew for more regulation of the drug industry. In 1932 the Committee on the Costs of Medical Care concluded that "the manufacture and distribution of medicines, because of their intimate relation to health and welfare of a community or nation, partake of the nature of public utilities." Consequently "the public interest may require 'regulation' of the industry."[35] The more immediate impetus to legislation followed the introduction of a new "Elixir Sulfanilamide" in 1937 by the Samuel E. Massengill Company. At least seventy-three people died from the toxic concoction, giving dramatic force to claims that Americans were being deceived and endangered by some of the medicines they used. Congress responded in the 1938 act by giving the Food and Drug Administration responsibility to make sure that new drugs were safe. Lilly regretted that the new legislation added another level of paper work and confusion, but the law had few other negative consequences for his company. Its major effects hit instead at the patent medicine makers. For ethical drug manufacturers like Eli Lilly and Company, the production of safe medicines had been a primary goal long before 1938, a goal that derived more from the Lilly family's sense of good business in making safe drugs than from the external pressure of government regulation. Indeed, sales for prescription manufacturers like Eli Lilly and Company may have increased as a consequence of the restrictions the 1938 act placed on proprietary medicine makers.[36]

The most important manifestation of what Lilly and many other American businessmen saw as the antibusiness policy of the Roosevelt administration and "the destruction of business confidence by the demagogues" came not in the 1938 law but in an outburst of trust-busting that began in 1939.[37] In the two years before Pearl Harbor the Justice Department's Antitrust Division brought approximately 180 cases against many of America's major companies. In April 1941 Eli Lilly and Company joined this group. The government charged that the Indianapolis firm had violated the Sherman Antitrust Act by combining with other insulin producers to "fix and maintain the prices of insulin" and thereby had "prevented and restrained free and normal competition in the sale and distribution of insulin." The indictment named not only the company but also President Eli Lilly. Similar charges were brought against Squibb and against Sharp & Dohme, the other two companies that sold insulin in the United States.[38] The charges followed an extensive investigation in which the "gestapo in Washington," Joe Lilly wrote his father, had extensively interrogated company executives "without, however, resorting to a rubber hose." Following a strenuous week of this questioning, Eli left for a weekend at Wawasee, telling Joe that "he was going to light a fire in the fireplace at the cottage and sit for three days without thinking about anything." Knowing his brother's energy, Joe added that "this would really be an accomplishment worthwhile for anyone with a mental apparatus which operates in a manner similar to a victim of the Saint Vitus's dance."[39]

The Justice Department's long investigation in the insulin suit wore heavily on Eli Lilly. The government had strong evidence that the three pharmaceutical manufacturers did indeed control the market for insulin, making sure that all insulin was sold at the same price. Lilly claimed that the charge was unreasonable. Avoidance of price competition had long been a tradition in the pharmaceutical trade. Moreover, the government, he asserted, did not give sufficient weight to the steep decline in the price of insulin since 1924, dropping to a cost of seven cents a day for the average diabetic. Claiming that the government's case was without merit, Lilly wanted to plead not guilty. But the company's legal experts urged a *nolo contendere* plea in order to avoid the costs and perhaps the negative publicity of protracted litigation.[40] Lilly might have sent another executive to Washington to make the embarrassing plea, but he decided to go himself. On learning of this decision his father wrote him: "Nothing you have ever done has leaped you more in the affection and esteem of your associates than your determination to be the goat in the case of the US versus us." Others in the company could have "gone to the martyrs block—your positive decision to go as the main spring really warmed the hearts of all and made your father very proud."[41]

The insulin suit was President Lilly's most troubling entanglement with the government. It revealed his difficulty in accepting the kind of regulation of the marketplace and protection of consumers that was becoming increasingly important in an economy dominated by a relatively small number of large corporations. Like many businessmen, Lilly accepted the rise of big business but not big government. In his understanding of the relationship between business and government, Lilly remained, as in other ways, a man of tradition, increasingly out of step as the twentieth century moved beyond its half way point. The insulin suit was his most difficult encounter with the government, but it was not the last. With war in 1941 came a much closer relationship with Washington, a relationship that included conflict but also cooperation.

All over the world the war changed everything and nearly everyone. In Indianapolis the struggle to defeat Germany and Japan meant a conversion of factories to war production, a large turnover of workers as young men went off to fight, and a scarcity and eventual rationing of sugar, tires, and gasoline. Like Americans elsewhere, Hoosiers struggled with housing shortages, new concerns about juvenile delinquency, and the loss of loved ones.[42] In his whimsical manner J. K. Lilly, Sr., captured the signs of the war on the home front. "A fire engine of brilliant hue occupies a stall in our garage," he wrote a relative in 1943. "Occasional blackouts bring a

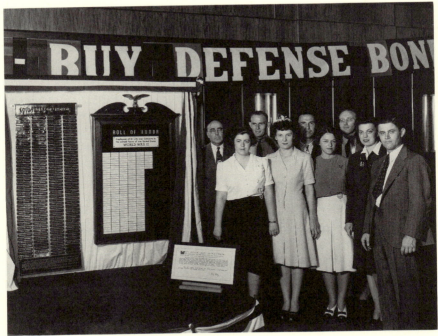

President Lilly (far left) and employees at World   *Eli Lilly and Company Archives*
War II defense bond rally.

swarm of civilian defenders, out goes the engine . . . and thrilling pande-
monium reigns." "Evie's beautiful husband, Mr. 'Shally-foo' [Francis B.
Chalifoux] is on a mission, per aviation." And there were "victory gardens
everywhere. It appears that Marion County is planning to feed the world."[43]

The Lilly family strongly supported the war. Even before Pearl Harbor
they had contributed financial and moral support to the Indiana Committee for National Defense, opposing those who advocated isolation from
international strife or cooperation with Hitler's Germany.[44] With American
entry into the war Eli Lilly directed the conversion of the McCarty Street
plant to making those products most necessary to defeat the Axis powers.
Often Lilly led by example. He spent long, hard days in the office, struggling
with a myriad of new problems and challenges, just as workers in the plant
extended their hours and eventually moved to double shifts in order to
meet the demands of war. Lilly's example of hard work and sacrifice extended
to the small details. In the face of wartime paper shortages he began to use

smaller and smaller pieces of paper for his letters and memoranda, causing comment and emulation in offices throughout the company. At home on Sunset Lane he closed off part of the house and turned back the thermostat to reduce heating oil consumption by 40 percent.[45]

In a talk to employees at the end of the war Lilly summarized the difficulties the company had endured. "We have not had the proper space. . . . We have been short in trained personnel. . . . We have had inadequate equipment and our material shortages have dogged us at every turn. The result has been exasperation and a nerve wracking strain. . . . "[46] Under these conditions output per worker declined sharply, causing special anguish for a company president who had always taken great pride in production efficiency. Profits also suffered. Although sales more than doubled in the war years, the large increase in taxes contributed to a balance sheet in which after-tax income as a percentage of sales dropped from 23.0 percent in 1940 to 10.5 percent in 1945. In addition to higher taxes there were more directives and controls from the federal government and its growing wartime agencies, particularly the Office of Price Administration, which closely watched drug prices. Research plans suffered, too, as scientists abandoned prewar programs in order to produce antimalarials, blood plasma, and penicillin.[47]

Blood plasma was one of the first major production challenges and provided evidence of Lilly's cultivation of a wartime patriotic spirit. A year after Pearl Harbor Lilly wrote a friend that he was struggling under "an enormous avalanche of business at the pill foundry," but that the important work included producing ten thousand packages of blood plasma a week. Lilly took great pride in this work, which was done in cooperation with the American Red Cross. He refused to allow any company profit because he "didn't think it was the right thing for anybody to make any profit on blood which had been donated." By the war's end the firm had dried over two million pints of blood, about 20 percent of the United States' total.[48]

War patriotism was evident also in the production of encephalitis vaccine. Not only did it require fifteen thousand white mice a week, but the vaccine was difficult and dangerous to produce. The risks were carefully explained to "our most careful girl operators in the Biological Department," Lilly wrote his father, and, with "real patriotism and bravery," all volunteered to do the job.[49] Lilly and the employees were particularly proud also of the Army-Navy "E" award granted for exceptional work.

The Indianapolis company made all manner of other drugs for special wartime demand. There was typhus and influenza vaccine, gas gangrene antitoxin, and Merthiolate. Merthiolate was an army standard issue, and twenty-two tank cars of this popular antiseptic departed from McCarty Street during the war.[50] Among the most important drugs and also among those causing the largest challenges were the old company standby of Iletin (Insulin, Lilly) and the very new antibiotic, penicillin.

The major difficulty in producing insulin was caused by the wartime shortage of pancreas glands from which the hormone was manufactured. In addition to difficulties in obtaining pancreas glands from meat-packers there was the tendency of some Americans to hoard goods they thought might become scarce. Doubtless swayed by shortages of all manner of goods, from tires to toilet paper, diabetics panicked and began to purchase insulin far in advance of their needs. By the spring of 1943 Lilly and Clowes were deeply worried that the company was reaching a point where it could no longer supply the amount of insulin diabetics needed. The two men struggled fiercely with the problem. Lilly was convinced that the most fruitful mode of attack was to encourage "some of the best men in the country to work on the synthesis of a substance having action the same as or similar to Insulin." Synthesis of insulin was one of the most important problems facing the research division, Lilly told Clowes, and "we must do something about it in short order."[51] Both men were convinced that development of a synthetic insulin would require interdisciplinary cooperation. "The problem," Clowes urged, "will never be solved by protein or biological chemists on the one hand or synthetic organic chemists on the other, working individually." Joint, interdisciplinary research, particularly by young scientists, they agreed, was required.[52]

The obstacles to producing a synthetic insulin were twofold. First, the scientific problem was exceedingly complex, requiring not only the best talent, but also large quantities of labor and luck. Second, as Clowes several times reminded Lilly when he pushed for research on the problem, the company's and the nation's university scientists were strained to their limits by war work already underway. Clowes and Lilly continued to fret over the problem but failed to find an answer. Like many other Americans in wartime they crossed their fingers and muddled through. Insulin hoarding and shortages continued after the war, and not until mid-1947 did Clowes report that the company had begun to build up its reserve stock.[53]

Many of the scientists most capable of working on insulin synthesis were fully engaged in twelve-hour days and seven-day weeks on a drug of major significance. Penicillin bore some resemblance to insulin in that it was soon proclaimed as a miracle drug, with powers beyond any imagined and with demand far outstripping the capacity to produce.[54] Like insulin, penicillin had its scientific origins outside the United States and in university and hospital laboratories, followed by development in the modern pharmaceutical company. Unlike the case of insulin, large-scale penicillin production involved the efforts and sometimes the collaboration of many pharmaceutical companies rather than one and the close involvement also of the United States government. Penicillin came to symbolize one of World War II's most important consequences—the close interaction of business, government, and the research university.[55]

British scientist Alexander Fleming published the pathbreaking article on penicillin in 1929. Not until 1940 did serious work to produce the antibiotic begin, however, led by Oxford University scientist Howard Florey. In 1941, with strains of Fleming's penicillin mold in his baggage, Florey traveled from a Nazi-besieged Britain to the United States. There he visited pharmaceutical companies and universities in an energetic campaign to persuade the Americans to attempt large-scale penicillin production. When Florey visited Eli Lilly and Company that summer before Pearl Harbor, researchers had already begun experiments with the antibiotic but had met no real success, partly because company scientists had little experience with the fermentation processes by which it was produced. Late in 1941 they converted to penicillin production a building that once housed rabbits at the company's Greenfield laboratories. The first yields in Indianapolis were obtained a few days after Pearl Harbor.[56]

Large-scale production of penicillin proved an immense challenge. The technical difficulties combined with the unparalleled potential of the new drug and the frantic wartime demand to bring about the involvement and the eventual cooperation of many pharmaceutical companies, universities, and the United States government. In Washington the Committee on Medical Research of the Office of Scientific Research and Development, headed by Alfred N. Richards, provided coordination and strong direction in the wartime development of the new antibiotic. The government's Northern Regional Research Laboratory in Peoria, Illinois, made major technical contributions that it shared with pharmaceutical companies, most notably in the development of the submerged or deep fermentation procedure, which gave much larger yields than the surface culture method first used. Eli Lilly and Company sent scientists to visit the Peoria laboratory as early as October 1941, and its scientists and executives, particularly Clowes and Lilly, had close written and telephone contacts with Richards and the Committee on Medical Research.[57]

Although the Indianapolis firm apparently lost enthusiasm for penicillin in 1942, contributing thereby to the lead of Merck, Squibb, and Pfizer in these early years, interest resumed on McCarty Street in 1943. Clinical tests of penicillin, including the rapid recovery from infection of soldiers wounded on Guadalcanal, convinced the government to urge pharmaceutical manufacturers to devote large resources to the drug. In spring of that year the Indianapolis company's Research Committee ordered that work be stepped up at once, leading to long hours devoted exclusively to penicillin. One of the first patients to receive the company's new antibiotic was J. K. Lilly, Sr., who was suffering from a serious infection. The solvent that remained in the solution given him in 1943 caused great pain, but the penicillin worked a miraculous cure. The penicillin produced in 1943 in Indianapolis was grown in thousands of milk bottles using the tedious and labor-intensive surface culture method. Some of the scientists and production men did not think penicillin could be produced in containers larger than five gallons. Scientist George B. Walden thought otherwise, and with Eli Lilly's strong encouragement he began to experiment with alternatives. As a result of Walden's work the company in 1944 changed over to large-batch production by submerged fermentation, using eight thousand-gallon tanks instead of two-quart milk bottles.[58]

Research in the last years of the war included not only a quest for improved methods of fermentation and purification but also a search for a synthetic penicillin. From Washington, Richards and the Committee on Medical Research exercised close control over attempts to synthesize penicillin, dividing the work between a group of eastern companies and a midwestern group, the latter composed of Abbott, Parke-Davis, Upjohn, and Eli Lilly and Company. Although there was conflict and secrecy as these private enterprises kept careful watch over their potential patents and profits, there was also sharing of information in the name of national good in time of war. The synthesis of penicillin never became commercially profitable, but this project did make important contributions to penicillin production while it showed the cooperative wartime spirit that prevailed in some of America's largest corporations.[59] Eli Lilly took great satisfaction in his company's contribution to the war through the work on penicillin, particularly when Richards testified before a congressional committee that the Indianapolis company president was "one of the most public spirited men that I know in industry."[60]

Peace brought an end to close cooperation between government and the pharmaceutical industry, but the search for new antibiotics continued.

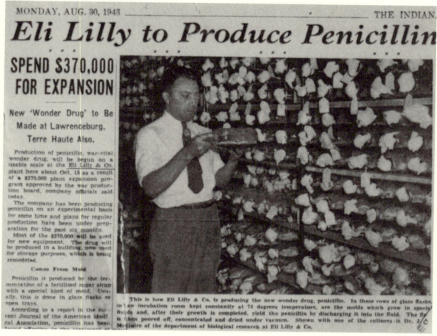

MONDAY, AUG. 30, 1943   THE INDIAN,

Eli Lilly to Produce Penicillin

SPEND $370,000 FOR EXPANSION

New 'Wonder Drug' to Be Made at Lawrenceburg, Terre Haute Also.

Production of penicillin, war-vital wonder drug, will be begun on a sizable scale at the Eli Lilly & Co. plant here about Oct. 15 as a result of a $370,000 plant expansion program approved by the war production board, company officials said today.

The company has been producing penicillin on an experimental basis for some time and plans for regular production have been under preparation for the past six months.

Most of the $370,000 will be used for new equipment. The drug will be produced in a building, now used for storage purposes, which is being remodeled.

Comes From Mold

Penicillin is produced by the fermentation of a fertilized sugar sirup with a special kind of mold. Usually, this is done in glass flasks or open trays.

According to a report in the current Journal of the American Medical Association, penicillin has been

This is how Eli Lilly & Co. is producing the new wonder drug, penicillin. In these rows of glass flasks, in an incubation room kept constantly at 74 degrees temperature, are the molds which grow in special fluids and, after their growth is completed, yield the penicillin by discharging it into the fluid. The fluid is then poured off, concentrated and dried under vacuum. Shown with one of the cultures is Dr. J.C. McGuire of the department of biological research at Eli Lilly & Co.

The Indianapolis press reports the penicillin story, 1943, showing Lilly scientist J. M. McGuire and some of the thousands of glass bottles used before development of the deep fermentation process.

Eli Lilly and Company Archives

As one of the Indianapolis chemists wrote in late 1945, "the whole field of antibiotics is before us."[61] And indeed it was, for penicillin was one of the first in a long line of antibiotics that brought better health to millions of people while contributing to the expansion and growth of the pharmaceutical industry in the postwar years.

The surrender of Germany and Japan did not bring a return to prewar conditions on McCarty Street. Shortages and price controls persisted after 1945, although the depression so many businessmen feared never came.

Instead, the late 1940s were years of prosperity and economic growth for the American economy generally and for the pharmaceutical industry specifically. New antibiotics and other drugs combined with a growing and more affluent population to cause rapid expansion and high profits for the industry, especially for the handful of large companies that now dominated in pharmaceuticals. Eli Lilly and Company was part of this peacetime prosperity. The company's sales increased from $71.5 million in 1945 to over $115 million at the close of Lilly's presidency in 1948. Aided by a reduction in high wartime taxes, the company's after-tax profits rose sharply, too, from 10.5 percent of sales in 1945 to 21.7 percent in 1948—profits that Lilly himself later believed were "unreasonably high."[62]

So large was the postwar growth in medical prescriptions that the Indianapolis company could not produce drugs in sufficient quantity to keep up with demand. Vice-President Joe Lilly told his brother in early 1947 that "a slow year would not be an unmixed evil for Lilly and Company. We might be able to get a little stock on the shelves."[63] In this kind of voracious market President Lilly's immediate postwar challenge was to expand the capacity of the plant, particularly in production of penicillin and other antibiotics. He supervised additions to the insulin, liver extract, and research buildings, construction of a new chemical pilot plant, and purchase of new warehouses. The major expansion came with the purchase in late 1945 of the Curtiss-Wright propeller plant on Kentucky Avenue, several miles from McCarty Street. Here the company moved a large part of its production, including its antibiotic manufacture. The Kentucky Avenue site also housed a new capsule plant and the shipping department. Lilly fretted over the move, as costs of construction and conversion escalated and as difficulties in obtaining the proper equipment mounted. Preparing for penicillin production at the new site proved especially worrisome.[64] Finally in mid-1947 his father wrote Eli at Wawasee with the good news that "the new Penicillin plant is blowing in with a gusto." Rather than "losing the first few lots down the sewer, . . . they are better than anything we ever got before."[65]

The growth of Eli Lilly and Company was not limited to Indianapolis or even the United States. The postwar years brought stepped-up interest in foreign markets for many American businesses, including the Indianapolis firm. Eli Lilly and Company had first shown serious attention to overseas markets with the development of insulin. In late 1923 Charles J. Lynn, a longtime supporter of Christian missions abroad, planned a foreign exploratory trip, "largely for the purpose of making Insulin available throughout the world."[66] Only cautiously did the company move abroad in the 1920s, however. A more aggressive overseas venture came in the 1930s, with the construction of a manufacturing plant in Basingstoke, England. This plant, the Lilly brothers hoped, would enable them to overcome differences between British and American standards in drugs, respond to "Buy British" sentiment, and provide access to markets in the British colonies and on the European continent. But the Basingstoke plant opened just as war broke out in Europe so that it was forced to concentrate on supplying Merthiolate, foot powder, and prophylactics for the British army. "It was a great blow for all of us," Lilly wrote in his review of 1939, "to camouflage that beautiful white building—it is now a dirty brown with great splashes of green."[67]

Peace brought a resumption of the overseas expansion begun in the late 1930s. By 1948 the firm exported 24 percent of its pharmaceutical output, compared to about 6 percent in 1938. Company employees worked in thirty-five countries, mostly in Latin America, Asia, and Africa. Most were salesmen, with the major overseas manufacturing remaining at the plant in England.[68]

In addition to facing the challenges of expansion overseas and in Indianapolis, Lilly remained closely involved in planning the company's research strategy. He continued his push for connections to universities of the kind that he had initiated in the 1920s. "Are we keeping in touch with fundamental research all over the country," he asked the Research Committee in 1945, "supporting it with fellowships, etc., as we should?"[69] The war had sidetracked systematic contacts with outside scientists as well as planning for long-term research. As early as the fall of 1944 the Research Committee that Lilly chaired planned for postwar resumption and expansion of visits, contacts, and fellowships. To communicate these activities to the larger scientific community the company began to publish and distribute *Research Today*, a journal that combined articles on major medical and pharmaceutical subjects, such as penicillin, with news of awards, lectures, and publications that emanated from McCarty Street. Support for fellowships and consultantships in 1947 totaled $306,814. Total research expenditures that year were $1,157,494, with much of this money assigned to development of new penicillins, streptomycin, and other antibiotics that were revolutionizing health care.[70] Lilly was determined to ensure that research remain "the soul of the enterprise."[71]

Expansion and change in the 1940s meant hard work for the management of Eli Lilly and Company. There was no doubt that President Lilly was very proud of the growth of the company, but as he admonished employees on several occasions, "the question is not how *big* we are but how *good*."[72] Indeed, he was acutely conscious of the potential disadvantages and the real problems "of having our business grow to too large a size."[73]

Prior to the 1940s problems of size had not been significant. Eli, Joe, and their father grew up in the business and were accustomed to close involvement in the details of pharmaceutical research, manufacture, and sale. The company had never developed layers of supervision. Rather, management was "lean" and closely in touch with production lines, laboratory benches, and sales offices. Eli or Joe approved all publicity before release to the press, for example, and a question about an individual employee's pension went all the way to the president's desk for an answer. Managers had "a sense of closeness to the seat of power," as one of them later recalled.[74] Growth in size made this simple form of management less adequate, however. Fritz Roethlisberger, the Harvard professor who visited the company in 1941, had warned of the need to ask "how large the organization may become before an increase in the levels of supervision is inevitable."[75]

In the mid-1940s Lilly decided it was necessary to respond directly to Roethlisberger's question. Lilly charged Earl Beck and Eugene N. Beesley to study the company's organizational structure. That structure had evolved organically over the decades and had left increasingly unclear lines of authority and various and confusing titles. The reorganization Lilly announced in late 1944, following Beck and Beesley's study, responded to past growth and prepared for future expansion by placing a vice-president in charge of each of the major functions of finance, marketing, production, research, and industrial relations. Each vice-president would report directly to the president. As Beck wrote Lilly, "By following a definite pattern in regard to various standardized levels of responsibility, it is possible to use the same terminology throughout the organization to denote the same level of responsibility."[76] The creation of functional divisions headed by vice-presidents led also to the splitting of research from production, with a new vice-president, Adam H. Fiske, placed in charge of research. Clowes, who had been due to retire at the end of 1942 but postponed that move because of the war, was now completely free to pursue his own research interests. The new organization chart also included an executive vice-president, who acted for the president in his absence and had special reponsibility for marketing. Joe Lilly filled this position, of course, carrying on in the new structure as he had for most of the previous two decades.[77]

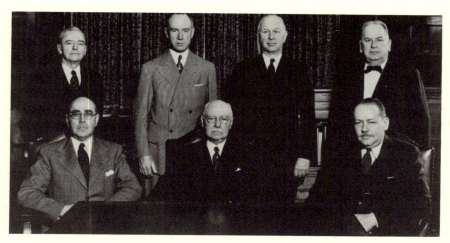

Eli Lilly and Company Board of Directors, 1945.   *Eli Lilly and Company Archives*
Left to right (seated): Eli Lilly, J. K. Lilly, J. K.
Lilly, Jr.; left to right (standing): J. S. Wright,
W. A. Hanley, N. H. Noyes, C. J. Lynn.

Signs of change appeared everywhere on McCarty Street as the company attempted to deal with growth in the 1940s. Formal, detailed organization charts became commonplace, and employees became familiar with job evaluation systems, progress ratings, written job descriptions, and formal grievance procedures. These new policies, according to the company's personnel experts, reflected "the necessity for formalizing certain relationships as size increased."[78] New faces appeared, too. There were more college and business school graduates. Even in some nonresearch areas the increasing complexity of the business required Ph.D. scientists who functioned as managers. The old production men who had taught young Eli Lilly the business of grinding and mixing were gone. He kept pictures of them in his office, reminders of a familiar but now distant past.[79]

Rapid growth very much concerned the three Lillys. J. K. Lilly, Sr., warned his sons in 1946 that the family must "not let the business get beyond our control."[80] Eli was so worried by mammoth size that he announced in early 1946 that construction at the McCarty Street location would cease. The company would expand in other locations instead.[81] In early 1947, just as the Kentucky Avenue plant was nearing completion, he appointed a committee to study "the advantages and disadvantages of decentralization of our manufacturing units, investigating the possibility and advisability of having smaller plants scattered throughout Indiana."[82] Headed by Earl Beck, the Plant Studies Committee considered the possibility of a "breakdown of the plant into the 15 smallest units that could logically be considered for physical decentralization." Such smaller units might be managed more efficiently than the sprawling McCarty Street and Kentucky Avenue plants. After more than a year of study, the committee concluded that the costs and inefficiencies of decentralization argued against such a strategic change and recommended that major production, administration, and research remain centralized in Indianapolis.[83]

A major stimulus to Lilly's formation of the Plant Studies Committee was "the personnel problems of bigness." By substituting a large number of smaller plants for two rapidly growing large plants there was the possibility that the traditional and familiar close-knit organization could be recreated in the new, decentralized facilities. But the Plant Studies Committee concluded that decentralization was a "dubious panacea for the personnel problems of bigness."[84] Those problems had to be addressed in other ways.

For President Lilly the issue was above all one of employee morale. He increased efforts begun in the 1930s to maintain the familial environment that Professor Roethlisberger had described in 1941. Roethlisberger had warned that expansion would bring administrative rationalization, which in turn would create more formalized relationships. Consequently, the company would need "to find ways of maintaining a morale as high as that obtained under the familial orientation."[85]

Lilly's major contribution to the problem of morale was through the force of his own presence and personality on McCarty Street. He moved out in front and became a familiar speaker at company gatherings. A surviving illustration of the force of his character came in a talk he gave to supervisors in February 1946. Lilly's remarks were recorded and later transcribed; they convey an informal and colloquial manner as he spoke from rough notes about recent and future changes in the company. His pride in the enterprise was brightly expressed but his own role modestly unstated. He spoke of "us" and "we" and "our company." Reporting sales figures for foreign offices, he admitted that the complexity of overseas sales "gets me all balled up, and everybody else." He addressed the difficulties of postwar plant expansion, saying that "we have got the bear by the tail and we will have to hold on for some years around these parts." But his manner of expression, backed up by figures and examples, left the clear impression that the company president had a firm hold on the bear's tail, knew just where he was going, and wanted everyone on McCarty Street to profit from the ride. In this talk and many others he left the impression of sincerity and honesty, of genuine concern about employee well-being, and of possible attainment of the highest ideals.[86]

In his recorded talk of February 1946 Lilly also expressed his explicit concern for employee welfare. He reported on wage rates and vacation policies and compared them with other industrial firms, including the unionized auto and steel industries, which showed the Indianapolis company "right-up-to date." He promised that we will "keep our ears to the ground and we'll not fall behind." Lilly also stated his distaste for the two work shifts necessary until new production facilities were brought on line: "these double shifts and working till midnight just aren't human and we ought to get away from that." The last half of his talk was devoted entirely to "the human end of the story," taking his text from Elton Mayo. He read from notes he had made of Mayo's writings and then commented on major points, translating the professor's thick social science vocabulary into everyday language. Mayo's arguments about the "disadvantage of large size" meant that "supervisors must train themselves in new social skills," Lilly told them. He advised them "to get the spirit and teamwork of an Indiana basketball team" in their own group, department, or division. He read his note on Mayo's advice that supervisors had to develop not only technical competence but the capacity to handle people by being patient and avoiding emotional upsets, and then added "I'm a good one to talk about that." He went on to explain in detail Mayo's advice for sympathetic listening to employee troubles and grievances. He closed not by citing profit figures, production quotas, or sales goals, but by stating his hope that Eli Lilly and Company would be "the finest place that anybody would care to work in."[87]

Lilly communicated his concern for employee morale also in the pages of *SuperVision*, a monthly publication begun in 1946 in response to his recognition that "the Company's present size calls for a strong line of communication extending to all levels of supervision."[88] Each month in "The President's Column" he conveyed a thought, idea, or suggestion in a warm, familiar way. In the first issue he restated his hope "to make this the best possible place in which to work." In later columns he advocated group management, good housekeeping, and economy in use of paper and pencils. The dominant threads running through "The President's Column" were those of human relations and employee morale. "One of the greatest problems of big business is how to stay little at heart," he wrote in mid-1947. Management cannot be "some far-removed, mythological Olympian group whose instructions and wisdom attempt to control us without the benefit of discussion or participation." Nor can employees "be dictated to by the old-fashioned, blustering 'boss.' His days are gone forever."[89]

In "The President's Column" Lilly addressed broader issues as well, for he clearly believed that the management problem was indeed a human problem. In one column he condemned materialism; in another he wrote of the Golden Rule, the Ten Commandments, and the Sermon on the Mount. Often he discussed the importance of examining one's personal relationships outside the workplace and encouraged readers to take stock of their own character and outlook on life, which, he argued, could be changed. "Each of us," he asserted, "is responsible for his own small sector in this life—his own personality." Several times he condemned anger and impatience. In a column noting the reinstatement of the company hobby show he wrote that "there is nothing so pathetic as the person who keeps his nose so close to the grindstone that when the time comes to adopt an easier mode of life, he has no other interests." This column on hobbies was one of the rare occasions in which Lilly used himself as a role model: "If I had any more hobbies, there would have to be one less person on McCarty Street, for between Indiana history and archaeology, farming, and sailing, the mortar and the pestle could be laid aside without too much of a jolt."[90]

"The President's Column" clearly reflected the personality and the interests of Eli Lilly, particularly as they had developed since the early 1930s. So, too, did a series of annual lectures on industrial relations inaugurated after the war. Some of the speakers came from industry, such as Charles Kettering of General Motors. But others were from universities, such as D. Elton Trueblood, a distinguished philosopher from Earlham College. Many provided elaboration on the kinds of themes Lilly addressed in his column.[91]

The challenges of size were not unique to Eli Lilly and Company. Large corporations across America wrestled with problems that derived from growth. In most of these big businesses management had already shifted away from family members to salaried managers.[92] The history of the Indianapolis company was less common, for it was a big business in the mid-twentieth century still owned and managed by a family. This challenge came to the forefront in the late 1940s.

J. K. Lilly, Sr., was intensely committed to family control and ownership of the company his father had founded. As early as 1922 he had begun to plan ahead, to look toward 1932, when at the age of 70 he thought he "may reasonably expect to drop out of business." The family must remain in full control, however. In 1926 he wrote his stepmother, the widow of Colonel Eli Lilly, to say that "I know that you will rejoice that I have provided as he provided, successors for management during the next generation." J. K. Lilly, Sr., always encouraged his sons' devotion to the business and to the family tradition. He was happiest, he wrote them in 1946, when the three men were in "their juxtaposition offices" on McCarty Street, for "the relations of our blessed trinity can only be described as a deep and tranquil harmony."[93]

The growth of the 1940s was not fully harmonious to the senior Lilly, however. At the end of the war W. M. Wheeler, the company's first full-time lawyer, proposed that the board of directors should expand the management force and adopt more careful and formalized methods of decision making and control—systematic methods of the kind that modern big business demanded. In a three-page rebuttal J. K. Lilly, Sr., explained why "Eli Lilly and Company has lagged so far behind in establishing up-to-date machinery for corporate management—executive committees, board of control, comptrollers, monthly, weekly, and called meetings, limiting actions by the president, etc., etc., etc." The reason for this lag, "as clear as a bugle call on a frosty morning," was that "the Lilly business was not born and raised that way!" The senior Lilly explained how the presidency had passed from Colonel Lilly to him to his elder son. "Without fanfare or 'resolutions by the board' Mr. Eli Lilly was voted the responsibilities of the office with the control that had descended from his father and grandfather." Like the two presidents before him, Eli consults with his associates—"a 'royal host' of scientists and business builders [who] have been invited into the family circle . . . but final decisions come, as ever, from him." It was a family enterprise and "not a creature of checks and balances, controlled by debating societies, executive committees, boards of control, and such modern methods."[94]

The two issues that J. K. Lilly, Sr., did not address in his 1946 memorandum were whether one man could continue to bear so large a responsibility and whether the company tradition of face-to-face, informal control would continue to suffice as the organization grew in size. Eli Lilly's direct response to his father's memo is not known, but his actions in initiating and approving the formalization and standardization of management on McCarty Street in the 1940s make clear that he did not fully share his father's view of the business. President Lilly did begin to introduce the kinds of committees and the more formal decision making and reporting that characterized modern big business. Eli Lilly remained, like his father, committed to family control of the company, but he wanted also to reduce the burdens that fell so heavily on him. Joe shared this hope of relief from the demands of McCarty Street, exacerbated in his case by deteriorating health in the 1940s.

The hope for the family future came to rest on the shoulders of Josiah K. Lilly III, Eli's nephew and the only great-grandson of the company founder. Since Eli's two sons had died in infancy and since brother Joe had only a daughter, Ruth, in addition to son J. K. Lilly III, there was only one male in the fourth generation of the business. The family assumed that young Joe, like all Lilly men, would enter the business and eventually head it. He joined the company in 1939 but soon left for war service. Eli was eager for his nephew to return to McCarty Street, writing him in 1941 that "I should like to have you here learning the business so I could quit sooner." Joe returned in 1945, and in early 1946 Eli proudly wrote J. K. Lilly, Sr., that he had appointed the young veteran superintendent of the new Kentucky Avenue plant: "This should give him a chance to show what he has got, amply backed by everybody concerned."[95]

Thus were the hopes and the burdens of being the heir to the family business thrust on J. K. Lilly III, just thirty years of age. He felt the load fall heavily on him, and he soon decided he did not want that kind of life. In late 1946 he resigned.[96] Uncle Eli was devastated. He wrote his nephew that "your letter of resignation was a great blow to family, hopes, and plans worked and thought over for many years. I cannot but think you have made a grave mistake."[97]

The company would have no fourth generation of family management. The future was drawn clearly by Harvard Business School Professor Melvin T. Copeland, who had been making periodic consulting visits to Eli Lilly and Company since 1925.[98] After a visit in 1947 Copeland reported: "The company is approaching a major transition—a separation of management and ownership. This is a very critical period." It was not only or even primarily the resignation of J. K. Lilly III that made separation of ownership and management inevitable. Rather, it was the fact, according to Copeland,

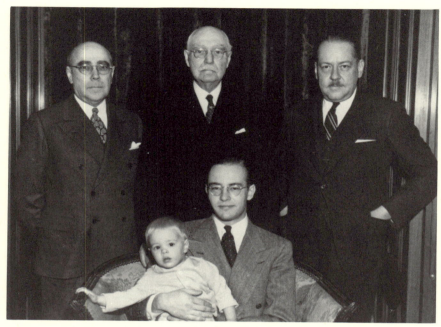

Four generations: back row, left to right, Eli Lilly,   *Eli Lilly and Company Archives*
J. K. Lilly, Sr., J. K. Lilly, Jr.; seated, J. K. Lilly III,
holding son, Eli Lilly, ca. 1945.

that the firm had become so large and so complex. As early as 1944 the
Harvard professor had predicted that "the biggest single problem ahead for
the company probably is that of developing administrative personnel"—
capable managers "to fill higher positions."[99]

Eli Lilly was aware of the problem. The new vice-presidencies he
created in 1944 provided the organizational chart and the boxes to be filled
in with names of managers. More important, Lilly had begun to identify
the most capable younger men in the organization and to give them larger
responsibilities. His favorite of the bunch soon came to be Eugene Beesley,
a graduate of Wabash College who had begun his career in sales. Beesley
played a major role in the 1944 reorganization. In 1953 he would occupy
the top box on the chart, the first nonfamily member to be president of
the company.[100]

The transition to nonfamily management occurred slowly, beginning
in the mid-1940s and continuing years after 1953. A major step came in
1948 with the death of the eighty-six-year-old J. K. Lilly, Sr., which occurred

on 8 February. Soon after, Eli assumed the position of chairman of the board of directors and J. K. Lilly, Jr., became president, a transitional position he held for the next five years. Eli continued to come to his office and to play a major role in company policy, but no longer after 1948 was he intensely involved in day-to-day administration. With the mortar and pestle less dominating, there was even more time for the "hobbies" he loved so intensely and the social responsibilities he felt so keenly.

There is no doubt of Eli Lilly's enduring attachment to the company his grandfather founded and of his pride in his own contribution, from his days as bottle washer to president and chairman of the board. That pride, always modestly stated, was well deserved. His presidency coincided with years of rapid growth, particularly in the 1940s, and with large profits. He oversaw the responses to the depression and to World War II, the development of new drugs, the expansion to Kentucky Avenue and to Basingstoke, England. He guided the family enterprise as it evolved to become a modern big business, and he gave it a reputation as one of the best managed of American companies. Professor Copeland thought so. So did respondents to a national poll conducted in 1947 by the magazine *American Business*.[101] But perhaps Eli Lilly's greatest achievement as president was his response to the human problem. His attention to the welfare of employees was unusually intense, sustained, and genuine. And it extended far beyond wages and benefits to include Lilly's growing fascination with the determinants of character and personality and the cultivation of respect and love. He set a tone of caring and raised a standard of human ideals that decades later would still bring a smile of gratitude to the face of those who remembered the days of his presidency.

Chapter 6

The Wider Horizons of Archæology

In mid-December 1929 Eli Lilly wrote to his eleven-year-old daughter, Evie, then living with her mother in Massachusetts. Like many of his letters to her, this one was filled with expressions of love for his only child and sprinkled with news of daily life that he hoped would interest her. This time he promised also a special project for their annual summer visit to Lake Wawasee. "Your Daddy has been having a lot of fun lately browsing in the State Library studying the history of the country around the lake. Lots of stories of old Indian chiefs." And, he promised Evie, "it will be lots of fun to see these places." In fact he was going to see "if there isn't an unopened Indian mound near the lake. If there is we will try to make arrangements to open it up next summer. Mr. [E. Y.] Guernsey, who knows all about those things and who visited us a day or so ago will tell us just how it should be done."[1] At Wawasee in mid-1930 Lilly followed through on his promise. Although he and Evie did not find an Indian mound that summer, they did visit with J. P. Dolan, a Syracuse lawyer who had a large collection of Indian artifacts.[2]

Evie never developed an interest in archaeology. Her father soon became passionately engaged in the study of prehistoric peoples. A forty-five-year-old man whose adult life heretofore had been spent largely in single-minded devotion to the pharmaceutical business now discovered a variety of interests that led to wider horizons. His success at Eli Lilly and Company in the 1920s, his termination of an unhappy marriage in 1926, and his joyful marriage to Ruth Allison in 1927 were followed by an unfolding of character and an expansion of interests that indicated a major shift in his life. Lilly remained a man of business, of course. He took great pride in the pharmaceutical company, but the pill factory no longer consumed his every moment. Indeed, he complained to an archaeology friend in 1933, "I should like very much to be able to consider jumping my job here permanently and go adigging, but unfortunately it seems impossible." And on another occasion he lamented, "I am so busy with Sales Managers this week that it will be impossible to have any fun at all."[3] Devoted to his duty, Lilly stayed at the task on McCarty Street, even after his retirement from the presidency in 1948, but other challenges attracted an increasingly substantial portion of the time and intellectual energy he once devoted to business.

Lilly's interest in prehistoric archaeology began with Indian artifacts. Like many amateur collectors, he was fascinated by the projectile points, blades, pottery, figurines, and other artifacts that were readily found in many parts of America. Lilly followed his summer visit to Dolan and his "Indian cabinet" with a visit to the collections of the Smithsonian Institution and the Ohio State Museum in November 1930, after which he exuded that he had "practically 'gone archaeology!'"[4] With the advice of Thomas Hendricks, an enthusiastic Indianapolis collector, he began building his own archaeology collection, eventually spending over $20,000. By early 1931 he owned all manner of artifacts and "several hundred problematical forms, including nearly a hundred bird stones."[5] Birdstones were particularly attractive; not only were they a delight to the eye but, because their purpose was, and remains, unknown, their mystery attracted the imagination as well. Lilly early on decided to specialize in problematical forms.[6]

As other collectors became aware of the Indianapolis businessman's new interest they wrote offering items for sale. The collection grew. In the new house he and Ruth built on Sunset Lane, birdstones, pottery, axheads, and gorgets took over the third floor ballroom. In 1932, soon after moving into the new house, Lilly wrote a dealer that his architect had warned him that "if any more weight is piled into the attic it is likely to smash the house, so I am not buying any more relics from anybody."[7] It was not the weight of the collection that stopped his purchases, however, but rather his evolution from a weekend collector to a serious student of archaeology.

Increasingly it was the mystery and the intellectual challenge of understanding prehistoric civilizations rather than the simple amassing of artifacts that sparked Lilly's imagination and energy. The transition was revealed in his changing relationship with W. A. McGuire, a colorful Missouri dealer in Indian relics. At first Lilly and McGuire poked fun at the silly pretensions of professional archaeologists. McGuire's interests were in the artifact itself and the price he could obtain for it, not in the cultural pattern it might reveal. Their relationship warmed to the point that Lilly proposed a joint digging expedition. But then in February 1932 Lilly wrote McGuire:

"For better or for worse, I have cast in my lot with the scientific archaeol-ogists and, as a result of that, I have stopped buying from all sources, and particularly those [like McGuire] from which I am unable to obtain the exact descriptions of the locations and manner of the excavation, with all details." Politely but firmly he concluded his relationship with the Missour-ian by saying "you stand on the other side of the fence."[8]

This maturing outlook between 1929 and 1932 occurred in part because Lilly discovered others in Indiana with serious interests in archae-ology. The prehistoric past had long attracted Hoosiers. The scientists of New Harmony, particularly Charles A. Lesueur, had undertaken archaeol-ogical investigations in the 1820s. And nineteenth-century Hoosiers shared the fascination of Americans in the myth of the ancient mound builders— the romantic notion that some vanished race of superior people had constructed the large earthen mounds of the Ohio Valley. Nineteenth-century archaeology had no serious institutional base in Indiana, however. There were no museums or university programs.[9] Not until the mid-1920s did a push toward organized, careful excavation, collecting, and study begin, directed by the Indiana Historical Society and the Indiana Historical Bureau. The former was a private institution, organized in 1830, the latter a state agency. Both were headed after 1924 by Christopher B. Coleman, a Ph.D.-trained historian, a skilled administrator, and a most likable gentle-man. In 1926 Coleman organized the first modern dig in Indiana, at Albee Mound in Sullivan County. The same year he formed an archaeology section of the Indiana Historical Society. The Society soon would become the major sponsor of archaeology in the state. Among the archaeology section's most active members were Elam Young (Dick) Guernsey, a state legislator from Bedford who had first interested Lilly in the subject; William Ross Teel, an Indianapolis stockbroker and the archaeology section chairman; and Glenn A. Black, a cost estimator for an Indianapolis company that produced industrial scales. All were amateurs, but their interests were serious.[10]

By late 1930 Lilly was part of this group. In December he attended an Indiana Historical Society lecture given by Warren King Moorehead. Moorehead had directed one of the first major digs in the state, near the Wabash River in Posey County in 1898. At the time of his Indianapolis lecture he was director of the Robert S. Peabody Foundation for Archae-ology in Andover, Massachusetts, and one of the most widely known of North American archaeologists. Moorehead greatly impressed Lilly and his associates, and they soon invited him to return for a serious tour of the state's archaeological sites. On 6 May 1931 Lilly joined Moorehead, Guern-

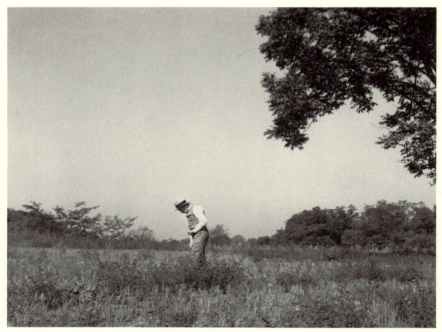

Eli Lilly, surface collecting between the Welborn   *Glenn A. Black Laboratory of*
mound and the Ohio River, October 1936.   *Archaeology*

sey, and Black for a three-day trip through southern Indiana, traveling in Lilly's Marmon to Martinsville, Worthington, Merom, Vincennes, New Harmony, Angel Mounds, and Boonville. In search of archaeological sites, Lilly tramped fields and woods alive with an Indiana springtime, talked with local collectors, and enjoyed the company of Moorehead, Guernsey, and Black. He ended the trip fully stuck to the prehistoric past. "The memory of the three delightful days in your expedition," Lilly wrote Moorehead, "will always be a happy one."[11]

Summer 1931 brought an intensity for archaeology that Lilly had shown previously only for the pharmaceutical business. As he would do for the next two decades, he spent much of his vacation at Wawasee in pursuit of the prehistoric past. He located what he hoped was an Indian burial at Cedar Point on Lake Wawasee. He planned its excavation and concentrated on "learning surveying for the purpose of helping make this expedition a real scientific attainment."[12] Not until the fall was he able to undertake the Cedar Point dig. It was "more or less a disappointment," he

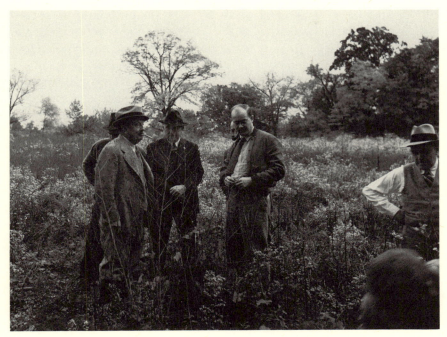

Left to right, front, Warren K. Moorehead, Henry Kersher, James B. Griffin, and Eli Lilly, Fort Ancient, Ohio.

Glenn A. Black Laboratory of Archaeology

concluded, for he found no skeletal remains. It was his first and last such dig.[13]

Lilly's interests were not those of a "dirt" archaeologist. He always enjoyed visiting sites and studying excavations. Even in his seventies he eagerly tramped over sites, though always with a coat, tie, and his felt hat. His major interest and talent developed not in the field, however, but in the library and the study. By early 1931 he owned several shelves full of archaeology books, and at Wawasee that summer he spent every morning reading, "trying to learn something about Indiana archaeological data by working up county bibliographies."[14] Lilly worked hard to prepare this bibliography and decided eventually to submit it to the Indiana Historical Bureau for publication. It was his first such effort. He learned the trials and tribulations of publication when Nellie Armstrong, the Bureau's meticulous editor, forced him to do two revisions. The Bureau published his "Bibliography on Indiana Archaeology" in 1932.[15]

In addition to work on the Cedar Point dig and the bibliography, Lilly also began in the summer of 1931 to contemplate the larger questions in American archaeology. In particular, he focused his attention on the question of time and the challenge of categorizing, dating, and arranging in chronological sequence the several cultures of prehistoric peoples who had lived in Indiana before the Europeans arrived. When he read of the recent success of A. E. Douglas in dating the Pueblo ruins of the American Southwest by studying tree rings in their wooden timbers, he wrote Moorehead: "I am all fired up with the possibility of finding a log in some of these mounds and burials, from the rings of which we might figure the age of some of these places like Douglas did in the Southwest."[16] Lilly's interest in time, in developing a chronological synthesis and taxonomy of prehistoric cultures in Indiana, would become the driving challenge throughout his life of archaeology.

To answer the questions of time, Lilly knew, required extensive excavations of sites and the intellectual power of professional archaeologists. In 1931 he put a new man to work in the field. Glenn Black would contribute more to Indiana archaeology than any other person. He would also become Lilly's closest friend.

Black was born in Indianapolis in 1900, fifteen years after Lilly. By the late 1920s he was actively collecting Indian artifacts and reading relevant books and articles. In 1931 the depression brought a reduction and eventually an end to his work with Fairbanks, Morse and Company. When offered the chance to serve as guide and driver for the Moorehead expedition in May 1931, Black eagerly accepted. Moorehead and Lilly were much impressed with the young, earnest, and unemployed Black. They concurred that he should be set to work in Indiana archaeology. Lilly agreed to pay his field expenses and a salary of $225 a month.[17] Black began work in mid-June 1931 preparing a map of sites in the state. While Lilly was reading archaeology at Wawasee, Black worked on the project in Lilly's Sunset Lane library and in his third-floor collections. By midsummer Black was in the field, digging in Greene County and sending frequent, detailed descriptions of his finds to Lilly. He and Lilly also began to correspond more broadly about archaeology. Lilly wrote Black of Douglas's tree-ring dating and advised him that if he unearthed any logs to "guard them as you would your life."[18]

Lilly took a risk in employing Black, particularly because he had no formal training in archaeology and only a high school education. Doubtless Black's earnestness, capacity for hard work, and determined interest in archaeology impressed Lilly. But Lilly recognized also the need for more formal education. So did Indiana Historical Society head Coleman and archaeology section chairman Teel. They knew that Fay-Cooper Cole at the University of Chicago had recently begun to train first-rate archaeologists. Professor Cole was pressuring the Society to hire one of his Chicago students. Coleman and Teel supported Lilly's preference for Black, but the three men agreed that the young Hoosier needed more academic polish. They wished, Lilly wrote Moorehead, "to avoid the scorn of one Dr. Cole in case he would say, 'Black, Black, who is this man Black?' So Mr. Teel is trying to make arrangements to get in some more scholastic education, probably this winter, so we can at least say he has been trained under Shetrone, or 'so-and-so.' This Black is willing to do and I still have hopes of making a good man out of him. He surely has the diligence and enthusiasm, which is a large part of the picture."[19]

From October 1931 through May 1932 Black studied with Henry C. Shetrone at the Ohio State Museum. Shetrone was the author of a book on the mound builders and directed one of the most active excavation programs in the state. He and the institution he headed were widely respected in archaeological circles. He had been reluctant at first to take on Black, advising Teel that the Society ought instead "to bring in a first-class scientifically trained man."[20] But Black eventually won over Shetrone, who later wrote Lilly that "we should be glad indeed to have him as a member of the Museum staff." In 1935 Black had the satisfaction of considering and rejecting a formal offer to join the Ohio State Museum staff.[21]

Lilly closely watched Black's progress. He visited him in Columbus and corresponded frequently. He asked Black's help in recommending titles "to build up a good modern library on the subject of Middle Western archaeology" and to expand references for the bibliography he was preparing.[22] Black responded fully to such calls, usually going beyond the specific request. The younger man remained a bit unsure of his relationship to his patron. Doubtless fearing disapproval, Black did not tell him of his marriage in late October 1931 to Ida May Hazard. Ruth Lilly read the marriage license application in the Indianapolis newspaper, and Eli wrote immediately: "You are not springing a surprise on us, are you? Here is hoping." When Black confirmed the marriage and expressed his "hope that this step will meet with your approval," Lilly replied with "the heartiest congratulations to you and to Mrs. Black."[23] The friendship between the two men would soon extend to a deep friendship between the two couples.

Black returned from Columbus in the spring of 1932 in time for summer fieldwork. Lilly continued to pay his salary, but now funneled it through the Indiana Historical Society so that "I can get credit on my income tax."[24] By mid-1932 neither Black, Teel, nor Coleman made significant decisions relating to the Society's archaeological work without first consulting Lilly.[25] His checkbook was always open for Black: "When it comes time for me to put any money into the Historical Society for the digging purposes, let me know and I shall send a check promptly."[26] Lilly's commanding role was formalized and expanded in 1933 when he agreed to serve as president of the Society, a position he held until 1947. Black remained in the employ of the Indiana Historical Society until his death, his salary paid by Lilly. The patron always insisted that the Society "make no announcement or publication or use my name in connection with the proposition in any way."[27]

Lilly's growing interest in archaeology soon expanded from a simple wish for self-education and distraction from the burdens of McCarty Street to development of a plan to push forward the field itself by adding to knowledge about Indiana's prehistory and by recruiting others to the task. A major step in that direction was his effort to synthesize and elaborate the main features of Indiana's prehistory. As he gathered references for his bibliography, as he corresponded and talked with Black and others, as his interest and questions grew, Lilly decided to write a book. He referred to the project facetiously as "my famous book" and emphasized that he was writing a "book for popular consumption" and did not "lay claim to any archaeological erudition."[28] Although he professed modest ambitions, Lilly worked long and hard on the manuscript, puzzling out a tentative chronology for Indian cultures, laboring over the use of stone, copper, bone, and shell, describing carefully earthworks and mounds, and sending chapters to Black and others for criticism. And he worked to improve his writing style, even to the point of following Benjamin Franklin's method of reading an essay in *The Spectator*, thinking it over, and then attempting to write the essay in his own words.[29]

Prehistoric Antiquities of Indiana was published in 1937 by the Indiana Historical Society. Lilly paid the publication costs, which were dear because the book was so handsomely produced, with 293 large pages and many well-done illustrations. *Prehistoric Antiquities of Indiana* was in no sense a vanity publication, however, for the content was most impressive and the scholarly reviews very favorable. The text was well documented, with an abundance of footnotes conforming to standard academic form and style and testifying to Lilly's wide reading. Like many proud authors, Lilly insisted that the footnotes be placed at the bottom of each page. The narrative presented a thoughtful and reliable synthesis of knowledge about Indiana's prehistory, often making broad, comparative references that ranged from stone axes used at the Battle of Hastings to bows and arrows in Mongolia. And the book was clearly and attractively written. The reviewer for the *Indianapolis Times,* doubtless no archaeology enthusiast, admitted that the "book is actually exciting reading." And so it was, for Lilly communicated to the reader his own enthusiasm for the subject, hoping, he wrote in the preface, "to interest more of the people of Indiana in the relics of our vanished predecessors, and to stimulate inquiry into the prehistory and archaeology of the state." And he added, "pursuit of this subject has led the author along such pleasant paths that he is desirous of sharing them with others."[30]

Perhaps the dominant theme in Lilly's *Prehistoric Antiquities* was the sense of mystery and of questions to be answered. He presented archaeology as an exciting voyage of discovery in which "certain vague, shadowy forms seem to be taking shape through the somber clouds obscuring the past." The object of the voyage was to identify the peoples who left behind the earthworks, mounds, burials, and village sites in Indiana and to classify them in ways that revealed the chronological sequence and patterns of their cultures. Lilly was confident that "some day the question will be answered." He briefly noted that "a group affiliated with the Indiana Historical Society . . . has been working intensively on this problem for several years. These investigators are attempting to approach the mystery from several different directions, triangulating upon the problem, as it were." Specialists in pottery, Indian languages, tree rings, skeletal material, and history were joining the archaeologists working at village sites. Lilly modestly neglected to note that the notion of a coordinated triangulation upon the mystery, the financial support for it, and the coordination and direction of it all came from the author of *Prehistoric Antiquities.*[31]

By late 1932 Lilly had decided that the questions of Indiana's prehistory were too complex for any single scholar to answer. As in modern industrial production, as he so well knew, complexity and scale required specialization of labor. Lilly formulated a "plan of attack on the Culture Problem" that called for the recruitment and organization of a group of specialized, professional archaeologists to triangulate upon the mysteries of prehistoric cultures in Indiana.[32]

As he moved closer to professional archaeologists, Lilly remained loyal to his amateur Indiana associates, giving moral and financial support to Dick Guernsey and others. In 1933 he hired a childhood friend, Paul Weer, who was financially hard up, to catalog his collections at Sunset Lane. Weer remained with him for the next two decades.[33] But Lilly's questions overran the more limited interests and knowledge of most of the archaeology section members. As early as August 1931 he had written Shetrone at the Ohio State Museum asking him to "recommend the best man or two in the United States who would come pay us a visit and teach us something."[34] Later that year Moorehead returned to Indiana to spend a weekend as Lilly's houseguest and to be the central attraction at a Sunset Lane dinner party for ten archaeology associates. A few months later Shetrone also visited for a weekend. These were the first of many such archaeology weekends at Sunset Lane. Sometimes they included large dinner parties, carefully planned in advance. More often they were informal gatherings. Lilly would write to Black, "If you have nothing else on to take you away Saturday morning we might have a confab."[35]

Lilly's contact with professional archaeologists expanded greatly in 1932 and 1933. Through his reading and growing correspondence he identified the leading institutions and scholars in the field and began to organize his attack. He was particularly impressed with an article titled "Time Perspective in Aboriginal American Culture, a Study in Method," published by Edward Sapir in 1916. Sapir's article suggested to him "how linguistics can be used to determine the time relations of various tribes."[36] In the fall of 1932 he wrote Sapir, then a distinguished linguist at Yale University, expressing his interest "in attempting to work out the time perspectives of the Mound Builders in Indiana." Coming quickly to the point in this brief letter, Lilly asked "if a fellowship could be founded under your direction" to study the languages of the tribes that once lived in Indiana "to see if any time relations could be scientifically proven."[37] It was the beginning step in his plan of triangulation.

Sapir was greatly pleased with this offer from an Indianapolis businessman he had never met. The Yale professor agreed to accept the fellowship and commended Lilly on his "unusually broad point of view" but asked for "more precise indication of the nature of the fellowship contemplated."[38] Lilly replied by emphasizing his interest in the tribes of Indiana and the possibility that if they "came in contact with one another . . .

certain effects might have been produced which would reveal something of the relative times that these contacts occurred, having in the back of our heads the solving of the problem of what tribes the different cultures of mound builders were."[39]

In reply to Lilly's query as to the appropriate amount for the fellowship, Sapir suggested at least $1,000 a year and ideally $1,500, with additional provision for summer field expenses. Negotiations then began. Lilly offered $1,500, to include field expenses. Sapir replied, pretending to hope that field expenses would be added to the $1,500 and asking Lilly to remit the money to Yale in early 1933, even though he had no one yet to nominate for the fellowship.[40] Sapir soon learned something of Lilly—a businessman with a decade of experience negotiating contracts with academic administrators and professors. Lilly responded in three curt paragraphs. In the first he wrote "the minute you say a man is available and ready to start work, the $1,500 will be forthcoming." The second paragraph read: "From my rather large acquaintance with medical fellowships of one kind and another, I know that in this day and time, a $1000 fellowship is very thankfully received and that is the reason I thought $1200 for the fellowship itself and $300 for traveling expenses would be adequate." Lilly closed his letter: "Perhaps the circumstances in connection with other sorts of fellowships and those connected with medical research are different. If so, please enlighten me." Sapir saw Lilly's point and accepted his terms.[41]

In the spring of 1933 Sapir wrote to nominate for the fellowship Charles F. (Carl) Voegelin, just finishing his Ph.D. degree at the University of California, Berkeley. Voegelin combined an interest in linguistics and ethnology. He accepted the $1,500 fellowship, to include field expenses, for the three-year period Lilly and Sapir had agreed upon. Lilly sent the money to Yale.[42] The Dean of the Yale Graduate School happily acknowledged the support and asked if the new program could be called the Eli Lilly Fellowship in Ethnology. Lilly replied: "Please do not give me any personal publicity on this fellowship. If you must have a name, simply call it the Indiana fellowship, or something of that sort."[43]

Carl Voegelin spent the summer of 1933 in the field, studying Shawnee language and culture in Oklahoma. He sent technical reports of his work to Sapir, but only a brief summary to Lilly. Then just before Christmas Carl visited at Sunset Lane, along with his wife Erminie W. Voegelin, who later would complete a Ph.D. in anthropology at Yale. Carl Voegelin came away from that visit impressed with Lilly's depth of knowledge and intensity of interest, for thereafter his letters to Indianapolis were not only more detailed but more academic in tone and content. Voegelin was particularly pleased with Lilly's openness to different methods and subjects. The pre-Christmas visit also enabled Lilly to form a high opinion of Erminie Voegelin so that when her husband was offered other means of financial support Lilly agreed to transfer the Yale fellowship to her.[44]

Lilly's long relationship with the Voegelins was generally pleasant and profitable. There were strains, however. Voegelin had a very high opinion of his abilities, even as a young scholar, and he pushed against Lilly's generosity. In early 1934 he wrote directly to Lilly asking that the fellowship be increased from $1,500 to $2,000. Lilly was furious at Voegelin's cheek but waited several weeks to reply. Noting that he had "handled somewhere between fifty and one hundred fellowships" at other universities, he grumped to Voegelin that "fellowships at Yale must come high!" However, "to show that there are no hard feelings," he agreed to increase the fellowship by $250 and then curtly closed debate by stating that "if you and Dr. Sapir do not think this sum is adequate, it will be perfectly satisfactory to have the fellowship dropped."[45] There were difficulties also because Lilly and Black thought Voegelin and Sapir were more interested in ethnology than linguistics and were straying too far from the prehistory of Indiana. After a meeting in Indianapolis in late 1935 to discuss these matters, Lilly informed Voegelin that he would not extend the fellowship beyond the original three-year period.[46]

Yet the Voegelin-Lilly relationship did not end, for Voegelin's linguistic strength was an essential element in Lilly's plan of triangulation. In 1936 he agreed to support Voegelin's appointment to the DePauw University faculty, paying his salary of $2,500 a year.[47] And five years later Lilly was a major force in arranging for Voegelin's apppointment to the faculty at Indiana University. Thus, with the Voegelins at home in Indiana, Lilly saw them often to talk over questions of prehistory.

The Voegelins were not the only scholars during the 1930s to benefit from Lilly's interest in archaeology or to test his patience. As part of his plan of triangulating on Indiana prehistory he established fellowships at other universities too, fitting the pattern he had used with Sapir at Yale. Following his interest in tree-ring dating, he set up a fellowship under Fay-Cooper Cole at the University of Chicago, held for a time by Florence Hawley. And at the University of Michigan he established a fellowship to work on pottery, directed by Carl Guthe and held by James B. Griffin, a student at Ann Arbor. Griffin became a longtime archaeology associate of

Lilly's and one of the leading scholars in the field. Like Voegelin he was a man of large self-confidence and sometimes a trial to Lilly's patience. Another fellowship at Michigan, begun in 1937, supported Georg K. Neumann's study of human skeletal material. Neumann, too, would be a lifelong associate of Lilly's.[48]

Lilly's relationship with Sapir, the Voegelins, Griffin, Neumann, and others showed a large tolerence for diverse interests and personalities. Generously he supported their work, even when he suspected they might be taking advantage of that generosity by following their own interests rather than his. Graciously he tolerated academic caution and procrastination even when he desperately wanted to know the results of a particular inquiry. Gently he rode herd over the professors, commending their work, inviting them to dinner, subsidizing their publications, financing their fieldwork, and contributing to their salaries. All this he did modestly and quietly.

In return Lilly was able to participate fully in his voyage of archaeological discovery, not as a distant patron but as an active pilot and contributor. The idea for a triangulated attack on the problem of time was his, and it was he who kept pushing and nudging the Indiana group, as they came to be called. He served as coordinator, making sure that reports, correspondence, and references circulated. He organized periodic meetings at Sunset Lane and at Wawasee. When Guthe and Griffin came down from Ann Arbor he invited the others to Sunset Lane for the weekend. They "went into a huddle early Friday evening and discontinued only for food and a little sleep until Sunday morning."[49] In 1937 he began to call an annual meeting at his Wawasee cottage, often a weekend in October, where the group would compare notes of the year's work. Usually invited to the lake were Guthe, Griffin, Black, Guernsey, Carl Voegelin, Weer, and Neumann. Those in or near Indianapolis would leave from Sunset Lane, piling into Ruth's Cadillac for the journey to the lake. Lilly sometimes encouraged each member to come with three small projects "in which you think our Wawasee group would be interested."[50] As a result of these conferences, Guthe wrote in 1937, "each member of the group is beginning to understand more clearly where his job fits into the general scheme."[51]

While Lilly's interests extended to many fundamental questions of prehistory, as indicated in the breadth of his *Prehistoric Antiquities of Indiana*, he gradually focused his energies on one particular body of evidence, the Walam Olum. The Walam Olum was a chronicle of the Lenni Lenape Indians, known to Europeans as the Delaware. This purported account of their history was painted in pictorial symbols on flat sticks, which were used by tribal patriarchs to recite or sing the story of their ancestors. Constantine S. Rafinesque claimed that he acquired the sticks of the Walam Olum from a man he described as "the late Dr. Ward of Indiana," who in turn had received them in 1820 from Delaware Indians living on the White River in the Hoosier state. Later efforts to identify Dr. Ward have been inconclusive. Rafinesque, however, was a prolific and well-known scientist of the early nineteenth century, though his reputation was, and remains, clouded. In the early 1820s he was teaching botany and natural history at Transylvania University in Lexington, Kentucky. Two years after acquiring the Walam Olum sticks Rafinesque claimed to have obtained from an unknown source a Delaware language version of the songs or verses that explained the pictographs. In 1836, after he had moved to Philadelphia, he published his translated version of the songs. Translations published by Ephraim G. Squier in 1849 and by Daniel G. Brinton in 1885 included the pictographs and the Delaware text and added to interest in this unique document.[52]

The significance of the Walam Olum rested in its potential to narrate the history of the Lenape from creation to the arrival of white invaders. As Lilly and others interpreted the Walam Olum, it recorded the Lenape migration from Asia across the Bering Strait and then south and east across the North American continent, encountering disease, enemies, and other challenges. About A.D. 1000, according to Lilly's interpretation, the Lenape moved into the Ohio River Valley, likely participating in the Hopewellian culture of the prehistoric peoples who built many of the great mounds. About three hundred years later they moved east again, crossing the Appalachian Mountains and arriving at tidewater near the Delaware River by about A.D. 1400.[53]

If genuine, the Walam Olum was a document of major significance. The challenge of understanding it might be to North America what Heinrich Schliemann's study of the Homeric epics was to European civilization—an exalted comparison that much appealed to Lilly.[54] Indeed, because the chronicle indicated that the Lenape had likely settled during the early centuries of the second millennium in what came to be Indiana and then returned to Indiana when pushed westward by white Americans at the end of the eighteenth century, Lilly referred to Walam Olum as "the Hoosier Iliad." His tongue may have been slightly in cheek, but Lilly was convinced that the document was genuine, and his long and compelling search to unlock the secrets he believed the Walam Olum held was most serious indeed.

In early 1932 Lilly wrote Black that he hoped to discuss with him "the Walam Olum, or what I like to call the Hoosier Iliad."[55] There followed an extensive correspondence in which they agreed, as Black wrote, that "the Hopewell mounds were built by none other than some branch of Algonquian stock and also that our own 'Hoosier Iliad' adds weight to that theory."[56] Both men were convinced that Black's excavations in Greene County in the summer of 1931 supported their theory. They knew too that it was an unorthodox theory and therefore would meet with much resistance from professional archaeologists. That may have been part of the appeal, for as Lilly wrote Black, who was then studying with Shetrone in Columbus, "It is a noble experiment to beard some of these old 'moss backs' in their dens." It was a noble experiment indeed, for Lilly and Black were setting out to connect the prehistoric people who had built the great mounds of the Ohio Valley with the historic Delaware tribe.[57]

By the fall of 1932 Lilly was ready to propose their unorthodox idea to others. He wrote Guthe at Ann Arbor: "Black and I have a hunch that the Walam Olum may possibly have in it the key that will open the riddle of the Mound Builders; we of course being particularly interested in the time perspective in connection with the aborigines of Indiana."[58] He also mentioned his hunch to Sapir at Yale, indicating interest particularly in the languages of the tribes mentioned in the Walam Olum. Sapir's enthusiasm for a fellowship did not extend to Walam Olum, while Guthe wrote more directly that "the Walam Olum thesis is a rather frail reed on which to lean in archaeological work."[59]

Lacking strong encouragement from the professors, Lilly nonetheless moved ahead with work on Walam Olum. During the next two decades he sometimes became discouraged and lost interest, but he could never shake off the ghosts of Rafinesque, Dr. Ward, and the mound builders. In his correspondence and meetings with the Indiana group he kept Walam Olum on the agenda. And in his Sunset Lane library and at Wawasee he toiled over the document, concentrating his energies on deciphering the pictographs and on sorting out the route and chronology of Lenape migration. By the fall of 1938 his laborious comparison of Brinton's 1885 book with Rafinesque's original manuscript had turned up forty-six errors in copying and more than twenty instances in which Lilly thought Brinton's interpretations of the pictographs were inaccurate.[60] Black was his constant support in this work. In correspondence and conversation they pored over the details of the document. The two men referred to their Saturday meetings as "Walam Olum day." Griffin, Neumann, Weer, and especially the Voegelins also toiled over special parts of the mystery. Others outside the Indiana group contributed occasionally. At least two scientists from the pharmaceutical company were briefly involved. K. K. Chen checked resemblances between Walam Olum ideograms and Chinese characters, while George Clowes gave an opinion regarding skull shapes. Most of the time Lilly worked alone, struggling over such questions as the location of the Fish River. He would sometimes spend a whole weekend "kind of Walum Olum-ing," as in the early spring of 1941 when, he wrote Black, "The old bug has bit me again!"[61]

World War II slowed the work by keeping Lilly tied closely to the business of pharmaceuticals, while the rationing of tires and gasoline made meetings of the Indiana group difficult to arrange. But Lilly continued his "weekend cogitations," often writing his absent colleagues afterwards. Following one such solitary weekend in the fall of 1942 he sent Voegelin a list of questions: "Wouldn't," he asked, "the pictographs with two chief's glyphs side by side indicate chiefs at the same time?"[62] In the midst of a Walam Olum vacation at Wawasee in the summer of 1943 he wrote that "before long my part of the job will be pretty well completed: (1) the remarks about each ideograph, (2) the concordance & (3) the bibliography—all checked 'n everything."[63] But as in any group project, not all members pulled oars at the same speed, and unanswered questions remained.

With the end of war Lilly began his campaign to push the Walam Olum project to completion. He resumed the fall meetings at Wawasee, inviting Griffin, Neumann, Carl Voegelin, Black, and Weer to the lake.[64] Soon the group doubled in size, for Lilly recruited new members by means of a fellowship program begun in 1946. The impetus for the new fellowships came from the Indiana group's need to know more about Delaware Indians in the Northeast, hoping that archaeological sites there would provide support for the migration route of the Delawares as interpreted in Walam Olum.

With this goal in mind Lilly wrote leading archaeologists or ethnologists in three states: Dorothy Cross in New Jersey, William A. Ritchie in New York, and Frank G. Speck in Pennsylvania. He offered to establish

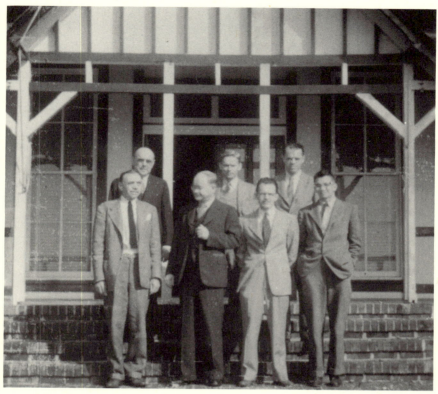

The Indiana group of archaeologists at Wawasee, late 1940s, in a photo probably taken by Glenn Black. Front, left to right, Paul Weer, James B. Griffin, Richard S. MacNeish, John Witthoft; back, left to right, Eli Lilly, Georg Neumann, Carl Voegelin.

Eli Lilly and Company Archives

two-year fellowships for graduate students under their direction to study Delaware sites in their respective states. The three scholars accepted Lilly's offer, recruited the students, and supervised their work. Supported by $1,000 a year fellowships, Catherine McCann in New Jersey, Edmund S. Carpenter in New York, and John Witthoft in Pennsylvania began work at Delaware Indian sites in the summer of 1946.[65] Lilly provided all the money and personally sent the checks, but he attached the name of the Indiana Historical Society to the fellowships. As he wrote Cross, "I do not like publicity and have covered up pretty well under the name of the

Indiana Historical Society."[66] More enjoyable to him than publicity was the pleasure of inviting the now enlarged group to Wawasee in October 1947 to discuss Walam Olum.[67]

Disappointment continued to mix with progress, however. The Delaware Indian work in the Northeast was slow in producing results and never provided the evidence necessary to connect firmly the archaeological record with the narrative of Walam Olum. The meeting at Wawasee scheduled for the fall of 1947 had to be canceled because Lilly wanted to stay close to his father, who was very ill. By early 1948 Lilly was unusually discouraged. The Walam Olum book was not ready to go to press, he wrote Carl Voegelin, and "I haven't the slightest notion when it will go, if ever." The fellowship work on the Delaware had not produced the desired results. Moreover, the linguistic work, which was Voegelin's responsibility, was going slowly. "We must know," he wrote Voegelin, "which dialect of the Delaware the Walam Olum was written or rather recited in, and if it is going to take six years to make a thorough digest of the various Algonquin tongues and dialects before this can be determined, the period will probably be carried beyond my normal life expectancy. So you see I feel rather discouraged about the whole proposition."[68] Some of Lilly's gloom doubtless derived from the fact that his father was on his deathbed and died in early February 1948.

By late 1949, however, Lilly was once more deeply engaged with the project, agonizing again over the location of the Fish River and writing Voegelin that "we have decided to go ahead on the publication of the Walam Olum."[69] Again, however, he fretted as his colleagues failed to produce their chapters for the proposed book. In the fall of 1951 he sent strongly worded letters to the Voegelins and Neumann, telling them he was coming to Bloomington to visit and that "it is now time for us all to 'fish or cut bait' on this Walam Olum matter as we want to get all copy together this fall for printing."[70] Fall passed to winter, and no copy arrived from Bloomington. Black, too, was slow in completing his sections. When he finally delivered his chapter in March 1953 Lilly encouraged him to "give Georg the psychological amount of speed elixir." Neumann at last delivered his essay in early September 1953, and the full copy went to the printer.[71]

While Lilly was prodding the professors along, another crisis developed. In the spring of 1952 Black returned from an archaeology meeting in Columbus, Ohio, shocked and angry—angrier than perhaps ever in his life. At the meeting Jimmy Griffin had stated, Black wrote Lilly, "that he had no confidence in the Walam Olum, & never had, and had told you so!!!!!"[72] Through the 1930s and 1940s Griffin had received Lilly's financial support and had worked on problems important to Walam Olum. He had attended many meetings at Wawasee and Sunset Lane and had expressed doubts but seemed supportive. His prickly assertiveness and ego sometimes caused conflict—Griffin was "a master of academic intimidation," one scholar noted—but Lilly's tolerance of academic personalities and respect for Griffin's large abilities smoothed over the tension. To Lilly and Black, Griffin's Judas-like outburst in Columbus was a depressing blow, however, not only because Griffin by this time was a major figure in American archaeology whose criticism of Walam Olum could not be brushed off easily, but also because they concluded now that he had deceived them and used them.[73]

Despite setbacks Lilly pushed ahead. In 1954, at last, the book appeared under the title of *Walam Olum or Red Score: The Migration Legend of the Lenni Lenape or Delaware Indians*. Printed by the Lakeside Press at a cost of $38,734 for 2,398 copies and published by the Indiana Historical Society, *Walam Olum* was a beautifully produced book. Lilly personally paid the printing bill.[74] The book contained Carl Voegelin's translation of the verses or songs, Erminie Voegelin's ethnological observations, Paul Weer's discussion of the history of the document, Black's analysis of the archaeological evidence, Neumann's consideration of the physical anthropological data, and Lilly's interpretation of the pictographs and his speculation on the route and chronology of the Lenape migration. The volume also contained a reproduction of Rafinesque's manuscript. The table of contents gave each author credit for his or her contribution, and the introduction acknowledged the many other scholars who had helped with the research. The title page might logically have carried the name of Eli Lilly, but the title page listed neither author, editor, or coordinator of the project. Nor did the acknowledgments or introduction indicate Lilly's dominant role in originating, directing, and financing the work. Instead, the enterprise was set forth as a group endeavor under sponsorship of the Indiana Historical Society. In presenting to the public the results of a project that had occupied him for two decades Lilly continued his policy of remaining modestly behind the cover of the Indiana Historical Society.

The scholarly reviews were mixed. Reviewers agreed that the Walam Olum document was an enticing riddle. They praised the interdisciplinary method of attempting to solve the riddle—Lilly's plan of triangulation. Robert B. Woodbury of Columbia University concluded it was "one of the most ambitious programs ever undertaken for unraveling the complex history and prehistory of an Indian tribe."[75] But doubts loomed over the validity of the document and the interpretations of it. C. A. Weslager was very critical: "To attribute historical validity to an English translation of a dubious transcription of a series of primitive glyphs obtained under mysterious circumstances by an eccentric investigator is unjustified."[76]

One of the longest and most thoughtful reviews came from Jimmy Griffin. Griffin had written Lilly when the book appeared, telling him he was reviewing it for the *Indiana Magazine of History* and indicating that although he recognized the large contribution of the work he had doubts about the interpretations set forth. Lilly sent Griffin's letter to Black, commenting angrily that "here is the opening gun from brother Griffin. . . . So far as I personally am concerned I am fed up with Jimmy."[77] When Griffin's review appeared Lilly wrote Black that "our friend has rather 'damned us with faint praise,' but what care we?"[78] Griffin's review was indeed mixed. It was filled with praise for the work as a "significant contribution," on the one hand, but, on the other, dismissed as wrong or unsubstantiated most of the major conclusions of the book. The archaeological, linguistic, and anthropological data conflicted with the legend and were open to many other interpretations, Griffin asserted. Lilly's analysis of the symbols of the Walam Olum was "painstaking" and "ingenious," and his chapter on the chronology of the migration was "stimulating" but not convincing.[79]

Griffin had another opportunity to evaluate *Walam Olum*. In April 1971 he came to Bloomington as the main speaker at the dedication of Indiana University's Glenn A. Black Laboratory of Archaeology. Griffin presented a lengthy paper on the development of archaeology in Indiana, focusing with much praise on the role of the eighty-six-year-old patron sitting in the audience: "There have been other research programs in American anthropology that have been supported by individuals, but I doubt that any had the breadth of view, the variety of personnel, or the continuity of purpose and tolerance 'for professional procrastination' that was always present in these endeavors." And Griffin added, "I also doubt that the patron of any other program of this nature ever participated as fully, shared discouragement with such compassion, or exulted more with each accomplishment." But in treating the Walam Olum project the tough-minded Griffin repeated the general criticisms made in his review sixteen years earlier.[80] Soon after the dedication ceremony Lilly wrote Griffin, thanking him for his work in preparing the paper and protesting that "you gave me entirely too much credit." Then in the last paragraph of his letter Lilly bit again at the Walam Olum bone, barking to Griffin that "a lot of us here in

Indiana still believe that there is some basic truth in the Walam Olum that will someday be more or less verified."[81] Soon after Griffin had revived the scent Lilly was once again on the trail of the Walam Olum riddle: he employed a researcher to examine the Rafinesque papers at the Workingmen's Institute in New Harmony for references to the late Dr. Ward, but again without success.[82]

The Walam Olum remains intriguing and controversial. The story deals with human origins in a way that crosses cultures, while the text, as an Italian scholar has written, "has a metaphysical profundity equal to any other sacred scripture."[83] The American poet Daniel Hoffman was so intrigued by Walam Olum that he attempted a poetic reconstruction of it and a fictional diary of Dr. Ward. Some scholars have suggested that Walam Olum was a source for the Book of Mormon, a position others have disputed. Some regard it as the creation of historical Delaware Indians, seeking to build a cultural tradition to resist European ways. Some scholars believe the document a likely fake, with Rafinesque the culprit. But even if, as its strongest critics imply, Lilly and the Indiana group were victims of a great hoax, their work produced large and positive results. More than a dozen young scholars in the 1930s and 1940s received from Eli Lilly financial support and morale-boosting encouragement that was critical in putting bread on their tables and launching them on productive careers. Archaeology in the eastern United States was a small, immature field in 1930, and Lilly's involvement over the next two decades made a substantial difference in hastening its development to maturity.[84]

Lilly's patronage of archaeology and anthropology had its most specific effect at Indiana University. As early as 1935 Lilly and Voegelin had begun considering the possibility of seeking an appointment for Voegelin in Bloomington. There, Voegelin suggested, "we could work in close collaboration."[85] With Lilly paying his salary Voegelin settled for a time at DePauw University, but in 1941 Indiana University hired him. Their general strategy, as Voegelin stated it, was "to (1) get me in the History Department, (2) get a physical anthropologist in another appropriate department, and then perhaps with one more person start an anthropology department."[86] The physical anthropologist they wanted in Bloomington was Georg Neumann. Lilly talked with him in the fall of 1941 and then began to lobby President Herman B Wells for Neumann's appointment. Lilly also raised the possibility of Glenn Black serving as a special lecturer. Wells agreed. Neumann joined the faculty in 1942 and Black in 1944. With Voegelin, Neumann, and Black on board they moved to their last step in the plan. In the spring of 1944 Lilly talked with President Wells and Graduate School Dean Fernandus Payne about establishing a Department of Anthropology. By mid-1947 the new department was in operation. Its newsletter was appropriately titled *Walam Olum*, reflecting the origins of its three members.[87] All thought of Lilly, Voegelin wrote, as "a *de facto* or *in spiritu* member of the Anthropology Department."[88] Lilly remained close to the department, visiting campus on weekends and even listening patiently to the jealousies and backbiting that eventually set in, particularly after Carl and Erminie Voegelin divorced in 1954.[89]

In addition to providing impetus for the department at Indiana University, Lilly's interest in Walam Olum also led him to pioneering efforts in encouraging interdisciplinary research. Walam Olum itself was an example of such research, with the disciplines of ethnology, linguistics, physical anthropology, history, and archaeology employed on one problem. In 1938, in his presidential address to the Indiana Academy of Science, Lilly presented a well-informed and sophisticated critique of university research. He criticized the "Departmental Pigeonhole System" in which scholars labored "in the gloomy recesses of a single department, heedlessly avoiding the sparkling sunlight of collateral branches of knowledge." Lilly urged combining branches of knowledge "to triangulate upon the most vitally important questions of the day." "Properly cooperative research work is synergistic," he concluded.[90] Whether in quest of the riddle of Walam Olum or of a new pharmaceutical product, Lilly could look at the university as a sympathetic outsider, less concerned with tradition and formalities than with results. Such quintessential academicians as Griffin and Voegelin recognized this strength early, commending Lilly's "refreshing interest in interpretation and not merely in academic formalism."[91]

The breadth of Lilly's interest in archaeology allowed room also for sustained attention to one specific prehistoric site. He had visited Angel Mounds on the trip with Moorehead in 1931. Moorehead told him that "it is the most important place archaeologically in your state" and suggested that Lilly buy the site in order to preserve it from the effects of continued farming and the encroachment of Evansville's population.[92]

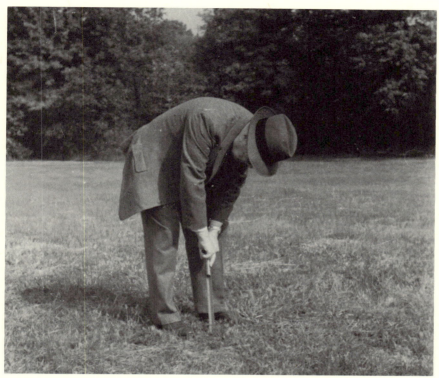

Eli Lilly taking soil samples at Mound C, Angel site, October 1959.

Glenn A. Black Laboratory of Archaeology

Lilly visited Angel Mounds again in 1935 and devoted several pages of his *Prehistoric Antiquities of Indiana* to describing the site, located on the Ohio, upriver from Evansville and just west of Newburgh. He noted the several large man-made mounds, particularly the central mound (Mound A), which he measured as 520 feet long at the base and 30 feet high, with a flat top that was 100 by 200 feet. He commented on potsherds, bones, chipped flints, human burials, and the high stockade that once protected the site from enemies. "What would we not give to reverse the film of prehistory to a view of the teeming life within this village, its boisterous play, sweat-producing work, revered ceremonies, bloody wars, and the general way of living?" There was no other site like this one in Indiana, yet no serious archaeological work had been undertaken. "Why do we sit idly by, letting these precious chances slip through our fingers?" It was time to act. "Here, baked in the glaring summer sun, frozen under winter snows, gradually wasting away under the plow and the harrow, is a site that the State of Indiana should rescue from oblivion, and so save to posterity another of our pre-Columbian heritages."[93]

Angel site was indeed worthy of preservation. But in the depths of the depression the state of Indiana was an unlikely candidate for assuming the responsibility. Nor were private contributors in the Evansville area forthcoming, despite the efforts at persuasion by Black and Lilly. As would happen so often when other means proved unavailable for a good cause, Lilly provided the necessary support. In 1938, acting again under cover of the Indiana Historical Society, he provided $68,000 of the $71,957 necessary to buy the 435-acre site. Black took primary charge of the project and in the spring of 1939 moved to a house on the site and began to supervise the newly arrived workers. Nearly all the men who did the surveying, digging, and cataloging at Angel site from the beginning in 1939 until work stopped in May 1942 were unemployed casualties of the depression, their wages paid by the Work Projects Administration (WPA).[94] Lilly and Black were staunch Republicans, vehemently opposed to Franklin D. Roosevelt's New Deal. But, after some initial reluctance, they decided that "we are crazy for not getting some of that easy money back that we are all paying out."[95]

In May 1939 Lilly made his first visit to Black's home at Angel site and returned again in September, writing Black, "When I go on W.P.A. will you give me a job?"[96] Though Lilly seldom if ever picked up a trowel or shovel, he was very closely involved with the work. He and Ruth often visited Glenn and Ida Black at their Newburgh home. And letters between Indianapolis and Evansville were detailed and frequent, with Black reporting each new discovery and the two men exchanging ideas and references to the literature and speculating on the cultural meaning of the particular artifact or burial. Both were particularly excited by the discovery in November 1940 of a fluorite figurine, carved in the likeness of an adult male. Lilly had special photographs made of their "Apollo a la Newburgh," as he called it. Their correspondence reached to the smallest detail, such as the question of repairing or replacing the office typewriter. Because Lilly's money was paying Black's salary and many other costs not covered by the WPA, Black carefully checked with him on expenditures. Black was very frugal and most resourceful in keeping costs reasonable, and Lilly always approved his requests, sometimes encouraging more spending.[97]

While Lilly derived large pleasure from Angel Mounds, he continued to seek ways to remove it from his and the Historical Society's responsibility. In 1941 he and Black approached Indiana University President Wells, who showed keen interest but could not offer financial support. As the depression waned, state aid seemed more promising. In 1941 Lilly lunched with Richard Lieber, the founder of Indiana's state park system, to encourage support for state purchase of the site and reconstruction of a prehistoric village. As the war wound down and a Republican returned to the governor's office, Lilly made a direct assault on the statehouse. In June 1945 he had dinner with Governor Ralph Gates and pushed hard for state purchase of Angel site.[98] As a result of Lilly's prodding Gates visited the site two weeks later, after which Black happily reported that "things do seem to be going the way we want them."[99]

For a short time they did. The state took title to the property in December 1946, but the conservation department, which was to administer it, failed to maintain and develop the site as promised. Indeed, in late 1945 Howard Peckham, the newly appointed director of the Society, telephoned Lilly to report that "the whole Conservation Commission has practically blown up, all the good men out and the politicians in full sway." The swing of Indiana's exceptionally sharp patronage ax had cut through the department, and the new party faithful—"the boys in the Claypool Hotel"—had received their rewards. Lilly forlornly concluded that they would have no choice but to try "to operate in a friendly fashion with the new banditti."[100]

The experience thereafter was "almost disastrous." Lilly and Black pushed for development of the site and construction of an interpretive center or museum, but without result. "No one [from state government] has ever visited the Mounds," Lilly grumbled in 1963, "in spite of hospitable invitations from time to time, and they have not at all fulfilled the agreement that the State has made." The state conservation department, Lilly wrote in his reminiscences, "was mainly interested in employing as many fish and game wardens as possible for political purposes."[101]

The shortcomings of a patronage-oriented state government did not prevent beneficial use of Angel site. The Society retained the right to continue digging and in 1945 agreed to join Indiana University in conducting a summer archaeological field school there under Black's direction. From 1945 to 1962 more than one hundred students spent a summer at the site, learning field techniques from Black and extending the work done by their WPA predecessors.[102]

Angel Mounds provided also the continuing point of contact between Lilly and Black. Their relationship began as student and patron, with the student doing all that was possible to please the patron. From the first Lilly

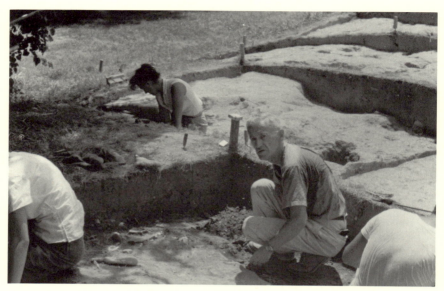

Glenn Black and students, Angel site, 1960.   *Glenn A. Black Laboratory of*
Archaeology

was very pleased. By the summer of 1932 he glowed, "Black is developing splendidly."[103] Not until late 1934 did Lilly change his form of address in correspondence from "Dear Mr. Black" to "Dear Glenn." And not until 1946, following a visit to Wawasee, did Black begin to use "Dear Eli" to open his many letters.[104] A year earlier Lilly had written one of his first direct statements of their friendship: "You know, I hope, that I love you like a brother—or more so."[105] Another oft-expressed relationship in their correspondence was father-son. Black's father died when he was a child; Lilly's two sons died in infancy. In the 1950s Black began to send father's day greetings. "You have been my 'father,' friend and councilor," he wrote in 1958. "More than anything else I have wanted to please you and give you no cause to regret that we ever took that first archaeological trip together in May 1931." Lilly replied, "Your fine 'father's day' letter touched me very much. . . . If I had a son I should wish him to have character and abilities equal to yours."[106]

The friendship with Black began with archaeology but expanded to include a wide range of shared interests. Black was a man of intense determination. His wiry frame and wavy hair conveyed accurately an image of single-minded dedication to a task. He was thorough and meticulous, honest and reliable, yet warm and caring, as his large popularity among Indiana University students indicated. He had a less formal side too. He made jewelry, built model race cars, listened to Dixieland jazz, and enjoyed photography. In the late 1950s he and Lilly proudly owned similar Ford Thunderbirds. Black dressed well, too, appearing quite dapper when not in the field. Lilly admired his abilities as a jack-of-all-trades and general handyman. He could fix things. He liked gadgets and often advised Lilly on setting up a new hi-fi system or working a new camera. And he encouraged Lilly's interest in woodworking. Black was also careful not to take advantage of Lilly's generosity and was protective of his privacy. He was especially reluctant to serve as a go-between by carrying requests from others for Lilly's assistance. [107]

Increasingly important were the trips the two couples enjoyed together. In 1949 they took a three-week trip on the *Delta Queen* steamboat down the Ohio and Mississippi, and in the 1950s they made excursions to Colonial Williamsburg, the Smoky Mountains, and the Ohio Mounds. In 1963 Black carefully planned a long automobile trip to the American West: their experiences ranged from painting the fence, made famous by Mark Twain and his character Tom Sawyer, in Hannibal, Missouri, to standing in awe at the prehistoric sites in Mesa Verde. By this time Lilly was amusing himself and his friends by writing poetry. After the Southwest trip he sent a three-page poem to the Blacks with stanzas such as:

> We attained the zenith of our trip
> As we camped on Mesa Verde's grand lip
> We viewed by the hour
> Pueblo and tower
> Not a stone did we ever skip[108]

Closer to home were the more routine diversions. The Blacks and Lillys usually attended a performance of the Metropolitan Opera when it made its annual tour to Bloomington. And they always attended together the spring workshops of the Indiana Historical Society, with Black routinely making the reservations. The Blacks usually visited at Wawasee in the summer; and the Lillys often visited at the Black home, which provided Lilly a chance to get away from the responsibilities of Indianapolis. Typical was a letter he wrote from his office in early 1946: "Have to go to that pestiferous Washington this afternoon. Would much rather come to Evansville." The house at Angel site was small and simple, but Ida was an excellent

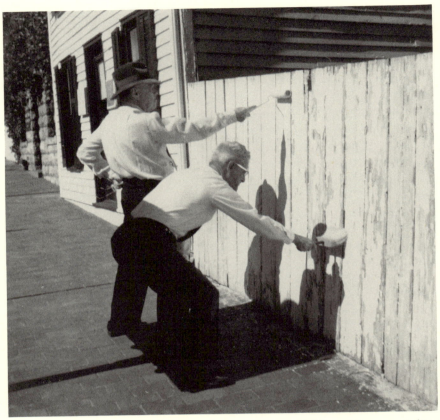

Eli Lilly and Glenn Black "painting" Tom
Sawyer's fence in Hannibal, Missouri, 1963.   *Eli Lilly and Company Archives*

hostess and enjoyed serving well-prepared meals with beautiful china and
silver. Lilly made her a fancy wooden back for her piano so she could sit
facing her guests while playing. Ruth and Ida usually remained in the
house while Eli and Glenn tramped over Angel site, or drove to a nearby
archaeological spot, or just sat and talked.[109]

Glenn Black died of a heart attack on 2 September 1964. A saddened
Lilly wrote Black's brother: "Glenn was almost as close to me as a son could
possibly have been."[110] Grief did not prevent action, however. At the conclusion of the funeral service, Lilly took charge of an impromptu gathering,
recording in his pocket notebook the things that needed to be done at
Angel site. Working closely with Black's secretary, he supervised the many

chores that Black's untimely death had created. One responsibility was to make sure that Ida had no financial problems by setting up a trust for her. Ida never recovered from the loss of her husband, however, and her personal difficulties and her request for even more money caused Eli and Ruth much distress as the long friendship withered.[111]

One major chore that remained was Black's report on Angel site. He had begun writing in 1962 and was nearly finished at his death. With Lilly's encouragement and financial support and some hard work by Black's former student, James H. Kellar, and by editor Gayle Thornbrough, the book was completed. The Indiana Historical Society published it in two handsome volumes in 1967. *Angel Site: An Archaeological, Historical, and Ethnological Study* was Lilly's and the Society's memorial tribute to Black.[112]

Another tribute came in the Glenn A. Black Laboratory of Archaeology on the Indiana University campus in Bloomington. Lilly's collection of prehistoric artifacts had remained in his Sunset Lane home since the early 1930s. Though he had given them to the Indiana Historical Society there was no place to put them. As early as 1941 he had discussed with President Wells the possibility of a museum at Indiana University. Black's death prompted Lilly to act. The Lilly Endowment provided most of the funding for construction of an impressive building on the Bloomington campus, although the state, through Governor Roger D. Branigin, made an important last-minute contribution of $218,600. The new structure housed Lilly's archaeology collection of artifacts and books, Black's Angel site materials and library, and other collections as well as display, office, library, and work spaces for archaeological teaching and research. Lilly insisted the building be named for Black and not him and proudly attended the dedication on 21 April 1971.[113]

The Black Laboratory retained a close tie with the Indiana Historical Society, continuing cooperative efforts in study of the state's prehistory. The laboratory received an important boost for this work in 1972, when Ida Black died and left most of her estate, in excess of $1,000,000, to the institution.[114] Reminded of distant quarrels after Jimmy Griffin visited him at Sunset Lane in 1972 and expressed an interest in participating in the archaeology program in Bloomington, Lilly wrote Kellar, the director of the laboratory: "Mrs. Black didn't want him to be connected with the laboratory. Did she make this legal in her will or not?"[115] Griffin never came.

One of the side benefits of the Black Laboratory was Lilly's developing friendship with its first director, James H. Kellar. Lilly counted on him to

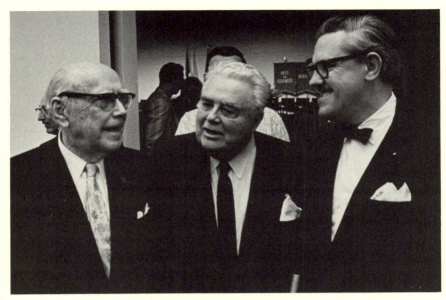

Eli Lilly, Herman B Wells, and Roll McLaughlin   *Roll McLaughlin*
at dedication of Glenn A. Black Laboratory of
Archaeology, Indiana University, April 1971.

keep informed of archaeological doings. In setting up a lunch meeting,
Lilly wrote Kellar: "I have nothing really serious in mind, only a desire to
occasionally meet with you and keep a little in touch with what is going
on."[116]

Lilly met often with Kellar to plan for change at Angel site. The long-
anticipated development from the state never materialized. But in 1968,
when Governor Branigin, whom Lilly very much liked, provided state
funds to complete the Black Laboratory, Lilly felt obliged "to get a little
even with the Governor." He gave, largely through the Lilly Endowment,
$750,000 to erect an interpretive center and to reconstruct several build-
ings at Angel site.[117] Lilly watched closely over the details of preparing the
site for visitors, suggesting, for example, that electricity be provided by
burying waterproof lines along the footpaths. When he learned that the
mayor of Evansville had proposed that the city lease the western two-thirds
of the site for a park and golf course, Lilly exploded, first in a telephone
call to his old friend, John G. Rauch, Sr., who was chairman of the Historical Society's Board of Trustees and then in a letter to Rauch. Lilly and
Black "had bled fighting the Pocket Politicians for thirty years," he wrote,

"and after the splendid help of Governor Branigin and Chancellor Wells had saved the day, I had regarded the property beyond the reach of the politicians." As for the mayor's veiled threat of political action unless the Society cooperated, "if our affairs are to be controlled by fear of political reprisals, I will quietly bow out from giving any further time or support to the Historical Society. . . . I will be firm in having nothing to do with fearing Pocket Politicians." Lilly's stand was sufficient to deter any further thought to the park and golf course. The site was developed as he and Black had long hoped, with an interpretive center and with reconstructed houses, a stockade, and a temple. The octogenarian spoke at the dedication, an unseasonably cold day in October 1972, and charmed the audience by offering to send free Lilly medication to anyone who caught cold.[118]

More than four decades of experience in archaeology left many happy memories for Eli Lilly. Over a long life he developed many other interests, ranging from Chinese art to historic preservation. And always there were the demands of Eli Lilly and Company, which were particularly heavy during the 1930s and 1940s. Yet Lilly determinedly made time to pursue his archaeological interests. Attracted to the intellectual challenge and to the company of fellow archaeologists, this amateur who never made a dollar doing archaeology became a scholar and a full participant in what Griffin called "an excellent research journey for all of us."[119] Lilly's legacy to the discipline included Angel Mounds, the Glenn A. Black Laboratory, and his publications. And less concrete but perhaps equally important, his legacy included financial and moral support for a generation of archaeologists who brought their field to professional maturity.

Chapter 7

The Wider Horizons of History
and Historic Preservation

Ely Lilly's initial interest in the past took form in his attraction to archaeology. Although study of the prehistoric past remained appealing to him
throughout his life, he developed, especially in the 1950s and 1960s, interests in the more recent past. Like his archaeological quests, these historical
pursuits focused largely on Indiana subjects.

The major institutional base for Lilly's fascination with the past was
the Indiana Historical Society, founded on the frontier in 1830, only fourteen years after statehood. The first decades were bumpy. Not until 1886
did the Society begin to hold regular annual meetings, and not until the
1920s did the organization acquire professional leadership. Sparked by the
statehood centennial celebration in 1916, membership grew to over one
thousand by the early 1920s. A major point in transition came in 1924,
when Christopher B. Coleman was elected secretary of the Society. Coleman was a professional historian, a Ph.D. holder from Columbia University,
a skilled administrator, and a genial and effective advocate of history. As
his successors would do until 1976, Coleman served simultaneously as
secretary of the Indiana Historical Society, a private institution, and as
director of the Indiana Historical Bureau, a state agency. The cigar-puffing
historian was a major force in expanding publications, including the *Indiana Magazine of History*, in building the library collections, and in attracting scholarly and popular interest in the past. Although Coleman widened
the scope and raised the quality of the Society's programs, the organization
retained some of its aura of a gentlemen's club for history buffs and old-
line Indianapolis families. The Society did not publicly solicit new members
because, Coleman explained, members wanted "to keep the Society representative of the very best citizenship of the state."[1]

It was the Indiana Historical Society that Eli Lilly bumped against
when he set out in 1929 to explore Indian sites as summer entertainment

for his daughter. Lilly came to like and respect Coleman, who encouraged the businessman's new interest in the past. Lilly soon became a major contributor to the Society. As noted in the previous chapter, he paid the salaries and expenses of Glenn Black and other Society archaeological workers. He donated his artifact collection to the Society in 1933, funded a new *Prehistory Research Series*, begun in 1937, and paid the printing costs of special archaeology publications.

Lilly's attraction to archaeology led him to the Society, but he soon expanded his commitments to the institution. In 1932 he agreed to serve as its president, an office he held until 1947. He remained until his death a member of the executive committee and the board of trustees. These were not honorary positions. Lilly worked hard, and he exercised his leadership as his concern for studying the past grew.

One of his major interests was book publication. Many of the Society's books were the result of his moral support to the author and his financial support to the printer. In addition to the archaeology publications and Lilly's own writing, the Society books he sponsored included *The Journals and Indian Paintings of George Winter* (1948); *Indiana Houses of the Nineteenth Century* (1962), by Wilbur D. Peat; *The House of the Singing Winds: The Life and Work of T. C. Steele* (1966), by Selma N. Steele, Theodore L. Steele, and Wilbur D. Peat; and *Sketches of Lake Wawasee* (1967), by Scott Edgell. The most well known Lilly-sponsored book was R. Carlyle Buley's *The Old Northwest: Pioneer Period, 1815-1840* (2 vols., 1950). The Indiana University historian had tried for five years to find a publisher before Lilly provided the necessary financial support. The investment brought a large return, for Buley's book won the Pulitzer Prize in 1951 and remains today as an outstanding example of the historian's craft.[2] Lilly and his colleagues on the Society's executive committee were proud of their support of serious scholarship and determined that the Society would continue such support.[3] But they found room also for amateurs and friends writing local history. When Charlotte Cathcart, who had been a childhood neighbor, told Lilly that she was compiling a memoir of Indianapolis, he wrote that if she submitted the work to the Society "I shall be glad to grubstake the venture." "Pink" Cathcart's delightful reminiscences appeared in print in 1965 as *Indianapolis from Our Old Corner*. Lilly paid the $12,100 printing bill.[4]

As president of the Indiana Historical Society Lilly attended to a variety of matters affecting the institution. One of his first tasks was to protect Coleman's tenure as secretary. The Democratic election sweep of 1932 had brought to the governor's office a very ambitious politician. Paul

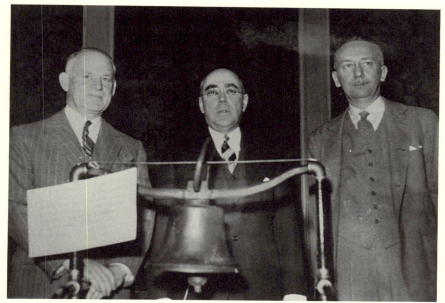

Indiana Historical Society leaders, December 1941, left to right, Cornelius O'Brien, Eli Lilly, John G. Rauch, Sr.

Indianapolis Star

V. McNutt was determined to replace Republicans with Democrats and to collect from nearly all state workers 2 percent of their paychecks for the party coffers. Because Coleman was head of a state agency, the Indiana Historical Bureau, as well as the Society, he was threatened by McNutt's political machine. The peril came not because of party affiliation—Coleman was a Democrat—but because of his principled refusal to pay collectors from McNutt's 2 percent club. Accompanied by Evans Woollen, Lilly's predecessor as Society president and a prominent Indianapolis banker and Democrat, Lilly called on McNutt. The powerful governor chose not to fight.[5]

Lilly also endeavored in the 1930s to produce larger returns on the Society's small endowment. As a member of the finance committee he worked out a strategy of investment in stocks rather than bonds, a shift that resulted in larger long-term growth. He retained a voice in the Society's investment practices for the next several decades.[6]

One of Lilly's most enduring frustrations at the Society was the long fight over publication of the diary of Calvin Fletcher. Fletcher was among the first and most prominent citizens of Indianapolis. The diary he kept from 1820 to 1866 recorded daily events, from births and cabin raisings to bank failures in the age of Andrew Jackson and Copperhead threats during the Civil War. The document is perhaps the most important historical source for the city's early history and one of the most interesting diaries penned by a nonliterary man of only local prominence. Lilly recognized its historical importance. He was also attracted to Fletcher's outlook on life—his strong Yankee character, his sense of duty and discipline, and his wide range of interests. Lilly soon became the dominant force in pushing for publication of the diary.[7]

Calvin Fletcher's granddaughter, Laura Fletcher Hodges, stipulated in her will that her estate should publish the diary. Delay and complication followed her death in 1923 as the family and the Union Trust Company refused to deliver on what Lilly and the Society thought to be the commitment of the bequest.[8] In 1940 the Society began to move on its own accord. Lilly chaired a special Fletcher diary committee, joined by Coleman and by John G. Rauch, Sr., a member of the Society's executive committee and Lilly's friend and personal attorney. They made plans to print the diary in six volumes, though some parts they thought should be left unpublished because they were repetitious, unimportant, "and in some cases unjustifiably derogatory to ancestors of present-day citizens."[9] Lilly twice had lunch with Fletcher Hodges, the great-grandson of the diarist. Lilly and Rauch also discussed the issue with the head of the Union Trust Company. Lilly indicated the Society's willingness to bear part of the publication costs, but he wanted financial support also from the estate of Laura Fletcher Hodges and full legal title to the diary. Fletcher Hodges and the trust company refused these compromise offers, arguing that the indefinite nature of the bequest made it impossible to execute and also expressing fears that the diary contained matter that was highly libelous. After prolonged negotiation, Lilly and the unanimous executive committee, backed by Governor Henry F. Schricker, decided to sue.[10] The controversy greatly pained Lilly, who abhorred even good publicity. An old family friend wrote him advising against the suit and telling him what he surely knew—that Indianapolis gossips were talking about Lilly and the Society and that the talk was not good. Lilly explained to his informant that he had tried hard to avoid the suit, especially because the Lilly and Hodges families had been friends for three generations, but that every offer of compromise had been rebuffed.[11]

The legal suit was not successful. The Marion County Probate Court decided against the Society in early 1947; the Appellate Court reversed

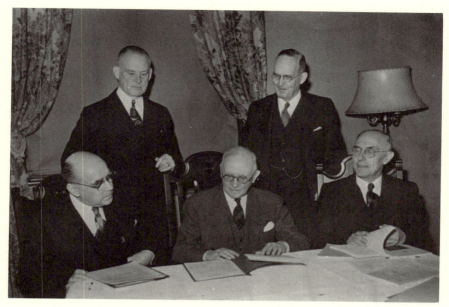

Members of the Indiana Historical Society executive committee at the annual conference, 1943; seated, left to right, Eli Lilly, Lee Burns, Albert J. Kohlmeier; standing, Cornelius O'Brien, Christopher B. Coleman.

Indianapolis Star

this ruling, holding that the trustees of the estate were obligated to publish the diary; and finally, in mid-1949, the Indiana Supreme Court decided that publication could not be forced. An unhappy Lilly remained convinced that the Society had the better case: "while it was a legal victory for [Hodges]," he wrote, "it certainly was not a moral victory." Lawyer Rauch was more direct. "Stink is the proper word!" he wrote Lilly, for this final ruling.[12]

Lilly retreated but did not surrender. Two decades later he wrote Gayle Thornbrough, newly appointed director of Society publications: "Just between us girls . . . what would you think of the Society gradually editing the Calvin Fletcher diary."[13] Lilly helped secure ownership of the diary from the heirs of the estate, and he provided the financial support necessary for the massive editorial undertaking. The first volume, dedicated to him, appeared in 1972, the ninth and last in 1983. The volumes totaled 4,657 printed pages, with unusually helpful explanatory notes and indexes prepared by Society editors Thornbrough, Dorothy L. Riker, and Paula Corpuz. The editors expurgated none of Fletcher's entries. Reviewers recognized immediately the diary's importance to scholarship. "It does not," one wrote, "seem to have any rival in its class."[14]

One of Lilly's most important achievements as president was finding a replacement for Coleman. Coleman's sudden death in June 1944 sent Lilly scampering in search of a new secretary. His choice among the candidates soon fell on Howard Peckham. The thirty-four-year-old Peckham was curator of manuscripts at the University of Michigan's William L. Clements Library of American History. He was energetic and filled with ideas about history. He was not a Hoosier, however, and Lilly had to call on Governor Schricker to discuss appointment of a Society secretary who would also hold state office as director of the Bureau. In joyfully telling a friend that "we have finally landed Peckham," Lilly confided that "the Governor had looked down his nose for some time because he was not from Indiana, but the Governor is a good sport, [and] finally gave up."[15]

It was good for the Society and for Lilly that Governor Schricker rose above his Hoosier provincialism. Peckham was a dynamic and productive secretary, and he soon eased the Society away from its club-like recluseness. He began to campaign actively for new members, taking the unprecedented step of setting up a membership booth at the State Fair. Peckham endeavored to make history more accessible and meaningful, even to the point of seeking publicity through newspapers and radio. He initiated weekend history workshops held in the spring at one of the state parks. To attract young people he encouraged high school history clubs. Lilly strongly backed Peckham in these new programs. A year after his arrival Lilly proposed that the Society add $200 a month to Peckham's salary, the money to be provided by the Lilly Endowment. On several occasions Lilly provided extra funds for Society programs in response to requests from Peckham. As with Glenn Black, however, Peckham was not extravagant in requesting or spending Lilly's money.[16]

Peckham became important to Lilly not only as head of the Society but also as a lifelong friend. Lilly welcomed Peckham to Indianapolis with a luncheon at the Columbia Club, and he and Ruth soon called on Howard and Dorothy Peckham. The young couple were much impressed by the Lillys' lack of social pretense and by their ability to make the newcomers feel welcome and at home in Indianapolis. The two couples eventually began to visit and to travel together, continuing after 1953 when Howard Peckham decided to accept the directorship of the Clements Library, where he would have more time for his own historical writing. Signifying their close friendship, the Lillys invited the Peckhams to Lake Wawasee every summer to stay in one of the houses on the Lilly property. There they would sail and read and talk. Howard, like Eli, did much of his writing at Wawasee. The Peckhams and the Lillys also traveled together several times to the Williamsburg antique show, where they could combine their interest in history with an appreciation for fine craftsmanship and especially the woodworking hobby that the two men shared.[17]

Howard Peckham was Eli Lilly's most important historian friend and advisor. The younger man became a distinguished historian, the author of many scholarly books. The two often discussed their work. At one point, in 1961, when Lilly was between writing projects, Peckham sent him a list of possible topics, the result of "ruminating about a new research project to keep you from becoming a juvenile delinquent." The relationship grew warmly personal, eventually matched only by Lilly's friendship with Glenn Black. Peckham was one of the few younger people to address Lilly as "Eli" rather than "Mr. Lilly." And as with Black there developed also a warm paternalism. In giving Lilly a copy of a book by Dwight Eisenhower, whom he knew Lilly much admired, Peckham inscribed it: "For Eli, with warm regards on Father's Day, 1967."[18]

Lilly's relationship with Peckham's successor was not so close. A native-born Hoosier, Hubert Hawkins had completed course work but not a dissertation for a Ph.D degree at the University of Pennsylvania and was teaching history at Butler University when Peckham decided to leave Indiana. Lilly was at Wawasee when the candidates were interviewed in mid-1953, but Peckham reported the strong support for Hawkins. The new secretary of the Society and head of the Bureau was an outgoing and convivial man, and he set out energetically to recruit new members. Hawkins enjoyed speaking to local history groups, schoolchildren, and service clubs and spent much time traveling the state. He made many friends for the Society and attracted new members.[19] Lilly came to regret, however, that, unlike Peckham, Hawkins was no scholar. Nor was he a good administrator, Lilly eventually concluded. In the margin of a copy of Hawkins's report of his activities in 1963, Lilly scribbled his terse judgments. Next to the secretary's brief statement about his research, Lilly commented, "Never writes." In the margin of the larger section reporting talks and field trips Lilly wrote, "Over done?" And at the beginning of the report he scribbled, "Starts & does not finish."[20] Lilly himself was a meticulous administrator, particularly in replying promptly to his correspondents. He became especially impatient with Hawkins when a simple request for information brought no response, necessitating a second request from Lilly.[21] When a fellow Society trustee proposed a large raise for Hawkins, Lilly hesitated, writing another trustee that Hawkins "has built up a large membership, [but] as an administrator he leaves much to be desired."[22]

Lilly maintained a polite relationship with Hawkins, and the two men conferred often about Society business, but Lilly did not rely solely on Hawkins for information or advice. Peckham continued to be his confidant about historical matters. A critical period of decision making for Lilly and the Society came in the late 1960s.

An increasingly pressing problem was space. As the Society added books and manuscripts to its library, which was housed along with Society offices in the Indiana State Library and Historical Building on Senate Avenue, quarters became more crowded. Hawkins clearly recognized the problem and worked to solve it. He began in the early 1960s to urge construction of a new building, not only to solve the problems of space but also to separate the Society physically from the State Library and the Bureau and thereby give it a more distinct identity. In 1966 Lilly, Hawkins, and three other members of the Society's Planning and Development Committee recommended raising an endowment of $2.5 million to be used in part for a new and separate building. Lilly soon expressed thoughts different from the committee's, however. He questioned the wisdom of locating the Society's library, editorial, and administrative work at a distance from the State Library. The collections of the two libraries had been developed so as to be complementary, and the staffs of the Bureau, Society, and State Library all worked together effectively in one building. Additionally, Lilly feared that a separate building would be more expensive to maintain and would drain money from library and publications programs. Other trustees, including Lilly's good friend, Governor Roger D. Branigin, came to share this view.[23]

In thinking about the problem of space Lilly began also to think about the total needs and purposes of the Society. One fact was clear. The Society was operating on a very small budget so that niggling and large-scale financial problems were omnipresent. Low membership dues and an anemic endowment were barriers to planning and development. The Society library was in particular need of help, with a small staff and a large backlog of books and manuscripts stacked about waiting to be processed and cataloged. The disorder in the library very much bothered Lilly. The publication program was of high quality, but with a small budget there could be no long-term planning, and worthy projects had to be turned away. Many of

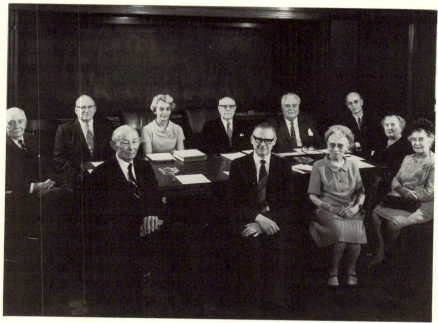

Indiana Historical Society trustees and staff, 1969: clockwise from left, John G. Rauch, Sr., John F. Wilhelm, Gayle Thornbrough, Eli Lilly, Herman B Wells, Hubert Hawkins, Mrs. George W. Blair, Elsie Sweeney, Mrs. John Quincy Adams, David V. Burns, William E. Wilson.

Eli Lilly and Company Archives

the Society's major programs and publications had resulted only because of Lilly's periodic financial support, often provided through the Lilly Endowment as well as his personal resources. In the spring of 1968 Lilly solved the immediate financial problem with one stroke by deeding to the Society 20,000 shares of Eli Lilly and Company stock, with a value of $2.2 million. As with most of his philanthropy, no publicity accompanied the gift, and very few people knew about it.[24]

Lilly's support for history and the Indiana Historical Society did not end with financial contributions. With his gift in 1968 came hard thinking about the institution's future. As a step toward broader and more efficient work in state and local history, Lilly prepared a detailed list of historical activities and programs in the state and indicated the person or institution responsible for each. He and Peckham talked over the subject at Wawasee that summer and decided that an outside evaluation of the Society was needed. Just as Lilly had brought Harrington Emerson, Fritz Roethlisberger, and other outside experts to the pharmaceutical company, he now decided that a historical expert should be brought in to advise the Society. On Peckham's recommendation, Lilly selected William T. Alderson, then head of the American Association for State and Local History. Lilly asked his friend John Rauch, who was then chairman of the Society's Board of Trustees, to write Alderson and invite him to Indianapolis. Rauch, though on vacation, acted immediately, and Alderson agreed to come to Indianapolis in September. Only after these arrangements were made did Rauch inform Hawkins of the forthcoming visit.[25]

Alderson visited the Society in September 1968 and soon submitted a generally laudatory thirty-five-page report. Lilly read his copy carefully, underlining important passages. He marked Alderson's conclusion that adequate space was the most critical problem facing the Society, with a particular need for "an improvement of housing conditions for the Society library." Alderson suggested that the recent Lilly gift should be used for programs and not on a new building, however. He did not report on the difficult question of how a new building should be funded or where it should be located, although he suggested that "there is no pressing necessity for the Society to be immediately adjacent to the State Library."[26]

Lilly remained adamantly opposed to "splitting off from the Indiana State Library."[27] Indiana University Chancellor Herman B Wells and others joined in this conclusion, but the Society's attempts to persuade the legislature to fund an expansion of the state library building failed. In 1973, once again, Lilly came forward, this time with a gift of $1 million. He suggested that this contribution be combined with another $1 million from the Society endowment (which, of course, was part of Lilly's gift of 1968) to construct a new building attached to the State Library and Historical Building. The state agreed to this offer, adding support to the construction costs and accepting responsibility for maintenance. The dedication ceremony occurred in October 1976, in time for Lilly to witness the physical expansion of the institution he so loved.[28]

These years of large gifts and building expansion also brought personnel changes at the Society. Lilly's first archaeology publication had given him a large respect for the talents of a good editor. Gayle Thornbrough had those talents in abundance. She joined the Society as the first full-time employee in 1937. One of her initial tasks was editing the *Prehistory Research Series*. In most of the later Society publications with which Lilly was involved,

Thornbrough served as editor. He soon developed a high regard for her character and dedication and was very disappointed when in 1967 she decided to leave for a position at the Library of Congress. Lilly wanted her back at the Society and soon proposed a job package that created a combined position of director of publications and of the library. He was delighted when in 1968 Thornbrough agreed to return to the Society to occupy the new position, where she reported directly to the Board of Trustees rather than Hawkins. It was at this time also that Lilly made his gift of $2.2 million to the Society. With Lilly's financial support and moral backing and with the encouragement of the Alderson report, Thornbrough brought order to the library and vigor to the publications program, most notably in the production of the Fletcher diaries. Her responsibilities expanded further just as the new Society building was nearing completion. In 1975 Hawkins, his health declining, announced his resignation, and the trustees selected Thornbrough to replace him. With new determination and financial strength, the trustees decided also to separate the job from the Bureau. Thornbrough was the first secretary able to devote full-time responsibility to the Society.[29]

A new full-time executive secretary, the new building, and the addition of new staff in the 1970s marked the most important changes in the institution's history. Lilly's money and guiding hand were at the base of all these changes. In the nearly half century of his association with the institution it had evolved from a small club of gentlemen historians to one of the largest and most effective state historical societies in the nation. Lilly's distaste for public recognition meant that few outside the executive committee knew of his role in this transition. When the Lilly name appeared several times in one of Peckham's first reports at the Society's annual meeting, Lilly gently reproached his young associate: "I was very much embarrassed to have such frequent mention made of the Lilly Endowment," he wrote. Accounts with the Lilly name attached should be changed to be called "gifts from members, or something of that sort." In other gifts, as that to construct the new building, he insisted that "there be no publicity."[30]

Reluctant for publicity, Lilly was also generally careful not to force his will on his Society colleagues. Certainly his voice was the most powerful one on the executive committee, doubtless from the beginning of his service until his death. When he chose to exercise that voice it was effective, as in the choice of a successor to Glenn Black as Society archaeologist. Hawkins and some trustees had a candidate. But Black before his death had expressed to Lilly major reservations about the man. Lilly felt obliged to honor Black's judgment and insisted that the Society trustees support him. They did, and they eventually presented a united front, for, as Hawkins wrote, "I think we are obliged to protect Mr. L in such a situation."[31] Lilly's voice also was heard in publication decisions. As he wrote one of his archaeology friends about publication of that friend's manuscript, "I am sure your and my wishes in the matter will be followed."[32] The voice could be powerful, but it was seldom loud. He encouraged discussion at executive committee meetings and sought consensus. Literally and figuratively he spoke softly.[33]

The Indiana Historical Society was one of Lilly's most treasured institutions. The level of his long-term financial support and the terms of his will (see chapter 10) indicated his intensity of commitment. But even more revealing was his personal commitment of time and energy. He thought seriously about the kind of institution he wanted it to be, particularly with the transition he initiated in 1968. He faithfully attended executive committee meetings, even in the busy days of World War II. He seldom missed a spring workshop, where he and Ruth would join the Blacks, the Peckhams, and others for a weekend of history. In the inn at McCormick's Creek or Spring Mill State Park with his history friends, he was most comfortable. There is every reason to believe his comment to Peckham that "my contacts with the Indiana Historical Society have been among the pleasantest that I have had in this lower mundane institute."[34]

Lilly's interest in the past extended to many hours of reading and writing as well as service to the Indiana Historical Society. He read with purpose and not simply for diversion. In the 1930s and 1940s he directed his reading and writing about the past largely to prehistoric archaeology. In the 1950s and 1960s his interests broadened. He bought large numbers of books, filling the shelves of his comfortable library in his home on Sunset Lane. When he made a rough inventory in 1973 he counted 1,800 volumes in the first floor library, 2,000 in the third floor ballroom, and another 250 at his home on Lake Wawasee. Unlike his brother, who became one of the nation's major rare book collectors, Lilly acquired books solely

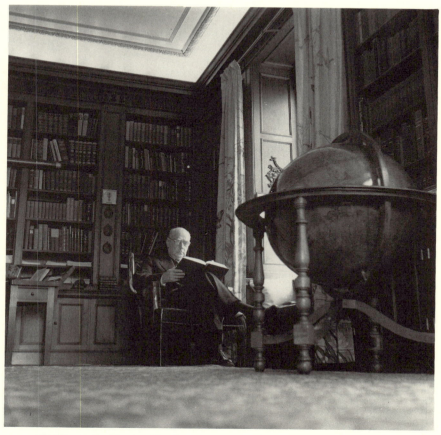

Eli Lilly in the library of his home on Sunset Lane, 1957.

Eli Lilly and Company Archives

to read, often underlining important sentences and scribbling comments in the margins.[35]

Sometimes Lilly made notes of his reading on five-by-eight cards. A collection of his note cards from the late 1940s, soon after he left the presidency of the pharmaceutical company, includes his jottings from books by T. S. Eliot, Arnold Toynbee, and Margaret Mead. Sometime in the 1950s he began to collect ideas, aphorisms, and words he found especially appealing and to record them in a notebook he called his "Shining Phrase Book." His entries included quotations from the writings of Edward Gibbon, John

Dos Passos, George Bernard Shaw, Anthony Trollope, Irving Stone, Lawrence Durrell, and Moss Hart. He delighted in recording such words and phrases as "clogged with learning," "gossip distilled from teapots," "snobocracy," and "a torch among tapers." As the notebook grew in size, Lilly made an index so that he could find specific quotations. Doubtless the project served primarily to record and fuel his simple delight in words and ideas, but the "Shining Phrase Book" also had a more utilitarian purpose. He drew entries from it for use in his own writings and speeches, testimony to his conscientious and continuing attention to building his vocabulary and improving his writing.[36] Lilly's attention to writing bore fruit, as a reading of any of his books demonstrates. In comparing Lilly with James Whitcomb Riley, Indiana University English Professor William E. Wilson concluded that "Riley is probably the only poet who ever became a millionaire by writing verse; Lilly is one of the very few millionaires who ever became a writer with a genuine literary style."[37]

In the 1950s Lilly's writing focused on historical subjects meaningful in his own life—Lake Wawasee, Indianapolis, and his church. With *Walam Olum* he finished his major archaeology publication and turned his attention to Christ Church, the Episcopal church on the Circle in downtown Indianapolis. He began work on the church history in 1951, taking up research in his usual thorough manner. He initiated a correspondence with the Church Historical Society (later the Historical Society of the Episcopal Church) that led to other sources of help. He hired a research assistant, Margaret M. Way, who spent months working through Indianapolis newspapers. He also employed a young historian (Thomas Vaughan) to copy the Jackson Kemper diary and letters at the State Historical Society of Wisconsin. Lilly himself dug in other sources. He made many notes from the Calvin Fletcher diary and used these references often in the book to give context to the early social and religious history of Indianapolis. He carried out an extensive analysis of membership, baptism, and confirmation trends at Christ Church, using statistical data he gathered and plotted on graphs to extract generalizations and larger meanings about demographic change in the congregation. With an accumulation of nearly six thousand note cards, he labored over the writing, working at Sunset Lane and at Wawasee. He finished his first draft in the summer of 1954. During the next two years he revised the manuscript, checked facts, and carefully watched over the copy editing.[38]

Eli Lilly's *History of the Little Church on the Circle: Christ Church Parish Indianapolis 1837-1955* appeared in 1957. Published by the church, the book was handsomely produced by Lilly's favorite printer, R. R. Donnelley & Sons. The dedication was to "R.A.L. and the Christ Church Family." This was Ruth Lilly's only mention in the book. Eli Lilly's name had only one index entry. He did make a few references to his father, who had served as a vestryman in the early twentieth century, but he often went out of his way to avoid mentioning the family and particularly his own role in the church. The fact that he served as a vestryman from 1927 to 1953 was ascertainable only from the list of vestrymen in the appendix. And while contributions of $500 and $1,000 merited Lilly's notice and praise, he gave only scant attention to the most important financial contribution in the church's history—an anonymous gift of $1 million in 1953, which, of course, came from Lilly.[39]

Lilly's modesty about his own role did not hide his presence in the narrative of Christ Church's past. His delight in words and humor appeared often in *The History of the Little Church on the Circle*. He wrote of a Christmas Eve celebration in Indianapolis in 1840, when "a large assembly of bad boys in an eruption of disorderly conduct," built a roaring bonfire in the middle of the main street: "Like the illumination, alas, many of the celebrants were probably lit up equally with spirits!" Evidence of attention to writing abounds throughout the book. In setting the scene for troubles in the 1870s, he began a paragraph: "During the winter when chill blasts of wind lashed around the Circle and the sky was often dove color with unshed snow, and many desired 'to go into a bottle, well corked and sealed' until spring, the new rector and vestry were tormented by many problems." He referred several times to Stephen Foster's songs, the songs he and his father so loved. And there were references to his distant heroes from Greek literature and his more immediate heroes: the Indianapolis banker Calvin Fletcher and the missionary bishop Jackson Kemper, both of whose diaries he used extensively.[40]

Lilly's presence in his history of Christ Church included also an interpretive framework for the book. Many church histories plod woodenly though the past, as their authors chronicle names and dates and assert constant progress and harmony in the congregation's godlike endeavors. Lilly's sense of history and scholarship resulted in a very different book. In addition to celebrating the achievements of Christ Church, he dwelt carefully on controversy and conflict, on disappointment and failure, on "those unfortunate misunderstandings that beset human flesh." And he paid particular attention to leadership. "The great lesson that has been learned in this study," he wrote in the preface, "is the *paramount importance of leadership!*" The church must attract rectors who are "men of enthusiasm, ability, and spiritual strength." There had been eighteen rectors in the church's history, but, he concluded, "only five of them have inspired an upsurge in the life and vitality of the Church." Lilly included the current rector, John P. Craine, among those five outstanding leaders. Craine's appointment had engendered great conflict in 1950, with "crosscurrents of misunderstanding running in several directions." Though Lilly did not admit this purpose, it is nearly certain that he saw his history as a calming influence not only on the controversy over Craine's appointment but also on the controversies to come. His prescription for his church was to recognize the hard fact of controversy in the past and to understand the importance both of careful selection of rectors and of dedicated service by vestrymen and other leaders. In the 1960s, as chapter 9 indicates, Lilly would have occasion to reflect on this goal as he stood at the center of the most bitter public controversy of his life and in the life of his parish.[41]

Lilly's next project after the Christ Church history was a collection of "little historical tales" about Lake Wawasee.[42] Reflecting his strong ties to the lake where his grandfather had built the family cottage in 1887, *Early Wawasee Days* was indeed a labor of love. Lilly worked through local newspapers and other written records, but his major sources were interviews with older residents and his own memory and experiences, sailing every square foot of the lake and walking the hills, points, and islands. He described the physical features of Wawasee but concentrated on the people—the Indians and first settlers and the fishermen, guides, hotelkeepers, sailors, and vacationing families. His sketches ranged from modes of travel to the lake and the variety of sailing races to "The Burning of Bob Epert's Barn" and "The Abduction of Laura Sargent," all told in sprightly prose sprinkled with humor, affection, and shining phrases.[43]

Lilly's *Early Wawasee Days* encouraged others, particularly Scott Edgell, who had been born on Wawasee's Buttermilk Point. Edgell and Lilly began a correspondence, exchanging memories. Lilly not only encouraged Edgell to write down his sketches for publication but actively assisted in editing and rewriting, even adding some gems from his shining phrases collection. When the manuscript was completed, Lilly took it to the Indiana Historical Society, which published it in 1967 under the title *Sketches of Lake Wawasee*.[44]

As he finished his own Wawasee book, Lilly began a more serious project, to edit the Indianapolis diary and letters of Heinrich Schliemann, famous as the discoverer of the site of ancient Troy. Lilly's interest in Greek myth and history began in childhood. His most vivid impression from his early schooling was reading a little book titled *Tales of Troy*, a book that caused young Lilly and his schoolmates to refight the Trojan War as they walked home. Much later, when he built the house on Sunset Lane, Lilly furnished the master bedroom in classical Greek style.[45]

Perhaps as attractive to Lilly as Greek history and myth was the romance of Heinrich Schliemann's life. The German-born merchant amassed a large fortune and then devoted his life to a passionate archaeological quest. Contradicting the wisdom of his day, Schliemann asserted that Homer's Troy was not a mythical place and set out to locate the ancient city. Schliemann's archaeological digs and publications, beginning in 1869, attracted immense popular and scholarly interest. His discoveries came to symbolize the romance and adventure of archaeology. More important, he became universally recognized as the founder of modern archaeology. This self-taught seeker of prehistory showed himself, in Lilly's words, superior to "the smug professionals" of his day. When Lilly discovered that the heroic archaeologist had lived briefly in Indianapolis, he set out to pursue the subject.[46]

Lilly's Schliemann quest began in May 1959 after reading Robert Payne's *The Gold of Troy*, a popular biography.[47] Lilly immediately wrote Payne to praise the book and to ask if he knew more about Schliemann's residence in Indianapolis. Payne suggested Lilly write the Gennadius Library at the American School of Classical Studies in Athens, where many of Schliemann's papers were deposited. Lilly soon learned that he needed personal help in Greece, and through the efforts of an Eli Lilly and Company international executive, he arranged for an Athens resident, John N. Pantazides, to represent his research interests at the Gennadius Library and with the Schliemann family. Pantazides secured the services of a research assistant, Peter-Nick J. Vavalis, who examined nearly twenty thousand documents in the Schliemann papers, pulling out for copying and translation those referring to Indianapolis. Meanwhile Lilly's associates at the Indiana Historical Society and the Indiana State Library responded to his requests and assisted in the work, as did his secretary, Eva Rice Goble. Margaret Way checked Indianapolis newspapers. Howard Peckham visited from Ann Arbor for a weekend to go over Schliemann material. Lawyer and friend John G. Rauch, Sr., became closely involved in the project also and advised Lilly on the legal issues of Schliemann's residence in the city. Gayle Thornbrough not only edited the manuscript but on a vacation trip to Greece in

June 1960 checked on certain items. Lilly himself labored hard on the project, especially at Wawasee in 1960 where he was often "Schlieman-ning," as he wrote Glenn Black.[48]

The Indiana Historical Society published Lilly's *Schliemann in Indi-anapolis* in 1961. As with his other Society publications, Lilly paid the printing bill. The volume included Lilly's introduction and a separate chapter he wrote on Schliemann's archaeological ventures. The core of the book consisted of Schliemann's diary kept while in Indianapolis and selections from letters he wrote while there, all with careful annotations. It is a most appealing compilation, for Schliemann was a man of wide-ranging interests with uncommon knowledge of languages, culture, and business. His observations about Indianapolis included complaints about the Sunday blue laws, the poor quality of servants, the heat and humidity, and the low level of intellectual life. Several times he visited the General Assembly, marveling at what he saw as "Democracy in all its roughness and nudity" with legislators "throwing paper-balls at each other and even at the speaker." Mingled with Schliemann's negative observations were expressions of marvel at the work ethic, pragmatism, and material prosperity of the city's people, particularly evident in the railroad trains that rumbled through Indianapolis and in the large numbers of healthy and happy children.[49]

The central theme of Schliemann's three-month Indianapolis sojourn was his divorce case. Long separated from his Russian wife, Schliemann learned that the quickest place to obtain a legal divorce was America and that Indiana's divorce laws were among the most lenient. He arrived in the city on 1 April 1869 and, aided by five of the city's best lawyers, obtained the decree he wanted on 1 July. While waiting for Indiana law to grant him matrimonial freedom, Schliemann initiated a courtship with a young Greek woman. This episode especially intrigued Lilly, who wrote his Greek correspondent Pantazides in late 1959: "The great point of interest here in Indianapolis in Dr. Schliemann's visit is the romance of his second marriage which led to such a congenial companionship and happy life."[50] Schliemann did find in his second wife a woman who, Lilly wrote, "always stood loyally by her husband and in difficult situations would always say the appropriate soothing words at the proper time." The "hard-driving, eccentric" Schliemann, in turn, "loved her sincerely and served her with the best intentions he could muster."[51] Perhaps among the elements that attracted Lilly to Schliemann might be included the shared experiences of unhappy first marriage, divorce, and happy remarriage.

Lilly's connection with Schliemann continued after the 1961 publication, particularly when the Schliemann family threatened to remove the papers from the Gennadius Library and also later announced that there were additional papers in the family's possession. In response to requests from the head of the Gennadius Library, Lilly began to provide financial contributions to obtain and keep the papers in the library. Between 1960 and 1967 he contributed $42,500 to this cause, and the Lilly Endowment gave another $24,000. In response to Lilly's request, and doubtless in return for his generosity, the Gennadius Library later agreed to place Schliemann's Indianapolis diary on permanent loan with the Lilly Library at Indiana University.[52]

Lilly had one other experience with the Greek past. In 1965 he wrote David Randall, librarian at Indiana University's Lilly Library, about a reference he had seen to drawings that Jacques Carrey had made of the Parthenon in Athens in 1674, a few years before the Venetian artillery destroyed it. Lilly asked Randall, one of the nation's most knowledgeable rare book men, if he could obtain a volume of the book in which the Carrey drawings were printed. Randall obtained the book for Lilly, who soon decided to support a new publication of the drawings. In late 1966 he sent a check for $48,500 to the Indiana University Press, to assist in publishing the volume. Two Indiana University fine arts professors, Theodore Bowie and Diether Thimme, began work on the project. As with the Walam Olum research twenty years earlier, the work took longer than anticipated. Three years after the project began, with no book in sight, Lilly complained: "Since I am eighty-four years old . . . I have quite given up hope of ever seeing the volume."[53] At this point Indiana University Chancellor Herman B Wells took charge, pushing Professor Thimme and the press to move the project forward. Wells and Lilly had a very high regard for each other, and Wells stayed in close touch, writing Lilly about the Parthenon book even from Duke University, where he was trying the famous rice diet.[54]

Finally, in August 1971 Lilly's secretary, Anita Martin, gave him a telephone message from Wells, saying that he would deliver the Parthenon book the next day. Lilly rose from his chair, threw up his arms, exclaimed that he was stunned into senselessness, and fell to the floor. It was all in jest, of course, but, Martin recalled, "it was quite a sight to see Mr. Lilly 'frolicking' on the floor that way. He was eighty-six years old."[55] The book, *The Carrey Drawings of the Parthenon Sculptures*, was worth such a reaction. It was an outstanding piece of bookmaking, produced by Lilly's favorite printer, R. R. Donnelley. And it was an important contribution to scholarship. Bowie and Thimme provided expert commentary on the provenance and history of the Carrey drawings, but the core of the book consisted of the color reproductions of the drawings, accompanied by photographs of the original fragments that remain (many in the British Museum). The reviewer for *Art Journal* concluded that the book was "indispensable for both classical scholars and historians of modern Greece."[56]

Lilly's interest in history extended beyond books and writing to include also preservation of the past. He believed in the importance of libraries and archives and, with his brother, organized the family and business archives at the pharmaceutical company. He actively supported development of a state history museum, but received little encouragement from the politicians.[57] He also became convinced of the importance of restoring old buildings and eventually made a major contribution to the developing field of historic preservation.

Lilly's first and most sustained venture in historic preservation came at Conner Farm, located along White River north of Indianapolis. The history of the farm and of the Conner family appealed to Lilly's sense of time and place. William Conner settled in the Indiana Territory in 1801 and soon became one of the major Indian traders on the frontier. His log house was an important landmark for Delaware Indians and for newly arriving settlers in central Indiana, serving, for example, as the meeting place for the commissioners who selected the site for the new state capital. As the government removed the Delaware Indians west across the Mississippi River, Conner shifted his attention to land speculation, agriculture, and mercantile trade with white newcomers. In 1820 he abandoned his Delaware wife and married a newly arrived white woman. In late 1823 William and Elizabeth Conner built a large, two-story brick home, one of the first brick houses in central Indiana.[58]

Lilly purchased the Conner home and about four hundred acres of farm land in 1934. He set out immediately to preserve and restore the house. Neglect and nature had left it barely standing. The walls bulged, and the roof leaked. Wooden beams were rotted, and the brick work was

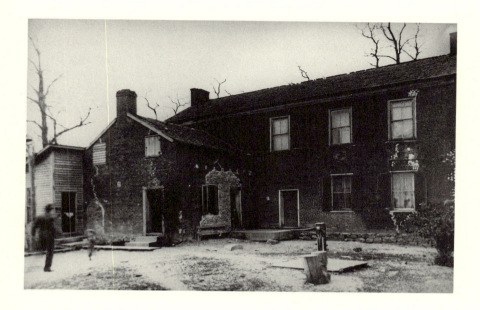

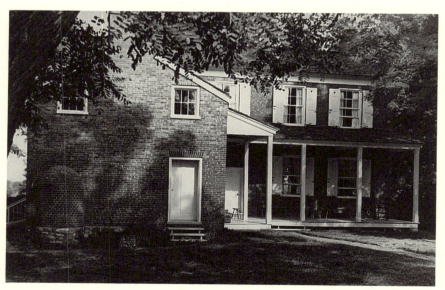

William Conner's house, before and after Eli
Lilly's restoration of 1934.   *Conner Prairie*

deeply cracked. The challenge was not simply to save the home but to restore it in a manner that would be historically authentic. With his usual energy Lilly set out to educate himself, seeking books and articles on historic restoration and corresponding with experts, such as Laurence Vail Coleman. He went to the statehouse and made a tracing of the original 1821 survey of the land. He began a detailed correspondence with his friend Elam Young (Dick) Guernsey, a state legislator, businessman, and dedicated amateur historian and archaeologist from Bedford, Indiana. Guernsey was then assisting in the restoration of the pioneer village in Spring Mill State Park, one of the first such projects of the kind. In early November 1934, after the dedication ceremonies for the new pharmaceutical research laboratories, Eli and Ruth traveled to Williamsburg, Virginia, where the first phase of the nation's leading historic restoration project had just been completed. At Williamsburg Lilly had his introduction to serious restoration: "If we didn't get eyes, ears, and brains full," he wrote Guernsey, "I don't know Arkansas!"[59] He was also pleased to find in Williamsburg an antique dealer who could supply hardware for the Conner house. With Guernsey advising on paint, woodwork, and bulging walls, and with architect Robert Frost Daggett and contractor Charles Latham supervising, twenty-five workers put on a new roof, repainted the brick work, shored up the walls, poured a new concrete foundation, and replaced the hardware, window frames, and glass.[60]

As restoration proceeded the Lillys set out to furnish the house. Ruth took major responsibility for this part of the project. She began her research with visits to the Indiana State Library, and she often accompanied Eli on business trips to search out antique shops. Guernsey continued to advise them, and at his suggestion they spent two autumn days with Drusilla Cravens in Madison, Indiana. Cravens had supervised the refurnishing and restoration of the antebellum Greek Revival mansion of her grandfather, James F. D. Lanier. From her they bought fireplace cooking utensils and several pieces of furniture, including a poplar bedstead. It was a delightful visit with "Miss Drusilla," Lilly wrote Guernsey, for "she was in unusually fine form with her tongue rattling along like a bell clapper, continually forgetting the thread of her conversation and running at tangents, not to say amuck." The drive through southern Indiana and Clifty Falls State Park "in full blast of color" and "in the soft Indian summer air" only added to their pleasure.[61] Lilly's satisfaction in furnishing the house was one of eagerness, even impatience. When his Williamsburg dealer failed to locate appropriate candlesticks, Lilly soon canceled the order, writing him that

"I designed a pair and had them made in our machine shop! I think you would be surprised at the favorable results."[62]

In addition to the work on the Conner house, Lilly also was hopeful "of restoring this place to its 'pristine' fur-trading post character."[63] During the late 1930s he began building an outdoor museum. He moved log cabins and buildings from elsewhere, principally Brown County in southern Indiana, and placed them so as to represent Conner's original home, trading post, stable, springhouse, and stillhouse. These he furnished, relying on his studies of pioneer inventories and the advice and help of several friends. Dick Guernsey, Glenn Black, and Jack Householder all provided assistance. Householder, a furrier at L. S. Ayres department store, obtained furs for the trading post to represent animals of early nineteenth-century Indiana. To find the right cougar skin Householder had to search as far away as Denver. Guernsey advised Lilly on log buildings and on distilled whiskey, which had been an important item in Conner's trade. He also joined the search for a still. Indeed, Lilly reported in mid-1936 that "all the Excise lieutenants in Southern Indiana are making special raids to find a still of the right kind!"[64] He soon had not one but two stills. Black joined in advising on Indian trade goods. By 1940 Lilly wrote Black that "the Trading Post is filling up in good shape."[65]

Lilly's re-creation of a pioneer past was not unique. Other wealthy men—many of whom had done so much to create modern America—were engaged in similar projects in the 1930s and 1940s, most notably Henry Ford at Greenfield Village and John D. Rockefeller, Jr., at Williamsburg. The historian of this movement has concluded that "these philanthropists all believed that something had been lost from the American scene and that it could be brought back only by the vitally important process of using objects, buildings, and crafts demonstrations for education."[66] Lilly doubtless shared such notions, hoping that the buildings and artifacts of frontier America would build character in modern Americans who saw them. The demands of the pharmaceutical business and the wide range of his active interests postponed a full step toward this objective until the last decade and a half of his life.

It should be noted also that Lilly shared with most others in the still immature field of historic preservation and restoration a proclivity to operate by instinct. He sought authenticity but not always fully or in ways later preservationists would approve. He and his associates, for example, failed to research thoroughly interior color schemes of the Conner house or to preserve paint samples. His most notable departure from authentic restoration was the addition of a large porch to the house simply because he enjoyed the view.[67]

As he attempted to re-create pioneer Indiana at the Conner Farm, Lilly developed another interest. Like not a few men born and raised in the city, Lilly wanted to farm. He wanted to know about animals and crops and to have the experience and challenge they brought. Soon Conner Farm was the home of Percheron horses, Shropshire sheep, and Berkshire hogs. These and other acquisitions were not ordinary farm animals, for Lilly endeavored to raise prizewinning stock. He took great pride in the farm, even writing a short history and description of the operation in 1940-41. The farm's horses provided shared activity for Lilly and his daughter, Evie. They took special pleasure in the horse *Jeb Stuart*, which the *Official Horse Show Blue Book* described as "one of the greatest five-gaited horses shown in 1938."[68] Lilly's cattle and hogs also won ribbons at state fairs, with hog breeding becoming the farm's most successful venture. Seldom inclined to boast, Lilly later recalled that "our hog breeding stock was surely not second to any."[69]

Lilly's farm experience was no Sunday afternoon dabbling. He sought expert agricultural advice, just as he did for the pharmaceutical company and for his archaeological research. Forestry consultants advised on woodland management, while soil scientists from Purdue University did an elaborate survey. Lilly was especially interested in animal breeding and read several textbooks on the subject and briefly employed the author of one, Dr. Laurence M. Winters of the University of Minnesota, as advisor to Conner Farm. Applying lessons learned on McCarty Street, Lilly instituted careful record keeping and insisted that farm employees "work with the team spirit of an Indiana basketball aggregation."[70] Major responsibility for executing these wishes fell to Tillman Bubenzer, who, beginning in 1942, was Lilly's farm manager. Bubenzer was a German immigrant whose stubbornness and cantankerousness often exasperated Lilly, but whose dedicated service to the farm caused Lilly to keep him on as long as he owned Conner Prairie.[71]

The effort paid off in fame but not fortune. Lilly's farm animals won ribbons, but they did not earn profits. Receipts from milk sales did not even pay the cost of dairy cattle feed. The major drain came in Lilly's pride and joy—the hog operation. Losses on the hog business were $21,691 in 1951 and $48,011 in 1952. As they continued to mount, Lilly became increasingly concerned not only about the direct financial drain but about the effect on his income tax. The situation came to a head in early 1955, when Lilly's accountant informed him that "the Conner Prairie farm has sustained losses in excess of $50,000.00 for four consecutive years, and is therefore in danger of falling in the 'hobby' loss category of the Federal Income Tax Regulations at the end of 1955 if the loss again exceeds $50,000.00."[72]

Lilly instructed farm manager Bubenzer to cut expenses. When the first quarter report for 1955 showed continued losses, he wrote Bubenzer that "if the situation does not look better by fall, I intend to change the whole procedure out there, and will suggest employing a farm expert to get us on the right track."[73] Bubenzer was hurt and replied innocently: "You have trusted me for 25 years. What have I done to lose your confidence?"[74] Lilly responded by asking for detailed reports on the hog business, which Bubenzer provided. The manager pleaded for Lilly's patience and argued that the farm's hog breeding experiments were in the position that Henry Wallace and associates faced in the early years of developing hybrid corn seed: "They had to go through trying years of development just like we are facing now."[75] Lilly kept pushing, suggesting that Bubenzer's bullheadedness and conceit prevented him from accepting the expert advice the farm needed. Bubenzer responded that Lilly's faith in experts was the cause of some of the farm's problems and that "I could have finished the job here successfully if left alone, but you do not want it that way." In anger, Bubenzer resigned. Lilly accepted the resignation and firmly rejected his manager's criticism of experts: "In our company down here, which you must admit has been a little more profitable than the Conner Prairie Farm, it has been our long-time policy to constantly call in your much despised experts to constantly improve our procedures, for nothing is done anywhere that cannot be done better."[76]

Despite these conflicts Lilly admired Bubenzer's knowledge and ability. Sometime in early 1956 the two men met and resolved their differences in a manner that suggests a surrender by Lilly: Bubenzer stayed on, and Conner Prairie Farms continued to show losses. Lilly gave up on turning it around. He wrote his lawyer in 1959 that the farm "was quite a financial drain and should be gotten rid of promptly."[77] As he and his accountant struggled to keep the farm classified as a business rather than a hobby, Lilly considered a course of action. For a time he thought of transferring it to the Lilly Endowment, the Indiana Historical Society, or Purdue University, but finally decided in 1963 on a different course, one that would provide above all for the future of the property as a historic site.[78]

In late 1963 Lilly decided to convey Conner Prairie Farm to Earlham College. The total value of the land, buildings, and chattels was $1,804,655. Lilly stipulated only one major restriction: the Conner house and the fifty-eight surrounding acres must be maintained in perpetuity and be open to the public. "The site and its structure," he wrote, "is one of the most important historical monuments in the State of Indiana." The rest of the property, including 1,370 acres of land, could be disposed of, though Lilly indicated his hopes that Earlham would continue to operate the farm, noting the college's distinguished record in biological sciences, its experience in operating farms of its own, and "its Quaker concern to serve mankind in practical ways." To lessen the financial burden, he promised a $50,000 subsidy in each of the next three years.[79]

It was a marvelous gift for the small Quaker-related college in Richmond, Indiana. Lilly was attracted to the institution for several reasons. He admired the traditions of Quakerism generally and respected the school's eminent theologian, Elton Trueblood. He was also impressed by Earlham president Landrum R. Bolling. Bolling was an intelligent, widely read, and widely traveled man, with broad interests and an energetic drive to serve the college. He and Lilly developed a close association, one that eventually led, in 1972, to Bolling's move to the Lilly Endowment. Tillman Bubenzer also played an important intermediary role. He had worked with Trueblood's Yokefellows project, a religious lay group, and first urged Lilly's consideration of Earlham. Bubenzer also assisted Bolling in preparing for the initial meetings with Lilly. When in October 1963 Bolling, Bubenzer, and Lilly gathered at Sunset Lane to discuss Conner Prairie, Bolling had worked out a detailed and orderly proposal that was very close to the final agreement. Earlham officials still had some doubts, perhaps even fears, that the gift might become a white elephant or an impossibly complex burden for the small college's administration. But Bolling astutely realized that the value of the farm land provided a financial cushion, and he grasped also the intensity of Lilly's commitment to the historical possibilities of the site. Bolling and Earlham took a risk in accepting the gift, but it was one that paid off handsomely for the college over the next fifteen years and beyond.[80]

The most immediate challenge facing Bolling and his colleagues was plugging the financial drain of the farm operation. The Earlham administrators felt obliged to Bubenzer, who stayed on as farm manager. It was a difficult situation, college business manager Harold C. Cope wrote, especially because Bubenzer thought that "everything should be done in a first-class manner."[81] To Cope's regret Bubenzer spent $14,000 to remodel a barn and leased one of the largest tractors available. Bolling reminded Cope that "without Tillman and his interest in Earlham I think there is no doubt we would not have this property," and then added, "unfortunately, we are doomed to be continually reminded of our debt to him as long as he lives."[82] Propelled by Bubenzer's spending, the farm debt in the first four years of Earlham's operation totaled $205,005, almost exactly equal to the $200,000 Lilly gave the college in those years to subsidize Conner Prairie. With Bubenzer's retirement in 1970, the college turned over responsibility to Halderman Farm Management Service.[83]

Much more interesting to Lilly than the farm was development of the educational potential of the property. The question was on his mind as early as 1935, when he invited the Society of Indiana Pioneers to stage a historical pageant at the Conner Farm. Lilly wrote privately in 1935 that he hoped "to present the property to the public in some form or other, but just how to do this is a serious problem, particularly so since our hitherto wonderfully handled state parks are now in the hands of the politicians."[84] He often invited guests to see the site and in the 1940s began to welcome school and other group tours. The WPA guide to Indiana, published in 1941, described the Conner homestead and advised prospective visitors simply to "obtain visiting permit from Eli Lilly, Indianapolis."[85] By the early 1960s making the site a more widely used educational resource for studying pioneer Indiana was foremost in his hopes. He had already made several trips to Williamsburg, the popular historic showplace of colonial Virginia. In 1961 he and Ruth joined the Peckhams and Blacks for a visit to Henry Ford's Greenfield Village in Michigan. Two years later the Lillys traveled to outdoor museums in the northeast, including Cooperstown, Mystic Seaport, and Sturbridge Village.[86]

Although he doubtless had these models in mind, Lilly carefully avoided dictating to Earlham any particular strategy of development. He did, however, make very clear how much the historic site meant to him. Soon after he and President Bolling reached their agreement in 1963 Lilly asked for a meeting at Conner Prairie to explain directly the historical associations of the home and its contents. Later he sent Bolling some of his research notes and correspondence. In late 1964 he expressed his strong pleasure that Earlham had begun regularly scheduled tours. Lilly, in fact, watched very closely over Conner Prairie in these first years. He visited often, asked questions, and knew well what was happening there. On the other side of the courtship, Bolling and his associates carefully kept Lilly informed. They soon came to realize the importance Lilly attached to responsible management. Thus, for example, the Earlham administrators quickly rejected the recommendation of an outside consultant that they

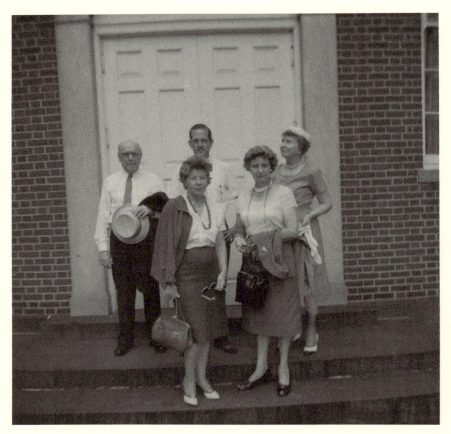

Glenn Black's snapshot at Greenfield Village,   *Howard Peckham*
1961. Front, left to right, Ida Black, Dorothy
Peckham; back, left to right, Eli Lilly, Howard
Peckham, Ruth Lilly.

sell large parts of the land to develop 190 single-family homes. James B.
Cope, brother of Hal Cope and an Earlham biologist and director of the
college's Joseph Moore Museum, became the liaison between the school,
Conner Prairie, and Lilly. He made sure, for example, that each Christmas
the Lillys received handcrafted items from Conner Prairie. A gift of a hand-
knit wool tie, made from hand-spun yarn and dyed with walnut husks
prompted Lilly to send the Conner Prairie staff a six-verse thank-you poem.
More important, Jim Cope visited Lilly often to keep him posted on developments. When a frontier era dugout canoe was discovered on the river,

Cope immediately told Lilly, who soon appeared at the site, camera in hand, questions ready. As the number of visitors rose, Lilly often told Cope and Bolling how pleased he was.[87]

By 1968 Lilly and the Earlham people had come to understand and respect each other. In February Hal Cope wrote Lilly that over the past four years the losses at the Conner Prairie Museum had totaled $33,154. The college had come to the conclusion that Conner Prairie could not "be profitably operated on a modest or 'middle ground' level. . . . We must develop the resource to its fullest potential or else not keep it open at all."[88] Soon the Conner Prairie Advisory Council was discussing the former alternative, in the form of a pioneer village depicting Indianapolis in 1825 or perhaps a hypothetical village of the early 1800s. The council, which included Lilly's close associate H. Roll McLaughlin, concluded that a feasibility study was needed. All this Bolling and Jim Cope discussed with Lilly.[89]

In January 1969 Lilly gave to Earlham College forty thousand shares of stock in the pharmaceutical company, with a value of slightly over $3 million. The gift was "to maintain and to operate the Conner Prairie Farm Museum complex . . . on a basis which will effectively and appropriately communicate to young people and to the general public the record of Indiana's early history."[90] In several conversations in the winter of 1968-69 Lilly told Bolling that he wished to protect Earlham against financial losses from the farm and museum, to provide for expansion of the museum, and to provide general support to Earlham. In a memo for his files Bolling noted that Lilly's delight with Conner Prairie had a positive effect on Lilly's attitude toward Earlham as a whole. Indeed, Lilly had already told Bolling that Earlham was now a beneficiary in his will, though he did not indicate the amount. Bolling also noted that Lilly was "extremely anxious to have no publicity," not "even the fact that it [Earlham] has received a gift of this magnitude from an anonymous donor."[91]

With this $3 million gift, planning for Conner Prairie Pioneer Settlement began in earnest. Jim Cope and Bolling continued to keep Lilly informed. Knowing that Lilly "constantly comes out to the Museum on his own, unannounced, to look and see what is happening," Earlham administrators and trustees believed that they had "a moral and ethical responsibility to do the right thing with this support."[92] Lilly clearly thought Earlham was doing the right thing in the early 1970s when it began a major expansion by moving buildings to Conner Prairie and laying out a village appropriate to the Indiana frontier of 1836. He even participated directly in creation of the village by locating a schoolhouse near Lake Wawasee and supervising its removal to Conner Prairie. Lilly's approval became even more clear one day in 1972 when he asked Cope to have Bolling stop in for a visit sometime. Bolling arrived the next day to learn, as Cope suspected, that Lilly wanted to make another gift to Conner Prairie. This second major donation consisted of twenty thousand shares of stock, with a value of $1,427,500. Lilly specified that the money be used to develop educational programs at the pioneer village and to support programs at Earlham, particularly the Joseph Moore Museum and the American history program.[93]

Lilly proudly attended the dedication ceremony for the Conner Prairie Pioneer Village in 1974. With this expansion of the early 1970s the number of visitors coming to learn about the frontier past grew from 1,500 in Lilly's last year of ownership to 127,140 during the 1975-76 season. At Conner Prairie visitors walked paths and entered buildings to talk with guides who wore period costumes and assumed a particular role from the Indiana frontier of 1836, ranging from storekeeper to housewife to schoolteacher. As they taught multiplication tables or carried on their spinning, candle making, or blacksmithing, the guides maintained a first-person conversation appropriate to the role they were playing.[94]

Conner Prairie was one of the great joys of Eli Lilly's life. Even into the mid-1970s he continued to visit frequently, usually arriving on a late Sunday afternoon. The weekend supervisor, Esther Linenberger, would drive him around the site in an electric golf cart. Mr. Lilly was "such a gentleman," she recalled. He almost always wanted to stop at the old schoolhouse and sometimes went inside to join in the role playing and to respond as a student when the teacher called on him.[95]

The development of Conner Prairie was Lilly's largest single historic preservation project. But there were many others. As early as 1933 he began to support restoration of the Vincennes home of William Henry Harrison. The Harrison project was undertaken by the Francis Vigo Chapter of the Daughters of the American Revolution, and Lilly made many contributions over the years.[96] He contributed also to the historic preservation work in Madison, Indiana. This town on the banks of the Ohio River had some of the finest early nineteenth-century architecture in the Midwest. In 1960, when it appeared that one of the most important homes in the town, the Sullivan house, was to be sold at auction, local preservationists wrote Lilly. He immediately sent $6,000 to enable Historic Madison, Inc., to purchase the house "with the understanding that the people of Madison would accept responsibility of taking over and caring for the house in the future."[97] Lilly's attempt to avoid a long-term commitment failed, as local fund raising proved inadequate to restore the Sullivan house. In 1962 he gave $10,000 and in 1964 another $10,075. Later he made more contributions to Historic Madison, Inc.[98]

Another historic site that attracted much more of Lilly's attention was Shakertown at Pleasant Hill, Kentucky. This Shaker settlement was a large and prosperous community during the first half of the nineteenth century but declined after the Civil War. The property passed to private hands in the early twentieth century and gradually deteriorated. In 1961 several private citizens determined to purchase and restore the village. Led by Earl D. Wallace, an energetic Kentuckian with a background on Wall Street, they formed a corporation, puchased the land and twenty-seven buildings, and developed a plan to restore and furnish the buildings and make them accessible to the public. Early efforts at fund raising met only modest success. In soliciting funds for a down payment on the surrounding farmland in late 1963, Wallace brazenly telephoned Lilly, whom he had never met. He knew, however, that Lilly had family ties to Kentucky and that he had visited at nearby Harrodsburg. After explaining briefly his plan for Shakertown, Wallace asked if he and Louisville newspaperman Barry Bingham could come to Indianapolis to present their case. Lilly then asked how much money Wallace needed. When told that it was $12,500, he promised to mail the check so that Wallace would not have to make the long drive to Indianapolis.[99]

The connection to Shakertown that began in 1963 lasted to the end of Lilly's life. He and Ruth made their first trip to the village soon after the $12,500 contribution. After Wallace took them through the dilapidated village and explained in detail his vision, Lilly asked him to write a letter outlining the project. The next day at breakfast, Lilly told Wallace that he had changed his mind. As Wallace's heart began to sink, Lilly went on to explain that he had decided that his original intention to present a request to the Lilly Endowment would take too much time. Instead, he gave Wallace at the breakfast table a personal check for $50,000, while Ruth wrote out a counter check for the same amount.[100]

In the following years Eli and Ruth usually visited Shakertown each spring and fall. With each visit they made a contribution, often $100,000. When restoration was completed, they stayed in the East Family House. After walking through the village, Lilly liked to sit in a rocking chair on the patio of the East Family House and talk with Wallace, discussing the progress of restoration and the steps ahead. Lilly was strongly attracted to Wallace's simple but difficult goal of authentically restoring original buildings without adding modern structures and without reconstructing buildings. He was interested in the practical side of the restoration and in the Shakers themselves, whose woodworking skills he especially admired. Lilly was always concerned too about the financial state of the project, and the alert Wallace kept him fully informed. The Lillys and Wallaces often ate together and went for long country drives, on one occasion attempting to find the home of a distant cousin. In between visits Wallace sent long letters describing the progress of the work. Often he included photographs of buildings and the landscape.[101]

Wallace and his associates made good progress and in the spring of 1968 opened Pleasant Hill to the public, providing food, lodging, crafts, and exhibits in restored Shaker buildings. But the major crisis was still to come. Operating expenses were high, especially in the winter months when few visitors appeared. By late 1970 Wallace sadly concluded that the anemic cash flow meant closing for the winter. Once closed, he doubted the village could open again, particularly because it was necessary at the same time to default on the corporation's government loan. With no other prospect in sight, Wallace drove to Lilly's Indianapolis office. After listening to the Kentuckian's description of the situation, Lilly asked how much was needed to make it through the winter. When Wallace said $100,000, Lilly replied that he'd better give enough for two winters, which he did in regular installments over the next two years. In addition, Lilly took Wallace across the hall to meet Eugene N. Beesley, president of the company and chairman of the Lilly Endowment. By insisting that the two meet and that Wallace inform Beesley about Shakertown, Lilly was ensuring that the Endowment would listen sympathetically to requests for aid, which it later did.[102]

With Lilly's support and Wallace's drive Shakertown survived the crisis of 1970 and soon flourished. Lilly continued his visits, even after Ruth died in 1973, and he continued his contributions. With a $300,000 contribution he gave for a rainy day, Wallace began an endowment fund in 1973. Sometime in 1973 or 1974 Lilly and Wallace talked about the odds and ends of restoration that remained, which Wallace estimated would cost $270,000. Lilly took the proposal to the Endowment, which made a contribution in that amount and added $90,000 for a survey of the original Shaker settlement area.[103]

Lilly's long and close association with Shakertown reflected his interest in historic preservation, in preserving the past for future generations. He and Wallace sometimes talked in such terms, with Lilly on several occasions saying that he wanted to contribute in ways that would survive him. Part of Lilly's interest in Shakertown derived also from his respect for Wallace. He was confident that this Wall Street man knew how to handle money. He never attached conditions to his contributions. Wallace seldom had to ask for money because Lilly usually asked how much Shakertown needed. It was clear to Lilly that Wallace was fully committed to the project, so committed that he began working full time for Shakertown, taking no salary, and paying his own very large travel expenses. The bond between the two men is indicated by the fact that Wallace was one of a handful of Lilly associates invited to the Wawasee cottage as well as the Sunset Lane home and one of very few in later years who addressed him as Eli. The two men were comfortable together, sitting in the autumn sun at Shakertown, telling jokes and stories, driving and walking through the country, and talking about the past and the future, about Conner Prairie and Shakertown, and about their hopes of leaving something important behind.[104]

Shakertown appealed to Lilly also because it gave him a chance to get away, to leave Indianapolis for a pleasant weekend. But Indianapolis was home, always. And it was in his hometown that he developed his most diverse historic preservation enterprise. Historic Landmarks Foundation of Indiana was incorporated in 1960, with Lilly and Indianapolis philanthropist Herman C. Krannert as cochairmen. As Lilly's interest became more apparent, Krannert gradually withdrew. Members of the newly formed Marion County/Indianapolis Historical Society and other Indianapolis citizens served on the board of directors and advisory committee and made important contributions, but two men provided the motivating force for the organization. Joining Lilly was H. Roll McLaughlin, an architect with James Associates who began to specialize in historic properties. After McLaughlin gave a talk on historic preservation at one of the spring history workshops, Lilly invited the young architect to breakfast the next morning, where they had a wide-ranging exchange about preservation. It was the beginning of an association and friendship that would last until Lilly's death, with McLaughlin serving as his primary advisor on preservation and enjoying an open invitation to lunch for a lively discussion of preservation and other activities. McLaughlin designed the Glenn A. Black Laboratory and the Angel Mounds reconstruction and visitors center, and he did the development study of Conner Prairie.[105]

Historic Landmarks Foundation began slowly, partly because McLaughlin and his associates did not grasp the rapidly growing intensity of Lilly's commitment. Lilly was unhappy, for example, when he learned that McLaughlin had deposited in a savings account a small contribution that he had made to HLF. Lilly wanted his money spent and the work begun. And when the Victorian-style Kemper house came on the market in 1962, McLaughlin and others concluded the price was too high, despite Lilly's urging that HLF purchase it. To save the house from destruction Lilly then bought it himself and set about restoring it on his own. He and Ruth actively directed the restoration and furnishing of the "Little Wedding Cake House," as they called it.[106]

Finally, after passing up a second house that Lilly had shown interest in, HLF in 1963 purchased the Morris-Butler house, located at 1204 North Park Avenue. This French mansard house was built during the Civil War of locally made, hand-molded brick and featured an imposing tower that rose nearly five stories. When McLaughlin and his associates agreed to purchase the house Lilly provided the money. And he made large financial contributions to the complex restoration work. McLaughlin, who served as restoration architect on the project as well as president of HLF, visited with Lilly often at the McCarty Street office or sometimes at Lake Wawasee. After listening to his progress report, Lilly would ask, "What's it going to take to keep the sheriff from the door?" To keep the sheriff from the Morris-Butler door in 1965 he made three contributions to HLF, totaling $58,000, and in 1966 four contributions, totaling $143,000. His role extended far beyond donor, however. Eli and Ruth actively searched for furniture and paintings for the house, and he advised on such details as placing a more durable iron fence around the front rather than the original wooden picket fence.[107]

HLF celebrated the grand opening of the restored Morris-Butler house in May 1969. This first project was a great success, showing Indianapolis the possibilities of historic preservation at a time when few people in the city had a knowledge of, or interest in, the subject. For Lilly the Morris-Butler house was a trial run, a test case to determine if HLF merited his continued support. He was thoroughly pleased. In early 1969, just as restoration was nearing completion, he called McLaughlin to his office. Lilly handed him an envelope, which the architect soon realized contained 40,000 shares of Eli Lilly and Company stock. Returning to his office, McLaughlin quickly estimated the worth at about $250,000. He was immensely pleased and surprised by this unanticipated gift, but when an associate joined him and they recomputed the value of the stock, McLaughlin discovered its value was in fact just over $3 million. "I nearly died!" McLaughlin later recalled.[108] Like most of Lilly's gifts to trusted associates, this one had few conditions. The deed of gift stated that the purpose was to enable HLF to purchase, maintain, operate, and restore historic build-ings, which "will effectively and appropriately communicate to the general public a record of Indiana's history."[109] With this financial security HLF gained a permanence and a reach that enabled it to expand outside Indi-anapolis, providing information, encouragement, and financial support for local preservation activity throughout the Hoosier state.

There were other Indianapolis preservation projects. In 1970, when Lilly learned that the Waiting Station at Crown Hill Cemetery was to be torn down, he initiated and financed its restoration. The Waiting Station eventually became the headquarters office for HLF.[110] He played a major role in the restoration of Lockerbie Square, the downtown residential area in which James Whitcomb Riley's home was the focal point.[111] He became interested in public buildings downtown, too. One of his favorites was the city market, which the Lilly Endowment saved from the wrecker's ball. He hoped also for the preservation of Union Station, and he supported gener-ally the Endowment's contributions to Mayor Richard Lugar's "great schemes for improving Indianapolis."[112]

Preservation was so important to Lilly that he even ventured toward the political battlefield, an area he abhorred. In September 1973 McLaughlin arranged a lunch with Lilly and former Indiana governor Roger D. Branigin. The two men very much enjoyed each other's company, not the least because of the historical interests they shared. The major issue they discussed at lunch was the drafting of a historic preservation bill to ensure that state-owned properties would be adequately funded and professionally staffed. In his struggles over Angel Mounds particularly, Lilly had suffered many frustrations dealing with state agencies dominated by party politics. Thus, for example, he refused to entrust Conner Prairie to state control. In discussing with Branigin and McLaughlin a plan to create a professional agency to administer state historical properties, Lilly indicated his willingness to contribute financially to setting up such an agency. But neither Branigin's political experience nor Lilly's financial strength was sufficient to bring about quick change. The bill they drafted failed.[113]

In the wide range of his historic preservation activities, extending from the Conner House and Shakertown to the founding and flowering of Historic Landmarks Foundation of Indiana, Eli Lilly had a fundamental effect on the development of the field. His interest in preservation when it was little known or appreciated made a crucial difference, especially in Indiana. Though he strove for anonymity, a generation of pioneer preservationists across the state knew of his dedication and support and took courage from it.[114] And long after his death thousands of visitors to the places he preserved take away some understanding of a different time. These physical reminders of a time past combine with the books he wrote and his guidance of the Indiana Historical Society to provide enduring evidence of Lilly's joy in discovering the wider horizons of history and his wish to share that joy with others.

Chapter 8

Philanthropy and the Quest for Character

Eli Lilly accumulated many millions of dollars. Most of it he gave away. In this he was like many other wealthy men in twentieth-century America, men who built large and very profitable corporations in steel, automobiles, oil, chemicals, and pharmaceuticals and then faced the challenge of living with far more money than they could possibly spend on themselves. Most of these men of great wealth believed in hard work and thrift; they professed economic and political ideas that emphasized individual responsibility, private enterprise, and limited government; many adhered to the practices of American Protestantism; most felt some obligation to honor the gospel of wealth by helping those less fortunate and by improving the community in which they lived. Eli Lilly seldom said much about such matters, but there is no doubt that he shared these basic values and objectives. Unlike many wealthy men, however, who often had a necessary but superficial interest in philanthropy, Lilly, from the 1930s until his death, devoted a major portion of his time and energy to giving money with purpose and direction.[1]

Philanthropy was hard work for Lilly. Advising his daughter, Evie, in 1939 to give part of her allowance to "worthwhile charitable and educational objects," he added: "This sounds easy, but the 'catch' is that it takes lots of time and study to know what objects of that nature are worthwhile and what are not."[2] Lilly's response, in part, to the challenge of responsible giving was to focus his philanthropy on people and institutions he knew personally.

Eli's grandfather, Colonel Eli Lilly, had played an important role in Indianapolis charities, particularly in response to the depression of 1893. The colonel's son, Josiah K. Lilly, Sr., was a lifelong benefactor of the city. On his deathbed he drew up a list of local organizations he wanted to support, ranging from the Indianapolis Symphony and the Children's Museum

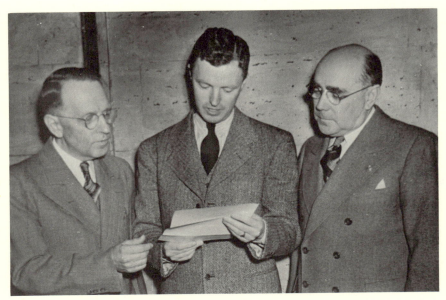

Marion County Tuberculosis Association leaders,   *Indianapolis Star*
1943. Left to right, Charles E. Lyght, E. O. Asher,
and Eli Lilly, chairman of the association's
annual Christmas seal campaign.

to the Community Fund, Red Cross, Wheeler Rescue Mission, and Tuber-culosis Association. "I must confess," J. K. Lilly, Sr., wrote, "a little prejudice in favor of Indiana institutions."[3] His son held to this prejudice throughout his life, not only as an inheritance from his father and grandfather, but also as the consequence of his deep affection for the city and state of his birth and of his wish to know more intimately the channels in which his philan-thropy would flow.[4]

Philanthropy at a distance did not much appeal to Eli Lilly. He told an interviewer in 1972 that in deciding about giving his "selection [was] simply made on the basis of personal interest and often on the basis of friendship."[5] His close, personal relationships with Howard Peckham at the Indiana Historical Society, Landrum R. Bolling at Earlham College, Frank Sparks at Wabash College, Glenn A. Black at Angel Mounds, Earl Wallace at Shakertown, H. Roll McLaughlin at Historic Landmarks, and John Craine at Christ Church constituted a major force in his decisions to give millions of dollars to the institutions these men led.

Lilly's decision to give money depended also on the depth of his knowledge about the cause as well as the leader. Most of his large contributions he made only after he had studied the subject and formed ideas about state and local history, private colleges, archaeology, preservation, or urban churches. In many instances, Lilly's largest contributions were made not because he was asked but because he actively initiated the gift. And that initiation came because he developed, often on his own, ideas and programs he believed worthy of support. Thus, his philanthropy was not only close and personal in the sense of giving to people he knew but also in the sense of giving for purposes he himself actively discovered and passionately embraced. Lilly did not give money simply to dispose of excess wealth or to respond to the requests of others. He gave because he had concrete objectives he hoped to accomplish.

Much of Lilly's philanthropy was private. An Episcopal clergyman would call at Sunset Lane and explain a new program in adult religious education. Lilly knew the subject and the clergyman, who would soon leave with a personal check for $25,000.[6] Much giving was also accomplished through the Lilly Endowment, organized in 1937. Lilly's strong feelings about the Endowment derived not only from the fact that his company had generated the profits that constituted the Endowment's assets but also from his active involvement in making grants. In an analysis of the nation's thirty-six largest foundations Waldemar A. Nielsen concluded that "on the whole . . . what the donors gave their foundations was a mass of resources and little else. . . . Only about half of them demonstrated any serious interest in philanthropy," Nielsen wrote. "Almost none had any serious concern with social problems."[7] Lilly was different. As with his private philanthropy, most Endowment grants reflected his personal interests and his own study and evaluation of the best ways to use money to improve the human condition. His interest in character education reflects this central feature of his philanthropy and reveals a major facet of his deepest and most enduring interests.

On a quiet summer evening in 1936 Lilly and his archaeologist friend Glenn A. Black talked, as they often did, about matters far removed from prehistoric pottery and burial mounds. Lilly raised the subject of children:

what factors shaped their character, the role of spiritual training, and the possibility of conducting experiments in character formation.[8] Lilly was on to a quest he would follow until his death. How do people, particularly children, develop character? How are moral and spiritual values formed? How can such values be strengthened?

Lilly had rigorously examined his own character and emerged in the early 1930s determined to develop a proper outlook on life. He expanded his interests, particularly in the fields of archaeology and history, devoted more attention to religion and to Christ Church, and became more interested in the morale and psychological well-being of his employees at the pharmaceutical company. And he began to think about the human condition. In his presidential address to the Indiana Academy of Science in the fall of 1938 he argued for the importance of developing more effective means of research, especially through interdisciplinary cooperation. He drew many of his illustrations for interdisciplinary work from science but turned in part of his address to other areas. "Our spiritual development has a hundred-year lag behind our material progress," Lilly asserted. The fields of education and religion were "far behind the times" and needed "all the power they can borrow, beg, or steal to stem the tide of materialism engulfing the world and to teach all humanity that it is not what we have but what we are that is of real importance." Lilly urged that "a coalition of talent" should attack "the gross, materialistic philosophy which occupies so many today."[9]

As he did in other areas of developing interest, Lilly began to read. Soon the shelves of his library at Sunset Lane were filled with books about religion, sociology, psychology, and philosophy, particularly books that emphasized moral values and character development. Lilly knew his limitations, especially in abstract thought and philosophy. In 1951 he explained to Indianapolis businessman Pierre F. Goodrich the frustrations "of my cruises into the uncertain areas of philosophy":

> Occasionally in the past, and even now, ambition leads me to set sail upon those entrancing waters, but unfortunately I never had any training in navigating the deeps of philosophy and have always promptly run hard aground on the reefs or mud flats of terms whose definitions I know not. Blowing a whistle blast for help from that staunch tugboat the Shorter Oxford English Dictionary, instead of one powerful unit coming to my help, three or four smaller variations of meanings show up, usually pulling in opposite directions, leaving me helpless and making it necessary to take to the life boats of history and biography.[10]

Despite these obstacles Lilly continued to read in his search for insight into the formation of values. In evenings and weekends at home and during summer visits at Lake Wawasee he underlined in red pencil as he worked, sometimes adding marginal checks and comments. Two authors were heavily represented on his shelves and assumed a large importance in extending Lilly's interest beyond reading to action.

Pitirim A. Sorokin was one of the most colorful and productive sociologists of the twentieth century. Born to a peasant family in northern Russia in 1889, Sorokin became a revolutionary and then an anti-Bolshevik. He was "imprisoned three times by the Tsarist Government," he later recalled, "and three times by the Communist government."[11] Expelled from the Soviet Union in 1922, Sorokin began an academic career in the United States, where in 1929 his publications on social mobility and sociological theory won him a professorship at Harvard University. Sorokin's distinguished career would eventually include election to the presidency of the American Sociological Association, but he was always, as one scholar commented, a "gadfly, iconoclast, scoffer at conventional wisdom."[12] At Harvard his writings ranged wider and wider, from art and law to science and religion to philosophy and psychology, all sweeping across the centuries of Western civilization. And rather than assuming the value-free and sterile social science mode increasingly in favor among sociologists, Sorokin became more and more a prophet and preacher, "a lone warrior, tilting his lance against the main drift of the times."[13] Some, in the 1950s, thought him a communist, but that was an absurdity of the McCarthy era. He thought of himself as a "conservative, Christian anarchist," but there was more yearning for stability and traditional values in his thought than in that of most anarchists.[14] The Sorokin that first appealed to Lilly appeared in 1941 in a book titled *The Crisis of Our Age: The Social and Cultural Outlook.* Western civilization was in crisis, Sorokin warned, and the cause was to be found in pervasive materialism and "ever-expanding appetites for sensory values." There must be, he warned, "a change of the whole mentality and attitudes in the direction of the norms prescribed in the Sermon on the Mount." Writing as Europe fell into war, Sorokin asserted that the only way to triumph over barbarian force was through development of "more familistic and altruistic relationships."[15]

Eli Lilly underlined in red these lines and many others in Sorokin's *Crisis of Our Age,* and he wrote the Harvard professor to tell him how much he liked the book.[16] In the fall of 1941, soon after Sorokin's volume appeared, the Indianapolis businessman wrote an essay titled "The Nemesis of Materialism." In ten pages he expanded on comments in his 1938 address to the Indiana Academy of Science, drawing heavily from Sorokin's book. Western civilization was threatened with "a total blackout of culture, a return to barbarism," Lilly warned. There was a growing percentage of "self-centered individuals," and "family loyalty has reached a low ebb." Art, literature, and music were in decline. In this "materialistic jitterbug dance," the average person could no longer "tell true from false, right from wrong, the difference between beauty and ugliness, or positive from negative." Lilly urged "quick remedial action":

> We must push back materialism into its real place and its right proportion. We must know that truth, goodness, and beauty are absolute values. The precepts of the Sermon on the Mount must take the larger part in the ruling of our lives. Familiar relationships must be established in all human relationships. There must be a spiritualization of mentality and an ennoblement of conduct. Expedience, pleasure, and utility must give way to duty. Licentious freedom must be given up for justice. Coercion and egotistic selfishness must be replaced by all-forgiving love.[17]

In "The Nemesis of Materialism" Lilly struck chords that would play through the remainder of his life. He was not alone in these concerns. In the midst of much chauvinistic boasting about the achievements of American civilization, some thoughtful observers began to suffer a crisis of confidence, a fear that the American people were losing direction in their blind concentration on the immediate, practical, and self-gratifying benefits of material progress. Since the 1920s, one historian has written, "the older American moral values of abstinence, frugality, and saving were challenged by a wider acceptance of promiscuity, high consumption, and living on credit." Parents, whose nineteenth-century grandparents had readily and forcefully taught their children right from wrong, now advocated freedom of expression for the child and relative rather than absolute values for themselves, leaving a "rubble of once imposing structures of ordained truths."[18]

To Lilly and to Sorokin the situation was one of crisis. In 1942 the prolific Sorokin published *Man and Society in Calamity,* calling for values rooted in "moral duty and the kindgom of God." Lilly eagerly read the new book and heavily underlined appealing passages.[19] World War II—powerful evidence for the spiritual crisis that so troubled Lilly and Sorokin—kept the pharmaceutical manufacturer busy with the challenges of insulin, antibiotics, and blood plasma, but he did not forget the Harvard professor.

In 1946 Lilly devoted his President's Column in the company magazine to a synopsis of Sorokin's writings.[20] More important, that first year
of peace he wrote Sorokin again and offered to assist financially in his
research. Sorokin welcomed this offer from a man he did not know. He
wrote Lilly that "unless human conduct and relationships become really
more altruistic and nobler, nothing can save humanity from the third World
War and apocalyptic destruction." Sorokin was committed to the cause,
but the problem would require a team attack from many disciplines with
"at least as great a concentration of the best brains as was done in the
invention of the atomic bomb." A few days after receiving Sorokin's letter,
Lilly sent him $10,000 to begin the attack, adding another $10,000 later.[21]

With Lilly's financial support, Sorokin outlined the challenge in his
book *The Reconstruction of Humanity,* published in early 1948. The first
sentence of the volume presented the problem: "Bleeding from war wounds
and frightened by the atomic Frankensteins of destruction, humanity is
desperately looking for a way out of the deathtrap." The route Sorokin
mapped was one in which individuals must serve "the God of Creation
and love" rather than "the Mammon of Enmity and Selfishness" and one
in which new techniques must be invented for "rendering human beings
more noble and altruistic."[22] Lilly read and underlined the book, declaring
that "it seems to be just what the world has been waiting for."[23]

Soon after he had read *The Reconstruction of Humanity* and while he
was visiting in Boston in late 1949, doubtless with his daughter who was
suffering a crisis of her own in her battle with alcoholism, Lilly telephoned
Sorokin. The Indianapolis pill manufacturer met the Russian revolutionist
and maverick sociologist for lunch. They got on exceedingly well. Lilly's
"sincerity, wisdom, common sense, and kindness impressed me most
favorably," Sorokin later wrote. "During the lunch I informed him that from
his fund of twenty thousand dollars I had spent some $248 to prepare the
Reconstruction of Humanity." Lilly responded, Sorokin recalled, "Can't you
put more steam into this business?"[24] Lilly took his enthusiasm for Sorokin's work back to Indianapolis. He explained the project to his brother
and urged that the Lilly Endowment support it. And he wrote Sorokin to
express his "great personal delight" in their Boston meeting and to ask for
a budget proposal to present to Endowment colleagues. As in some other
instances of eager enthusiasm Lilly promised Sorokin that if the foundation
did not "back the project to the tune of $20,000 a year for five years, I will
do it myself, so you can pursue your plans." J. K. Lilly, Jr., eventually agreed
to support his older brother's notions, and in January 1949 Eli wrote the
president of Harvard, committing the Endowment to $20,000 a year for

five years to support Sorokin's new Harvard Research Center in Creative Altruism. The benefactor's only request was "that the name of Lilly be left out and also that there be no printed publicity as to the source of the fund."[25]

In its ten-year existence the Harvard Research Center in Creative Altruism sponsored symposia and collaborations of nationally known scholars, including Paul Tillich, Gordon Allport, F. S. C. Northrop, and Erich Fromm. From Sorokin's typewriter books tumbled; more than a half dozen appeared in the 1950s, most with the word "love" or "altruistic" in the title.[26] Sorokin sent copies to Lilly, who dutifully read and underlined each one. The two continued to correspond, and on at least one occasion Sorokin spent two days as a guest in the Lilly home on Sunset Lane. Knowing Lilly, Sorokin wrote, "has been one of the most significant events of my life-experience. If, in so-called capitalist society, there were more 'capitalists' like Eli Lilly, there would be no need for the appearance of powerful anti-capitalist movements!"[27]

J. K. Lilly, Jr., and others at the Lilly Endowment did not share Eli's enthusiasm for the Russian-born sociologist. In 1951 Joe sent his brother a report from American Legion headquarters, located in Indianapolis, which charged that Sorokin was associated with people who had questionable ties to communism. Sorokin was a signer of a peace petition thought to be a communist device, and he was one of the sponsors of a banquet honoring W. E. B. Du Bois, a black historian thought to be pro-communist. Eli Lilly refused to change his views about the Harvard professor.[28] Nor did he accept charges made against Sorokin from another angle within the Endowment. In October 1956 Endowment staffer Manning M. Pattillo suggested to Lilly that Sorokin, who had retired from teaching in 1955, was not "in a position to make an important contribution to social thought." Lilly disagreed, and in the following year the Endowment made a grant of $15,000 to help Sorokin continue his writing in retirement. In conversation with Lilly in 1962, Pattillo again raised doubts about the quality of Sorokin's work and then proceeded to obtain evaluations from six sociologists. "You will note that the reaction is somewhat mixed," Pattillo reported to Lilly, "but it seemed to the staff that there was a basis here for an additional grant if you are so inclined." Lilly was so inclined, and the Endowment awarded Sorokin $5,000 for secretarial assistance, adding to a similar grant of $9,000 made in 1960. Through these years Lilly also provided some personal assistance for Sorokin's projects and in 1967 contributed $10,000 to the American Sociological Association to establish the Sorokin Award and

Lectureship.[29] When he learned in 1967 that Sorokin was dying of cancer, Lilly wrote him: "The most overwhelming thought is what a wonderful gift you are to the human race, a mighty warrior in the front ranks of those who have dealt telling blows for the higher things of life. To have known you and to have been inspired by your personality and work ranks among the greatest blessings that Ruth and I have had."[30]

Sorokin was a prophet and preacher. He provided inspiration and warning, but not much direction in practical measures to restructure humanity. Lilly stayed the course with Sorokin but needed more concrete results. Just as biological science led to the profitable production of pharmaceuticals so too should social science lead to practical applications for improving the lives of humankind. Lilly thought he found in Ernest M. Ligon the scholar who could assist in the more applied side of his quest.

Lilly discovered Ligon through his reading. Sometime in the late 1930s he read Henry C. Link's *The Return to Religion.* In this and later books Link, like Sorokin, lamented the decline in moral values. He placed even more emphasis on the urgency of revitalizing religious belief as the basis for moral behavior, and he placed special emphasis on child rearing. In a chapter titled "Children Are Made," Link wrote that "minds are not born, they are acquired by training. Personality is not born, it is developed by practice."[31] Lilly underlined those sentences and then went in search of the author. He visited with Link, but for unknown reasons this meeting did not lead to collaboration. Instead, Link suggested that the person best suited to match Lilly's interests was Ernest Ligon, director of the Character Research Project at Union College in Schenectady, New York.[32] Lilly wrote Ligon in February 1939 asking for publications about "the education of young children so as to inculcate 'character' or 'personality.'" [33] It was the beginning of a relationship that would last into the 1970s.

Ernest Ligon was born in 1897 and educated at Yale, where he earned a divinity degree and then, in 1927, a Ph.D. in psychology. He studied for a year in Switzerland with Jean Piaget, whose analysis of moral development in children became a classic in the field of child psychology.[34] In 1935 Ligon published *The Psychology of Christian Personality.* Combining science

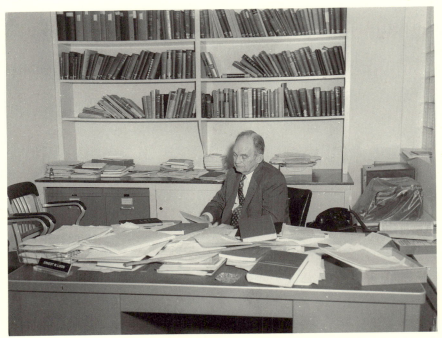

Ernest M. Ligon in his office, ca. 1960.   *Schaffer Library, Union College*

and religion, Ligon attempted "to interpret the teaching of Jesus in terms of modern psychology," particularly in ways that would help parents develop character in their children.[35] The book provided, one reviewer wrote, "definite techniques for applying the principles of Jesus in character education."[36] Even more so than with Sorokin, the Sermon on the Mount was Ligon's central theme. For the next four decades Ligon expanded on this theme, concentrating on eight character traits that he drew from the Sermon on the Mount: vision, a dominating purpose in the service of mankind, love of righteousness, faith in God, sympathy, democratic sportsmanship, magnanimity, and Christian courage. To put these lofty ideals into action Ligon and his associates studied values of children to discover at what ages they could learn particular religious and moral concepts. They then prepared curriculum materials to be used in homes and Sunday Schools, appropriate to different age levels and focused on concrete and everyday behavior, such as sharing, truth telling, and respect for elders. At the nursery level they would teach "the friendliness of Jesus" and how not to be afraid of the dark or of thunderstorms. At a higher level a lesson might focus on "the concept of returning good for evil" or of building self-confidence. Thousands of parents participated in Ligon's Character Research Project, teaching their children about good character and filling out questionnaires to be analyzed at the Union College laboratory.[37]

The Lilly Endowment made its first grant to Ligon and his Character Research Project in 1946. In the next ten years the Endowment awarded another dozen grants totaling just under $1 million, making this one of the most generously funded Endowment projects in these years.[38] With this support Ligon and his growing number of research associates produced books, pamphlets, and articles, written in increasingly dense scientific language, with discussion of hypotheses, laws, and taxonomies, to which were added large amounts of psychology and even larger amounts of religion. Ligon's book *A Greater Generation*, published in 1948, asserted that "it is certain that there are laws of character development which are just as inviolable and powerful as the laws of nature." The challenge was to discover these laws through scientific research. Ligon was convinced that religious belief was central to the quest. "Character education must find its central dynamic in religion," he wrote, especially in the Beatitudes, which specified "eight general character traits." These and other passages Lilly underlined as he read.[39]

By the early 1950s the Character Research Project was the primary center of character education in America. The Endowment assisted in publicizing Ligon's work, including distribution of his 1956 book, *Dimensions of Character*, to more than 1,500 scholars. Endowment funding also enabled Ligon to carry out experiments across the country with curriculum programs for character education. By 1952 forty-six churches and several YMCA groups were testing Character Research Project materials, monitored and supported by Ligon's staff of forty-two at Union College. The Character Research Project also carried its message through annual youth conferences and workshops. A knowledgeable visitor to the summer workshop in 1952 reported that "more research money and brain power are going into this project than into any other research program in Christian education."[40] A reviewer in 1957 asserted that Ligon and his associates were "blasting new pathways in the almost trackless area of scientific appraisal of religious education."[41]

Lilly stayed in close touch with this work. From Ligon "Dear Eli" letters arrived often, and on several occasions the Ligons were guests at Sunset Lane and at Lake Wawasee. At least once, in 1948, Lilly visited with Ligon at Schenectady, when Union College awarded him an honorary degree. In correspondence and in conversation the two men struggled over ways to develop character. Lilly's direct participation was not as deep and personal as it was in his collaborative archæological projects, but it extended far beyond the level of simply giving money.[42] When others threatened to cut off that money, Lilly showed clearly his intense dedication to the project and his loyalty to Ligon.

Ligon's work was controversial, partly because his scientific approach to religion fell between the stools of social science and theology. He was, a religious authority wrote, "a storm center for religious educators in the churches, some of whom viewed him as a sort of devil's advocate challenging the church school to more scientific approaches, and some of whom viewed him as the devil himself."[43] Even friendly religious critics charged that "his theology is a bit too facile," and "he tends to oversell the usefulness of scientific method in religion."[44] Ligon's personal charm and his enthusiasm and commitment attracted many zealots to his cause, but he often displayed a stubborn insistence that his way was the only way and thereby alienated many leaders in the main line Protestant denominations. A Congregational Church official charged in 1949 that his program "has a degree of pontifical finality which is alien to the genius of our churches, and which is not justified by any evidence of scientific infallibility or even of enduring Christian fruitage."[45]

Social scientists were less impressed than religious educators. Their work after World War II moved in different directions than Ligon's, away from a search for character traits and toward psychoanalytic and behavioristic orientations. Articles, conference papers, and bibliographies reporting on academic research in areas combining the social sciences and religion often did not mention Ligon or cite his publications.[46] And among public school teachers and administrators the appeal of character education declined also because of the perceived need for more classroom time for science, vocational training, foreign language, and other subjects and because of a growing uneasiness about teaching traditional and absolute verities in a pluralistic and more tolerant modern world. Many schools thus moved toward neutrality or silence regarding issues of morality and character. In this modern environment Ligon appeared old-fashioned.[47]

J. K. Lilly, Jr., and other Endowment board members were not enthusiastic about Ligon's work either. In late 1958 the board decided to cut back on grants to the Character Research Project for 1959 and 1960 and to make 1961 the final year of support. Eli Lilly wrote the Endowment's executive director, G. Harold Duling, "I am not at all happy about this reduction." And to Ligon he promised that if the Endowment did not "continue the $100,000 for 1959 and 1960, I will make up the difference." In an additional show of support a few weeks later he gave Ligon 5,000 shares of Eli Lilly and Company stock, which, he told his friend, should yield income of about $10,000 a year for his retirement, due in 1962.[48]

In October 1960, as the termination year of 1961 approached, the issue heated up again. Lilly strongly objected to ending support, asserting that "the improvement of character in the world is the most important thing to accomplish. Here we have a group of twenty persons dedicated to this job and making some progress. It is the only group that we know of in competent hands so doing."[49] Lilly's will prevailed, and the board reversed its decision and agreed to provide $115,000 for 1961 and for 1962. Endowment staffer Duling refused to let the issue rest, however, and in late 1961 he appointed five consultants to investigate the Character Research Project and report to the Endowment. Lilly wrote Ligon that this move "is repugnant to me but I cannot help feeling it will turn out for the best."[50] The consultants' report of May 1962 noted strengths in the Character Research Project but concluded that the staff had not used the best and most appropriate methods of research and data gathering and had not reported their findings in a way that reached large and appropriate audiences. The consultants recommended that the Endowment terminate support.[51] Lilly was not surprised by the report, he told Ligon, and had "been against that plan from the start but Ruth and I fought alone against board and staff and had to give way."[52] At Lilly's urging, in July Ligon came to Wawasee, where Lilly assisted him in preparing a written response to the consultants' negative report. Soon after the visit Lilly wrote Ligon to advise him to send his response directly to Sunset Lane and not the Endowment office: Duling "will be told that I am handling the project from here on in and if anything comes to the Endowment office in connection with it he is to turn it to me with suggestions but that I will determine the final action in each case." In an undated note to Duling, Lilly informed him of this decision and asked for all the files on the project and all future correspondence, adding that this "is the one project of the Endowment nearest my heart."[53] In September Lilly sent all board and staff members copies of Ligon's formal response to the consultants' report, along with a cover letter recommending continuation of funding. Lilly agreed that Ligon and his associates must do more to get their work known in the social sciences and among experts in character study. But he stated clearly that he and Ruth would vote to continue funding the work at Union College. Three weeks later Lilly happily informed Ligon that the board had cast a unanimous vote to continue support for two more years.[54]

Lilly's victory did not go unchallenged. A year later Duling made another strike, writing Lilly: "I wonder whether the CRP staff have not become ingrown, complacent, and self-indulgent about its own importance." And Duling added, "In all the literature in the field of religion and psychology, I constantly search for references to the CRP and find few if any." Duling had just finished Ligon's new book, *The Marriage Climate*, and reported to Lilly that "I found it a chore to read this book."[55] By this time Lilly shared some of these doubts, particularly about Ligon's writing, which was so filled with thick jargon that at times it read like a parody of social science style. Lilly read *The Marriage Climate*, too, and with his red pencil, now sharpened by several decades as a writer of clear, vigorous prose, he circled the more ridiculous of Ligon's usages, including the dozens of times he used the word "dynamic" in a near meaningless context. And in the front of his copy of the book Lilly wrote one of the little poems that so amused him:

> *Any one with eyes that could look*
> *would see this a wonderful book*
> *But I continue to plead*
> *It would be easier to read*
> *If it contained less gobbledegook!*[56]

Lilly had some success and satisfaction working with Ligon's associate, Leona J. Smith, on, in Lilly's words, "a book for parents on the attitudes they should take with their youngsters at various age levels."[57] Smith sent him drafts of the manuscript, and Lilly worked over them carefully, paying particular attention to removal of gobbledegook. The book appeared in 1968 under the title *Guiding the Character Development of the Preschool Child*. In her inscription to Lilly, Smith wrote: "The only true title for this book is what we have always called it—the Lilly Book. We all bless you for it."[58]

Lilly was nonetheless growing frustrated and disappointed with the Character Research Project. He sometimes expressed his frustration to Ligon, particularly criticizing his reluctance or inability to present his research in more accessible form. In 1971 Lilly acknowledged receipt of a publication from the project but told Ligon: "I am not sure I can make heads or tails of it. . . . I wonder after CRP's 30 years of experience if they wouldn't have some very important ideas on how to approach families on a practical basis."[59] Yet Lilly, as he often did in such circumstances, remained stubbornly loyal to an old friend. Endowment support continued through 1974, and Lilly himself sent Ligon a personal contribution of $10,000 each year from 1966 through 1974.[60]

Lessening of enthusiasm for Ligon's Character Research Project did not include a lessened concern for the subject itself. Indeed, in the late 1960s Lilly showed a new burst of energy in continuing his search beyond the Ligon project. He urged the Endowment board and staff to think of new projects, and he began to write about the subject to friends and associates. Lilly was particularly pleased that Landrum Bolling, the president of Earlham College with whom he worked on transferring his Conner Prairie property, had ideas on character development. In correspondence and in visits at Sunset Lane and Lake Wawasee the two often discussed such subjects as peer pressure, permissiveness, and the needs of youth for role models. And they talked about possible projects for the Endowment to support.[61]

In 1971 the eighty-six-year-old Lilly was still pushing hard for character education and even hopeful of introducing it into the public schools. "We do not dare use the words 'religion' or 'morals' or 'church' (!!!)," he wrote Endowment board member Eugene N. Beesley, "but character education leads in the same direction and there cannot be objection to it." After decades of reading the assertions of Ligon, Sorokin, and others, Lilly believed that "facts governing human character are as certain as the multiplication table. Children should be taught from the cradle that following the right path is the only way to develop a happy, successful and rewarding life." Character could and should be taught just like other subjects were taught.[62]

Lilly's forty-year struggle with the challenge of character education produced mixed results. Compared to his activities in the pharmaceutical business or in archaeology, history, and preservation, his efforts in character education were perhaps less successful, certainly less visible and enduring. Sorokin's work in altruism and Ligon's in character research made slight lasting impression.[63] Character education and larger questions of morality and religion nonetheless remained very important to Lilly. The intensity and personal involvement with which he pursued the quest testify to his concern for humankind, to his hopes that traditional values might exert a larger influence in the world. It was a Quixotic quest, some might argue, but many good men and women have joined the search. And perhaps the world is better for it, even if the windmills still stand.[64]

Lilly's exact motives in this quest remain unknown. His own religious belief and his sense of stewardship doubtless played a major role. So too did his own personal and family history. Sorokin's and Ligon's studies often pointed to the importance of family love, and Lilly often underlined such passages in their books. He knew the very positive influence of his father and Ruth in his own life. And he knew that families could also exert negative influences and produce unhappiness and disappointment. He remembered the hurt of not knowing full maternal love. He suffered greatly over his own failed first marriage and especially over the troubled life of his daughter. Evie's two marriages ended in divorce; she struggled with alcoholism; and she never developed passionate interests or settled into a career or home life. She never developed a proper outlook on life. In 1968 Lilly set down on paper his side of the unhappy first marriage and the effects on Evie. His divorce in 1926 and the granting of custody to Evie's mother, Lilly wrote, "haunt me to this day as a betrayal of Evie to an affectionless mother, to be raised by nurses until 15 or 16 years old, in a group of youngsters down east of not too high a type. To this denial of love and security I attribute most of Evie's troubles. I pray for forgiveness for my part in this sad affair."[65]

Soon after Lilly's death, the board of directors of the Lilly Endowment adopted a memorial resolution. Documents of this sort sometimes exaggerate, obscure, or mislead, but in this instance the memorialists expressed accurately and well a fundamental facet of Lilly's character:

> The Endowment's commitment to programs to support a broad range of activities in the field of religion, and to encourage education directed toward ethical, moral and social values, was a reflection of his own deep personal interests. He was profoundly concerned with the strengthening of human character. While he saw no magic formula for accomplishing this difficult goal, and was sometimes disappointed in those who seemed to promise more than they could accomplish toward that end, he persisted in his conviction that this was a major direction in which we should move.[66]

Lilly's long quest in the realm of character development and moral values indicates his very large influence in forming Endowment policy but suggests also that others played important roles too. His brother and father, other members of the board, and the staff all helped shape the Endowment so that in surveying the institution's history it is not possible to separate fully Lilly's contribution from that of others. But at the core, the Endowment was Eli Lilly's idea and his creation.

Lilly was uncharacteristically immodest in recalling in 1967 the origins of the Endowment:

> I would like to set straight that I was the first person to suggest the Lilly Endowment. A year or two before it was finally organized, I suggested to my father and brother that we should form such an organization if we wanted to continue the family tradition of being generous in public affairs. The rising income taxes would otherwise make such a course impossible. . . . After a year or so the Messrs. J. K. Lilly finally agreed that it was wise to do so.[67]

Lilly's claim that tax advantages were a major factor in the establishment of the Endowment is not surprising. The decade of the Great Depression was a time of considerable resentment toward wealthy Americans. President Franklin D. Roosevelt called them economic royalists, and his New Deal policies threatened a leveling of wealth. That did not happen, but new taxes in the 1930s did take a larger bite from the 1 percent of Americans who earned over $10,000 a year and encouraged them to seek ways to reduce the burden by means of tax-deductible, charitable contributions. Philanthropic foundations provided a special advantage for successful family businesses, since donors could give appreciated stock to the foundation without paying a capital gains tax. The number of foundations increased substantially in the late 1930s and 1940s.[68]

Foundations also provided an advantage for Americans wishing to maintain control of their family businesses. This problem was very much on Lilly's mind by 1934. J. K. Lilly, Sr., was seventy-two, and Eli worried how he and his brother would pay the inheritance tax on their father's pharmaceutical company stock without selling large portions of it and thereby risk losing control of the company. In June 1934 Lilly discussed this problem with Albert E. Bailey, a professor at Butler University. Bailey set out to study foundations, even meeting with Frederick Keppel, the respected head of the Carnegie Corporation. Bailey concluded that Lilly should form a corporation called the Lilly Educational Foundation, transfer to it all his father's stock, and "appoint you, your wife, and your brother Trustees of the Foundation." "By this act," Bailey advised, "you have not diminished your own or your brother's personal incomes; you have escaped the necessity of hoarding against the payment of 50% inheritance tax; you have riveted the family hold on the ancestral business; and you have created a Foundation that will link your name to a great benefaction for generations."[69]

The Endowment was formed in 1937, as Lilly later remembered, so that money instead of "going for income tax could be put to charitable use" and because it "gave control of the business to the Lillys as long as one was alive."[70] These were commonplace motivations in the formation of America's large foundations, combining genuine charitable impulses with desires to reduce tax burdens and maintain control of family-owned businesses.[71]

From their beginnings America's large foundations roused the attention of critics. They were elitist and nondemocratic, some charged, using money that ought to go to the public treasury for purposes decided on by a small group of white, Protestant, Anglo-Saxon males rather than elected representatives of the people. The donors and staffs of foundations constituted a ruling elite, an "unregulated and unaccountable concentration of power" that had "a corrosive influence on a democratic society." Those foundations closely tied to the business of the donor, with all or most of their assets in the family company, tended to generate relatively small financial returns and were susceptible to responding more to the good of the business than the good of society, critics asserted.[72]

Lilly was certainly aware of such charges, for they burst out periodically in government investigations and other public arenas. He took some steps to diminish the force of criticism. Although he had initially supported the practice of using Endowment grants for medical research, he moved away from medicine and related fields so as to avoid the charge of mixing philanthropy with business profit. Fundamentally, however, Lilly differed radically with foundation critics. He saw nothing wrong with the Lilly Endowment's assets consisting almost entirely of Eli Lilly and Company stock and with the Lilly family and company executives alone constituting the board of directors. It was a family foundation built on the wealth of a family-owned and -managed company. Like many philanthropists, he believed giving was the responsibility of those who made the money.[73]

Over the years the three Lillys gave a total of more than 32 million shares of Eli Lilly and Company stock to the Endowment, with a value at the time of the several gifts of nearly $94 million. J. K. Lilly, Sr., was the largest contributor, giving $86.8 million in stock; J. K. Lilly, Jr., gave $4 million; and Eli Lilly gave $2.8. The pharmaceutical stock increased in value so that the market value of the Endowment's assets exceeded $500 million by 1968 and $1 billion by 1972.[74] By the late 1960s the Endowment was one of the five wealthiest foundations in the country, a fact the institution usually did not publicize because Eli Lilly thought such bragging was "not in good taste."[75]

Eli Lilly ran the Endowment from the left-hand drawer of his desk for the first dozen years after the founding in 1937, taking it upon himself, his brother wrote, "to be the chief administrative officer of the organization, investigating requests for contributions and making recommendations to the Board." The board was composed of the Lilly family, including, in addition to Eli, his father, brother, and wife, plus Nicholas Noyes, who was treasurer of Eli Lilly and Company and related to the family by marriage. In December 1937 the board approved its first grants, the largest of which was $10,500 to the Indianapolis Community Chest, constituting about two-thirds of income available for grants that year and setting a pattern of concentrating support within the Hoosier city and state. In these early years the Endowment was largely an extension of the Lilly family's traditional charitable activities, with little attention to expanding or developing new initiatives.[76]

In the late 1940s the Endowment began to change. A major bequest of stock from J. K. Lilly, Sr., quadrupled assets, which increased from $9 million in 1947 to $39 million by 1948. Grants, which had averaged less than $200,000 a year in the previous ten years, now in the years 1948-57 averaged over $2 million.[77] Eli Lilly concluded that managing an institution of such size required a full-time professional staff. "We are all looking forward to the time," he wrote in early 1949, "when very much more thought and study can be put in on the proper expenditure of this money."[78] Such an opportunity came when his nephew, J. K. Lilly III, decided he did not like working at the pharmaceutical company and agreed to become secretary of the Endowment. Young Joe Lilly studied the policies and procedures of other, more mature foundations and began to effect change. He hired an assistant, G. Harold Duling, an ordained Methodist minister, and he opened an office in the Merchants Bank Building in downtown Indianapolis. Joe began in 1951 to publish annual reports, which included thoughtful and well-written accounts of Endowment policies and procedures. And he initiated a requirement of written rather than oral requests from organizations and individuals asking for support.[79]

J. K. Lilly III brought more system and direction to the Endowment in the early 1950s, but his efforts along these lines were not entirely successful. In 1954 he resigned and moved to New England, feeling that he needed "to construct a useful life for myself in different surroundings."[80] His father and his Uncle Eli were reluctant to adopt more formal procedures. Eli had surrendered the contents of his left-hand desk drawer to young Joe but remained very influential in all aspects of the institution. He blocked his nephew's efforts to make more grants outside Indiana, and he was reluctant to allow the staff to follow up after a grant was made, fearing this would lead to undue control or direction of a recipient's activities. At board meetings Eli Lilly sometimes introduced proposals not on the agenda. Although tactful and solicitous of the opinion of others, he usually had his way, particularly in granting money. When he suggested support for a particular item, the others would usually agree. Often Noyes would respond "Well, it's your money."[81] The annual report for 1952 proudly stated that "the operations of this foundation through the years have been closely supervised by its board of directors rather than by a highly specialized staff employed by the foundation."[82]

Eli's brother played a smaller role in the Endowment, even though he was president of the foundation from his father's death in 1948 until his own death in 1966. Through the Endowment J. K. Lilly, Jr., supported some of his special interests, including scholarship that produced a catalog of Thomas Jefferson's library and a bibliography of American literature. After 1966 Eli Lilly made sure that the institution continued funding some of his brother's projects. Eli paid close attention, for example, to the Endowment's annual grants to the Lilly Library at Indiana University, to which his brother had given his outstanding collection of rare books. When in 1973 the university's president, Herman B Wells, made an appeal for an increase in the $250,000 that the Endowment annually gave the library, Eli readily agreed: "Since that library was Joe's pride and joy, I'd be willing to double the amount we give Indiana University as a minimum."[83] While his brother was alive, Eli was usually careful to consult him before making large commitments. Eli decided while editing the Heinrich Schliemann diary, for example, that the Endowment should purchase the Schliemann papers for the Gennadius Library in Athens, but he carefully obtained his brother's approval before instructing the Endowment staff to make the $20,000 contribution.[84]

J. K. Lilly, Jr.'s, influence can be seen in a few specific Endowment projects, but Eli was a far larger presence in each of the Endowment's three major areas of activity during the 1950s—education, religion, and community service. He continued the family tradition of support for local charities and played a major role in bringing more system and efficiency to voluntary giving in Indianapolis. In 1954 the Endowment funded a detailed, three-year study of philanthropy in the Hoosier city, focusing on problems plaguing the loosely structured Community Chest. At the same time Lilly himself worked with the city's large corporate givers to encourage them to agree to limit the number of charity drives by joining a consolidated fund drive. The result of these efforts was the United Fund, formed in 1957 and generously supported by the Endowment in the following years. Local institutions such as the Children's Museum, the Indianapolis Home for the Aged, the Day Nursery Association, and the Boys' Club also received direct grants from the Endowment.[85]

Lilly's concern with strengthening traditional moral values was especially influential in funneling Endowment support toward religion, not only in the work of Ligon and Sorokin but in support of many other projects and institutions. Lilly directed the Endowment toward major contributions to Christ Church, the family church in downtown Indianapolis, and to many Episcopal causes. But the Endowment also supported many other religious endeavors, such as a program to strengthen Protestant theological seminaries in the nation; a research and training project to develop a plan for adult religious education; and an interdenominational organization called Yokefellow Associates, headed by D. Elton Trueblood of Earlham College and designed to prepare lay church members for leadership roles. The Endowment's very strong presence in religion was unusual, since very few American foundations shared this interest. By the 1950s the Endowment had emerged as the foundation perhaps most strongly identified with religion.[86]

The Endowment's programs in education reflected Lilly's special affection for church-related, liberal arts colleges in Indiana. As with his other serious interests, he did his homework, educating himself by reading. On his shelves were books about liberal arts education by the presidents of Carleton, Kenyon, and the University of Chicago, and by the dean of the Harvard Business School, all with Lilly's customary underlining of important passages.[87] The pharmaceutical manufacturer was loyal to his alma mater, the Philadelphia College of Pharmacy, and made large contributions to it, but he showed little interest in technical or professional schools.[88] He thought professors should be "men who have had some practical experience and not simply one hundred percent theoreticians," but he believed firmly in the values derived from a traditional liberal arts education, especially at "small liberal arts colleges like Wabash *without too much government influence in them.*"[89] In 1947 he established four scholarships at Wabash College in Crawfordsville, Indiana. Eli Lilly and Company funded the scholarships and provided summer employment for the students selected. Lilly hoped they would continue with the company after graduation, but he stipulated that "the student's education is to be in liberal arts rather than in vocational training for work in a specific business."[90] Near the end of his life he regretted that too many of America's universities, "once the conduit for our cultural heritage, have now largely declined into the mere training of specialists for career roles."[91] Occasionally Lilly raised the question of character education on college campuses, but he seems not to have pursued this systematically, in part because he believed that character education "probably will have to be done before the college age," and doubtless because he thought character would be strengthened simply by a good liberal arts education.[92]

Wabash College was Lilly's favorite. Founded by Presbyterian Yankees before the Civil War, it remained a men's school with high standards and, under President Frank Sparks, aggressive leadership. Lilly became a trustee of the college in 1946 and seldom missed a meeting until his death. Over the years he gave large sums of money to the institution. By 1961 his gifts totaled $1,639,375, most of it in Eli Lilly and Company stock. Many millions would be added later, making him the most important benefactor in the college's history.[93] As with other causes important to him, Lilly gave more than money and the prestige of his name. Often he wrote Sparks to report news from other campuses—an innovative fund raising strategy, a college president's report, a new lecture series, a revival of religion on campuses. Sparks, of course, kept Lilly fully informed of events at Wabash. The two men met often for lunch in Indianapolis, usually at the Columbia Club, where they discussed matters ranging from building a new library to bleachers for the football field to the student-faculty ratio and methods of instruction. After Sparks's retirement in 1956, Lilly warmly welcomed his successors, inviting them to lunch and continuing his close attachment to the school. Asked about this relationship in a 1973 interview, Lilly responded that he liked the men who served Wabash as trustees and presidents, especially Sparks, and then added, doubtless with a smile, that perhaps his large support was due also to the fact that Wabash was the first college to give him an honorary degree, which it did in 1938. Lilly also liked the school's strong liberal arts curriculum and its graduates.

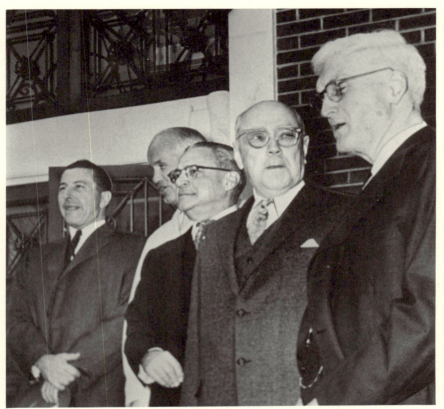

Left to right, Wabash College President Byron K. Trippet and trustees Ivan L. Wiles, Norman E. Treves, Eli Lilly, and Pierre F. Goodrich at the dedication of the Lilly Library, Wabash College, 1959.

Indianapolis Star

Several Wabash alumni became associates in his activities. One, Eugene Beesley, was the first non-Lilly to become president of the company and later the president of the Lilly Endowment.[94]

Eli Lilly was the driving force in the Endowment's campaign to improve Wabash and Indiana's other independent colleges. This long-term endeavor initially focused support on ten institutions: Butler, DePauw, Earlham, Evansville, Franklin, Hanover, Manchester, Rose Polytechnic Institute, Valparaiso, and Wabash. By 1957 the Endowment had granted these schools approximately $6 million for operating expenses and building programs.[95]

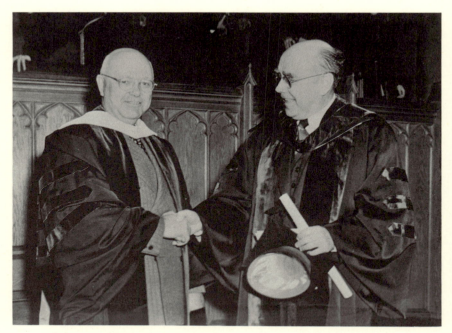

Clyde E. Wildman, left, president of DePauw   *Indianapolis News*
University, awards an honorary degree to Eli
Lilly, 1948.

In 1956 Lilly, his brother, and the Endowment staff discussed "a general overhauling of Endowment policy," with the purpose of "actively seeking good projects for the placement of Endowment funds."[96] One result of these discussions was a decision to concentrate even more heavily on higher education. In the years 1958-62 approximately $8.5 million was given to Indiana colleges. The unrestricted grants to the ten Indiana schools continued, although beginning in 1961 the Endowment required matching contributions from alumni or the sponsoring church. And the Endowment supported faculty development grants, programs to improve foreign language teaching, and requests for special projects, expansion of library collections, and new buildings. What college president would not respond eagerly to a letter like the one Earlham's president received from the Endowment in 1959, asking him to submit "a list of the four or five most urgent nonrecurring needs of Earlham College, arranged in order of priority." President Landrum R. Bolling listed a new library first in order of priority, and in 1963 Earlham's new Lilly Library was dedicated. Perhaps because educa-

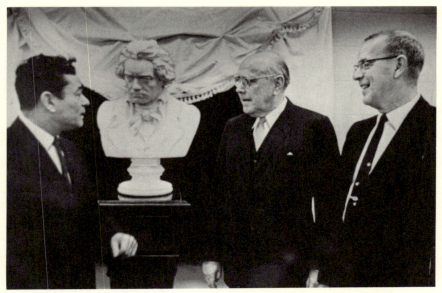

At dedication ceremonies of Lilly Hall, Butler
University, 1962, left to right, Izler Solomon,
Eli Lilly, and J. K. Ehlert.

Indianapolis News

tion was so important to him, Lilly eventually allowed the family name,
though not his own, to be attached to campus buildings. At Wabash,
Franklin, Indiana Central, Butler, and other campuses buildings bearing
the Lilly name sprouted.[97]

Endowment support for Indiana's private colleges extended also to
helping them help themselves in fund raising. Under the leadership of
Frank Sparks of Wabash and Thomas Jones of Earlham, the schools joined
in 1948 to form the Associated Colleges of Indiana. Based in Indianapolis,
the organization developed cooperative approaches to fund raising. It
particularly encouraged corporations to provide financial support for private
colleges, for "if free enterprise and free education were to continue, these
small schools should not turn to the Federal government with its possible
encroachment and control of what would be taught and how it would be
taught."[98] The Endowment was a major force in the Associated Colleges of
Indiana, underwriting the organization's administrative expenses by providing
$412,500 in support in its first decade and a half. The Indiana program
was so successful that it became a model for other states.[99]

While Indiana's independent colleges received the largest and most sustained support from the Endowment, several other institutions of higher education also attracted Lilly's interests. His research on Walam Olum led to support of Transylvania University in Lexington, Kentucky. In Kentucky also he developed an affection for Berea College, a school that emphasized Christian values and the work ethic.[100] There was also long-term support for predominantly black colleges in the South. In 1945 the Endowment began contributing to the United Negro College Fund. Lilly became a sponsor of the fund in 1951 and served in 1959 as honorary chairman of the organization's national convocation.[101]

There was one rapidly growing form of higher education that Lilly did not support. When the president of Purdue University asked him to contribute to a new library Lilly refused, arguing that "state institutions should be supported by the broad base of taxation." And he added, "the private colleges deserve more help because of the handicap they suffer under the competition with state institutions." Because of this belief the Endowment generally did not support state universities.[102] There were exceptions, for Lilly personally and for the Endowment. Indiana University's archaeology program received substantial support as a consequence of Lilly's interests and friendship with Glenn A. Black. And his brother's donation of his collection of rare books to the Bloomington school led to generous and continuing support of the Lilly Library there. There were a few special projects at state schools, such as the program begun at Indiana University in 1960 to provide more academic training for teachers of American history and another program at the University of Wisconsin to fund research in midwestern regional history.[103] And late in life Lilly urged Endowment support for a program in science and theology at Purdue in order "to smash up this monolithic objection to teaching morality and character in our public institutions."[104]

The patterns set at the Endowment in the 1950s persisted to the end of Lilly's life. The foundation continued to concentrate on the three areas of education, religion, and community service. And Indianapolis and Indiana received primary attention. Personal knowledge of recipients remained highly valued. A decisive comment at a board meeting, especially if it came from one of the Lilly brothers, was "Look, these are good people trying to do a good job. Let's help them."[105] There were, however, some slight twists and modifications within the Endowment in the 1960s and again in the 1970s.

The 1960s was a decade of unusually rapid change in America, affecting every aspect of life, including philanthropy. Reacting strongly against major social and political changes, the Lilly Endowment in these years took on a tone of strident conservatism, combining anticommunism, free enterprise, and religious fundamentalism. During the McCarthy era of the early 1950s, when many Americans found communists hiding under every bed, the Endowment had remained moderate in its reactions, as evidenced by Eli Lilly's continued support of Professor Sorokin. Beginning in the early 1960s, however, the Endowment began to make grants to right-wing and fundamentalist organizations. The amount of such support was relatively small: in 1964 the staff estimated that "10.3 per cent of our grants went into the support of the free society, plus another $306,000, or 6 per cent of our grants into projects designed to combat communism."[106] Thus, for example, in that year community service grants included not only $210,000 to the United Fund of Greater Indianapolis, $20,000 to a local home for unwed mothers, and $150,000 toward construction of Clowes Memorial Hall on the Butler University campus, but also $44,900 to the All-American Conference to Combat Communism, $15,000 to The Truth About Cuba Committee, and $10,000 to the Christian Anti-Communist Crusade.[107] The Endowment's annual reports in the early 1960s began to preach aggressively the virtues of free enterprise and evangelical Christianity. The report for 1963 claimed that philanthropy "should strengthen the foundation of liberty, which we interpret as including a belief in God and His Son Jesus Christ, a limited constitutional republic, the right to own property, and the freedom to engage in enterprises designed to maximize creative energies and their exchange."[108]

Just why the Lilly Endowment embarked on this path to the right in the early 1960s is unclear. Especially unclear is Eli Lilly's part in this departure. One certain source of the change was John S. Lynn. A graduate of DePauw University and the Harvard Business School, Lynn was the nephew of Charles Lynn, Eli Lilly's old nemesis during his early days in the pharmaceutical company. John Lynn had worked on McCarty Street for two decades before he joined the Endowment in 1961 to become general manager and director of community services. Soon after his arrival he was urging the need "to involve larger amounts in the defeat of Communism and the bolstering of the free market economy."[109] Lynn believed in the real and present danger of "the internationalist communist conspiracy"— an "evil conspiracy to take over the world."[110] And he held to a fervently fundamentalist brand of Christianity. John P. Craine, Lilly's close friend and the bishop of the Episcopal Diocese of Indianapolis, believed that Lynn was the cause of the Endowment's new face. "John Lynn is a real right winger in every respect," he wrote a colleague seeking Endowment support in 1966, and "I must warn you that they have consistently turned down almost every forward looking social or theological enterprise."[111] To another correspondent Craine commented on the appointment in 1964 of Charles G. Williams as the Endowment's director for religion. Williams was "a former Free Methodist minister, which tragically tells the story of the direction of the Endowment—ultra Conservative. . . . I have no particular influence with the new direction they have taken."[112]

Lynn had worked in market research with J. K. Lilly, Jr., who shared Lynn's political views and actively encouraged his transfer to the Endowment. J. K. Lilly, Jr., had shown only limited interest in politics before 1960. Sometime in the early 1960s he read Barry Goldwater's *Conscience of a Conservative*, which so greatly impressed him that he bought some 250 copies for associates. Soon after, he obtained from Goldwater a list of conservative organizations, from which he selected several for Endowment support.[113] J. K. Lilly, Jr., died in May 1966. The Endowment board memorialized him in a resolution, stating that "until ill health overtook him, he maintained a keen personal interest in many of the grants, particularly those in support of the preservation of liberty in the country he loved."[114] It may not be coincidental that during the late 1960s the Endowment purposefully reduced its grants to right-wing political and religious organizations and cooled the heated rhetoric that marked the annual reports of the early 1960s.[115]

Eli Lilly was never far from the center of the Endowment. He certainly knew about the new path to the right in the early 1960s and trod part of it himself, coming to share his brother's attraction to Barry Goldwater in particular. His personal financial contributions in the 1960s included some small gifts to the Christian Anti-Communist Crusade and a few similar organizations. Ruth Lilly's personal giving included gifts to a much larger number of such organizations, particularly those with religious orientations. While Eli's contributions of this sort declined and disappeared, Ruth continued this kind of philanthropy until her death. She was occasionally vocal in her support of conservative causes at Endowment board meetings and among friends, though her primary philanthropic interest was the Indianapolis Children's Museum.[116] The support Eli gave to ultraconservative political and religious organizations was not only small in dollar amounts but also distant in personal commitment. John Lynn later recalled the warm ideological support he felt from J. K. Lilly, Jr., and Ruth Lilly but not from Eli. In fact, Lynn eventually concluded that he had pushed his interest in the trinity of free markets, anticommunism, and fundamental Christianity "further than Mr. Lilly wanted to go." There is no evidence that Lilly read about and pondered these causes as he did those truly close to his heart. Strident anticommunism and emotional, rock-ribbed fundamentalism did not much appeal to Lilly.[117]

In areas within his major interests and affections, however, Lilly did react defensively to the liberal political and social changes of the 1960s. Senator Estes Kefauver's attack on the pharmaceutical industry in the early 1960s (discussed in chapter 10) doubtless helped bring about a more alert conservative political orientation for Lilly and his colleagues on McCarty Street. The social and political activism at Christ Church and within American Protestantism greatly distressed him, too, as the next chapter elaborates. Lilly was also upset by the upheavals occurring on college campuses, which by the mid-1960s were alive with protests of all sorts. Approximately 50 percent of Endowment grants in these years were made to education, mostly to higher education. In early 1965 Lilly became concerned that the political and social climate on many campuses did not allow sufficient voice to conservative professors. He asked Endowment staffers what could be done. Lynn and his associates responded by outlining policies already in place that supported the research of conservative scholars, especially those at "institutions which are not readily susceptible to being torpedoed by liberal administrators and faculty members."[118] Thus, the Endowment funded the research of economists Milton Friedman at the University of Chicago and Donald L. Kemmerer and his Committee for the Study of Individual Freedom at the University of Illinois.[119] And Endowment staffers reminded Lilly of the new visiting scholars program, which could be used to bring conservative academics to left-leaning campuses.[120] Lilly favored such programs, but after reading the reports from the Endowment staff suggested another response: "It seems to Mrs. Lilly and me that probably we have gone a little too heavily on colleges, especially in view of their leftist tendencies, and if something really good and promising in either of the other two fields [religion and community service] is presented we would be willing to see the 50% go down toward the 40%."[121] Such a shift did occur. In the period 1949-66 education received about 50 percent of Endowment grants, while community services and religion each accounted for about 25 percent. During the years 1967-76 the proportions changed, with community service grants increasing to 40 percent and education declining to a near-equal percentage. Religion accounted for the remaning 20 percent of Endowment grants in these years.[122]

Lilly also became more concerned in the 1960s about the growing presence of the federal government. He favored grants to organizations not beholden to Washington and was very much opposed to assisting colleges and universities that sought federal aid.[123] When he learned in 1965, for example, that the Indianapolis Symphony was "flirting with the Federal Government for a contribution" he thought such action would "change our attitude toward them."[124]

Most American foundations supported traditional and conservative causes, but the shift of the Lilly Endowment in this direction in the early 1960s was particularly noticeable. A major study, written by Waldemar A. Nielsen and published in 1972 under the title *The Big Foundations*, concluded that the Lilly Endowment was "a unique example of retrogression in development: after a steadily productive period of more than twenty years, it has more recently become highly ideological and as a result has now lost much of its good reputation in the swamps of the far Right."[125] Nielsen's criticism exaggerated the shift by failing to note clearly the relatively small proportion of Endowment funding going to conservative causes, but his attack stung nonetheless. Indeed, soon after the book appeared Lilly telephoned Nielsen from his Wawasee cottage. It was a weekend, and Lilly first apologized for disturbing Nielsen at home but said that he had just finished reading *The Big Foundations*. His initial reaction was anger, because Nielsen's account was unfair to the Endowment. Yet, Lilly admitted, there had been embarrassing support for some organizations and too much negativism and hostility to government. On balance, Lilly told Nielsen, his book was useful. Nielsen had never met Lilly and was not only surprised by his telephone call but also by his thoughtfulness and quiet modesty. A few months later Nielsen met Endowment board member Beesley at a social function. Beesley was more aggressive and brusque than Lilly but admitted that Nielsen's book had helped bring a resolution of difficulties that he and others had perceived at the Endowment. Both Lilly and Beesley told Nielsen that Lynn had to go.[126] Lynn did resign at the end of 1972, soon after Nielsen's book appeared, but in fact change had begun months earlier.

In July 1971 Lilly sent a memorandum to the Endowment board. "We should have broader and more important projects for the Lilly Endowment to back," he wrote. With this call to action he enclosed a list of the areas of interest of major foundations. Rockefeller, Ford, Danforth, Mellon, and others worked in such areas as the conquest of hunger, problems of population growth, quality of the environment, housing, equal opportunity, and conservation. "The opportunities," Lilly wrote, "for much broader and important studies to back are just waiting to be seized. Let's seize some! Let's go after some of these large and important projects."[127] A change such as this, Lilly always believed, required good leadership, and he set out to find someone who could provide that at the Endowment. He soon settled on Landrum Bolling. In working on Conner Prairie and Earlham College projects, Bolling and Lilly had often visited informally at Sunset Lane and Wawasee and discussed all mannner of issues. Lilly liked and trusted the fifty-eight-year-old Quaker. In August 1972 he offered Bolling the position of executive vice-president of the Endowment.[128] A new era in the institution's history began.

The 1970s brought change not only because Lilly willed it. So did the federal government. The large foundations had always generated mixed feelings among Americans, ranging from pride and gratefulness to envy and mistrust. Calls for government investigation and regulation had produced periodic outbursts that had little effect on their operations until the late 1960s. At a time when all institutions were under scrutiny and when the tendency to distrust wealth and power was unusually large, Congress began to investigate foundations. The leader in what evolved into a major attack was Representative Wright Patman, a maverick populist from Texas who uncovered a variety of financial abuses among some foundations. After hearings and debates Congress passed the Tax Reform Act of 1969, which had significant effect on all foundations. Critics had charged that many foundations were too closely tied to the business interests of their donors, creating a relationship that benefited the family and the business but not philanthropy or the American people. The Lilly Endowment was subject to this charge. Until 1968, when Eli Lilly's Sunset Lane neighbor, Byron P. Hollett, joined the board, all its directors were either members of the Lilly family or company executives. Nearly all Endowment assets consisted of Eli Lilly and Company stock. In 1971, of the approximately $4 billion worth of pharmaceutical company stock, Lilly family members owned about $1 billion and the Endowment about $900 million, an arrangement that reduced significantly the threat of outside influence in the company.

Because cash dividends on Lilly stock were not large, the Endowment's grant payouts were less than they might have been if its assets had been more diversified. The 1969 act forced several changes on the Lilly Endowment. In 1972 the Endowment was required to sell three million shares of Eli Lilly and Company stock and to place the proceeds in other investments. In addition to this step toward diversification the new law also forced the institution to increase its grant payouts, which rose from less than 2 percent of the market value of Endowment assets in the late 1960s to over 6 percent by the mid-1970s.[129]

It was Landrum Bolling's job to respond to these new regulations and their consequences and also to Eli Lilly's wish that the Endowment support broader and more important projects. Bolling had to manage the rapid rise in grant payouts caused by the 1969 act and also by an increase in assets due to a large payment to the Endowment in 1972 from a trust established by J. K. Lilly, Sr. Annual grants increased from less than $9 million in the late 1960s to over $50 million by the mid-1970s. To accomplish this the staff grew from six to seventy-five in a few years and moved to a large office building on North Meridian Street. The board expanded, too, with the addition of members not part of the Lilly family and company, including Indiana University president Herman B Wells, former Indiana governor Roger D. Branigin, and Wabash College president Byron K. Trippet. The Endowment retained its emphasis on education, religion, and community services and its support of Indiana and Indianapolis institutions. Lilly's interest in character development continued to have effect, too, as he periodically asked Bolling for an update on "the efforts with children" and "our effort to improve character." But character development evolved toward more support for applied research, counseling, and social work in juvenile delinquency, drugs, sexuality, and other specific problems of youth. Bolling visited the Character Research Project at Union College, and soon after the Endowment terminated funding. Religious programs remained important and expanded to support special seminary training for ministering to black and Hispanic Americans. While building on earlier concentrations Bolling and his associates also developed new initiatives. As he had suggested in early discussions with Lilly, Bolling began to encourage more grants outside Indiana and the United States, including support for programs to promote international understanding and to assist disaster relief in Africa. And there were grants made to organizations that received tax dollars, modifying some of the early fear of entanglement in the Washington tar baby.[130]

There was also in the early 1970s a modest beginning toward a new role in the city of Lilly's birth. Unlike the Colonel, Eli, his brother, and father had always been reluctant to take a commanding part in Indianapolis. It was nonetheless no surprise that when local newspaper reporters studied "Indy's movers and shakers" in 1964 and again in 1976 they discovered that Eli Lilly belonged to the handful of most powerful men in town.[131] His support of major cultural and social institutions in Indianapolis was essential to their well-being. Sometimes he was willing to use the power his wealth allowed. Annoyed by the Indianapolis Symphony's program selection, for example, he wrote Beesley in 1972: "We will undoubtedly have to make larger annual contributions to the Indianapolis Symphony if it is to survive. I am in favor of doing this provided they will have at least one program out of three like the Boston Pops. We won't give a cent otherwise!"[132] Lilly was generally reluctant, however, to impose directly or forcefully his will on his hometown. Because he believed that broad community support was an essential prerequisite for responsible philanthropy, he seldom took an aggressive public leadership role. In moving the community toward support of historic preservation, for example, he waited until a group of dedicated preservationists formed before committing his money and prestige.[133]

In the summer of 1972 Lilly met with Indianapolis Mayor Richard Lugar, a young and ambitious Republican with progressive ideas about improving the city. The two men discussed the quality of life in the central business district, which like many cities was becoming largely a place for suburban commuters to serve out their eight-hour days. One of the projects the two men discussed was the old city market, then standing in danger of the wrecker's ball. Lilly was eager to help, writing Beesley that "I have had in mind for a long time that we should be doing something for the city." Three days later Lilly wrote Lugar to tell him that the Endowment would likely provide support to renovate the city market.[134] Soon restored and alive with patrons, the market became one of the first signs of a revitalized downtown. Lilly was greatly pleased. When a threat developed that fast-food franchises might drive out local sandwich, fruit, and vegetable stands, he wrote an Endowment officer that his secretary, Anita Martin, "and other oldtimers are very much worried about allowing the Kentucky Chickens and the Burger Biggies to invade the market house. Is there any way we can influence the authorities in this matter to keep the foreign interlopers from having stands in this place?"[135]

A few months after Lilly and Lugar met to discuss downtown development, Lugar's chief aide, James T. Morris, moved to the Endowment to oversee Indianapolis projects. And in 1976, a year before he died, Lilly called Endowment leaders together to consider patterns of philanthropy. At a retreat in Nashville, Indiana, he suggested that perhaps the Endowment was scattering its resources too widely to be effective. From this meeting came a renewed commitment to Indianapolis, a commitment that, after Lilly's death, would lead the Endowment in partnership with others to transform the city's core.[136]

Eli Lilly was eighty-seven years of age when he selected Bolling to manage the Endowment. Confident in Bolling and in Gene Beesley, Lilly told the Endowment board in October 1972 that he was resigning as president: "Changes are coming too thick and fast for me to handle, and you all know that for the last several years I have lacked the training, experience and inclination to take an active part in the rough and tumble of increasing government control and other difficulties."[137] Despite this decision Lilly did not turn his back on the institution he had created. He not only supported the expanded programs Bolling initiated but also played a major role in a new commitment to the city of his birth. Until Lilly's death, Thomas Lake recalled, "nothing was done of major consequence about the Endowment unless he was involved." Even after his death decision makers in the Endowment offices often asked, "What would Mr. Lilly think of this?"[138]

Lilly's philanthropy was personal, thoughtful, and ambitious. He gave most of his money in areas that personally interested him. Thus, he concentrated on Indiana and Indianapolis and on history, archaeology, private colleges, religion, character education, and other areas of direct involvement and personal enthusiasm. He was aware of the dangers of philanthropy, of helping too much and thereby diminishing the potential for self-help. He knew the obligations of thoughtful giving, and he did his homework, though at times, as during the later years with Ligon, his heart ruled his head. He did not avoid risk taking. He challenged fundamental human problems in ways that practical people might regard as hopelessly romantic and idealistic. And in an age when many wealthy Americans gloried in displaying their affluence and power, Lilly insisted on anonymity. Even his close friends knew little about the extent of his generosity.[139] Although intensely engaged in giving, his was never a selfish, self-centered philanthropy.

On a rainy gray day, driving south on Meridian Street in Indianapolis, Lilly stopped at a traffic light next to a young woman riding a motor scooter.

Impulsively, he rolled down the window of his Rolls Royce and offered her his raincoat. She politely refused. At the next traffic light, Lilly repeated the offer, more insistently. This time she accepted, doubtless wondering about the identity of this unusual person. A few days later Lilly purchased several folded plastic raincoats, ready thereafter for simple, personal, rainy day philanthropy.[140]

Chapter 9

Pillar of Christ Church

There were few institutions Eli Lilly loved more than Christ Church. He was baptized in the church in 1885 and sang in the choir as a boy. In 1900 his family dedicated a new altar in memory of his grandfather, Colonel Eli Lilly. In young adulthood the grandson was only an occasional churchgoer, but in 1927, the year that he married Ruth Allison, he became a vestryman of Christ Church, serving in that position until late in life. Eli and Ruth were nearly always present in the family pew for Sunday services. When in 1928 the Lillys established the church library in memory of Eli's beloved Aunt Margaret Ridgely, Ruth immediately took charge of organizing and supervising it. Eli soon took a strong interest in financial affairs, persuading the church in the early 1930s to shift part of its small endowment from bonds to stocks.[1] In the early 1950s he served as junior warden, responsible for the property of the parish. A newly arrived rector later recalled his astonishment when he "discovered Mr. Lilly, taking his duties as junior warden very much to heart, in the furnace room of the church cleaning out an awful accumulation of debris."[2] Lilly's larger labor of love during the 1950s was his *History of the Little Church on the Circle*, published in 1957 (see chapter 7). This detailed, sprightfully written, and carefully argued book reflected on every page Lilly's strong attachment to the institution and its heritage.[3]

Lilly's love for Christ Church was an intensely personal attachment that grew as the years passed. It was the church of the Lilly family. When a young grandniece sat apart at a Sunday service Lilly sent her a note, kindly admonishing her to "ask to be seated in your Lilly pew."[4] Christ Church was part, too, of Lilly's personal religious conviction. His privacy and modesty kept him from outward displays of religiosity, and he had, as his rector noted, an impatience "for conventional religious small talk." But there was little doubt as to his fundamental belief in God, in the divinity of Jesus, and in the essential goodness of human beings. Nor was there doubt of his commitment to making religion a greater force through his philanthropy generally and particularly through his study of character development. His religious convictions, social beliefs, and family ties bonded him to Christ Church.[5]

From these bonds Lilly developed two special objectives for Christ Church: it must remain on the Circle in downtown Indianapolis, and it must attract strong leadership. During the 1950s he struggled mightily to achieve these two purposes.

In vestry meetings and conversations Lilly talked of the paramount importance of leadership in institutions generally and Christ Church specifically. The great moral of his history of the parish, he wrote, was that "leadership is the pearl without price." The church would survive only if led by rectors and vestrymen "with the qualities of knowledge, wisdom, dedication, and courage."[6] Lilly took an active part in pushing the appointment of John P. Craine as rector in 1950, preferring him over a local candidate Lilly considered too weak for the job. The thirty-eight-year-old Craine was well educated, with experience in several urban parishes, serving at the time as rector of Trinity Church in Seattle, Washington. He had a commanding presence and the kind of administrative talents that enabled him to accomplish tasks. Many in the congregation preferred the local candidate, however, and about half the members signed a petition to Craine urging him not to accept the rectorship. Lilly was convinced that Craine was the strong and experienced leader the church needed and, along with others on the vestry, stood firm, "trying to pour oil on the troubled waters of an incipient church row," while at the same time reassuring Craine that "the situation here is quieting down."[7] Craine accepted Lilly's reassurances and came to Indianapolis. He soon brought vitality and growth to Christ Church and became Lilly's lifelong friend.

Although Christ Church grew and prospered in the early 1950s, Lilly knew that population shifts in Indianapolis threatened its future. Many other downtown churches had already moved with their congregations to the rapidly growing suburbs. In the very center of the city, where churches had once ringed Monument Circle, Christ Church now stood alone. Lilly was determined that Christ Church must "hold the line."[8] In 1953 he gave to the Episcopal Diocese of Indianapolis securities worth approximately $1 million. This anonymous gift was probably his largest personal contribution to that date and represented his commitment to keeping the little

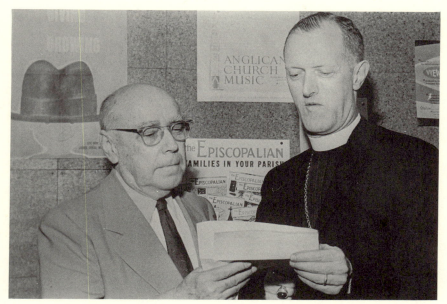

Eli Lilly presents his report as diocesan histo-
riographer to the Rt. Rev. John P. Craine, bishop
of the Episcopal Diocese of Indianapolis, 1962.

Indianapolis Star

church on the Circle. Lilly's deed of gift stipulated that the income from
the endowment was to be used to maintain the church in repair and to
continue its ministry to the community in the event that the congregation
became unable to bear the financial burdens. Christ Church was, as Lilly's
deed of gift noted, not an ordinary church of a few hundred Episcopalians,
but rather "a precious possession of the City of Indianapolis and of the
State of Indiana, standing in the very heart of the City and State as a visible
witness for Jesus Christ and as a symbol that the spiritual values of His
revelation endure while all material values perish."[9] Lilly included in his
gift a provision that the diocese could use excess income beyond the needs
of Christ Church for other purposes, and in the following years he carefully
watched to be sure that no one used this flexibility to the detriment of
Christ Church.[10]

Lilly's 1953 gift also included a suggestion from him that Christ
Church be made the procathedral of the diocese. In 1954 this was accomplished. John Craine assumed the new office of dean of the cathedral as

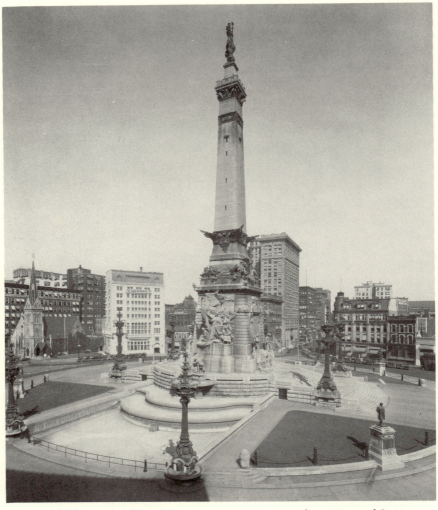

Christ Church, on the Circle, 1925.   *Indiana Historical Society*
                                             [93416-F]

well as rector of the church, and Lilly became one of the seven proctors responsible for governing relations between the diocese and Christ Church parish.[11]

Christ Church was now an even more prominent and permanent part of downtown Indianapolis. The Early English Gothic structure would stand heroically, enduring even as new bank buildings and hotels rose around it. "The symphonic lines of the little church, the sound of its beautiful chimes playing the old familiar hymns at noon and at five o'clock," Lilly wrote, would be "a blessed influence far beyond our imaginations to conceive."[12] But Lilly was not content with the symbolic influence of limestone and mortar nor with the sentimental appeal of hymns played on the new carillon he had given in memory of his father and mother. He wanted Christ Church to be a church of action in the community.

In 1956 Dean Craine was elected bishop coadjutor of the Indianapolis Diocese. Lilly was proud of this affirmation of his earlier judgment of Craine's leadership ability, but he knew also that this change would necessitate a search for a new person to serve as dean and rector of Christ Church. Lilly chaired the selection committee and gave the task the thorough and careful attention that was his nature. He wrote letters to many senior Episcopal clergymen, seeking advice. Typical was his letter in late 1956 to James A. Pike, notable dean of New York's Cathedral of St. John the Divine. Lilly wrote Pike that "we know the secret of the Church's success lies in this matter of leadership." And he emphasized that "we are agreed that the man should have a background of interest and concern in community affairs, as he should be able to speak out and work in these areas in Indianapolis."[13] In reading the replies from Pike and others Lilly carefully underlined and noted their main recommendations. One man very much appealed to him, and in early 1957 Lilly and his selection committee agreed that Paul Moore, Jr., should be called to Christ Church.[14]

Paul Moore might have seemed an unusual choice for an Indianapolis Episcopal church. Moore was born to a wealthy east-coast Episcopalian family and educated at the best schools, including Yale. He joined the Marine Corps during World War II, received a serious bullet wound in combat on Guadalcanal, and later was awarded the Navy Cross, Silver Star, and Purple Heart. What made Moore unusual, however, was that after graduation from the seminary he sought out an inner-city church, settling in Jersey City, New Jersey. There, from 1949 to 1957, he and his wife devoted their immense energies to problems of homeless and needy resi-

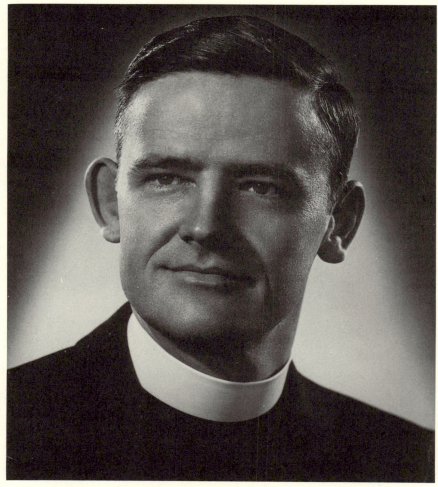

Paul Moore, Jr., dean and rector of Christ   *Christ Church Cathedral*
Church, ca. 1962.

dents, to issues of public housing and racism, and to organizations such
as the National Association for the Advancement of Colored People. Moore
soon developed a large reputation as a liberal, human-rights activist, an
energetic, inner-city clergyman, an Episcopal priest far removed from the
staid, conservative stereotype—long before the 1960s, when such a reputation would become commonplace among many young Protestant clergy.

Moore's long career in the church certifies his firm Christian belief and his consistent and enduring social action convictions. He did not hide these convictions from Lilly and the selection committee who interviewed him at Christ Church. Moore's experience in Jersey City appealed to them as just what Christ Church needed in Indianapolis, although it is possible that Lilly did not understand the full implications of Moore's commitment.[15]

Paul Moore and his family arrived in Indianapolis in the fall of 1957. Ruth and Eli Lilly were among the first to invite them to dinner. Moore had known Lilly's daughter at summer dances and parties on Boston's North Shore. He was thirty-eight in 1957, almost exactly Evie's age, and a handsome man, six feet, four inches in height. *Newsweek* later described him as a person of "immense personal charm, instinctive kindness, and a seemingly complete lack of guile." Lilly and Moore soon developed a close friendship, one that Moore thought approached that of father and son. They often had lunch together, usually next door to Christ Church at the Columbia Club and usually beginning with Lilly greeting Moore with the title "Mr. Dean!"[16]

Moore came to Indianapolis to continue the kind of community work he had done in Jersey City. He soon discovered, however, as he noted in a book he wrote while in the Hoosier capital, that "the spirit of the community, and therefore of the Church, is rather suspicious of progress and leery of anything which might seem 'liberal.'"[17] One issue on which the city was especially conservative was race. A survey by the Race Relations Committee of the Church Federation of Greater Indianapolis reported in 1955 that none of the main line Protestant congregations in town were racially inclusive. Well into the 1960s few blacks would have felt comfortable attending the city's white churches.[18] The new dean's first crisis came after he delivered a sermon condemning school segregation in Little Rock and after he had baptized several black babies at a Christ Church service. Some members of the parish were furious and let Moore know of their feelings. Lilly reacted differently. In the midst of the controversy he appeared at Moore's office with a "Good morning, Mr. Dean" and an apology for interrupting him, saying that he just wanted Moore to know that even "if you want to paint the church blue with pink polka dots, fine—I'll stand by you."[19]

Lilly backed up his supportive gesture with direct action. He told Moore that he wanted to make a special financial contribution so that Moore and Christ Church could help the city. The Episcopal dean, whose experience in large gifts had heretofore been in amounts of several hundred dollars, raised his hopes that the wealthy Lilly might be thinking in terms of several thousand dollars. Later, when Moore began a discussion with Lilly about how the church might spend such a sum, Lilly interrupted to say that he was not talking about "chicken feed."[20] Indeed not, for the discretionary fund Lilly established in 1958 and named in honor of one of his heroes, Christ Church's nineteenth-century rector Joseph Talbot, began with 5,000 shares of Lilly stock, worth $387,500. He stipulated that the Talbot Fund be used for salaries of clergy and for missionary and social welfare work in the city. He explained his wish in the deed of gift:

> The vocation of Christ Church Cathedral is not only to minister to its own, but also to serve the City of Indianapolis. The history of Christ Church Parish shows that the effectiveness of this dual voca-tion over the years has depended upon sound and inspired leadership by the clergy. In order to attract to the service of Christ Church Cathedral men imbued with the spirit of Christ it is important that they be paid adequately and provided liberally with the means with which to carry on their work. Christ Church Cathedral of the Diocese of Indianapolis, as administered by its clergy, should have a profound effect upon the life of the Church in the whole Diocese. By virtue of its location in the heart of the City and the State, and its vocation as the last Christian church standing in the downtown district, it should exert a leadership not only in the Episcopal Church, but in the spir-itual life of the whole city. Let no man ever suggest that this church be moved from its present location.[21]

With the Talbot Fund of 1958, Lilly gave Moore the financial base necessary to develop programs of the kind he had begun in Jersey City. Among these was the Cathedral House program, a ministry situated in a ramshackle building in the inner city which opened in 1960 to serve the physical, emotional, and spiritual needs of children in the neighborhood. The Cathedral House experiment attracted national attention. With the income from the Talbot Fund, Moore initiated other social programs, too, in planned parenthood, urban renewal, and intergroup relations.[22]

Moore and Lilly talked often about the social problems of Indianapolis and urban America. By the early 1960s many other Americans—journal-ists, scholars, church leaders—were also discovering the problems of the cities and seeking remedies. Moore was reading widely in the rapidly grow-ing literature on cities, partly in preparation for writing a book, published in 1964 under the title *The Church Reclaims the City*. As a result of their discussions Lilly and Moore agreed that Christ Church should undertake a systematic study to identify the special needs of residents and workers in downtown Indianapolis. With Lilly's backing Moore set up a three-year research program and in 1962 brought Peter Lawson, a young clergyman from Trinity Cathedral in Newark, New Jersey, to carry out the work.[23]

The social programs Lilly and Moore began in the late 1950s ended tragically. Indeed, Lilly's experience at Christ Church in the 1960s became one of the most unhappy events in his life. Two factors sparked the tragedy. Moore resigned in 1964 to become suffragan bishop of Washington, D.C. His successor was Peter Lawson, whose relationship with Lilly quickly turned bitter. Moore later recalled that had he stayed at Christ Church through the 1960s he might have been able to maintain Lilly's friendship, but of that he was not fully confident.[24]

The difficulty that would have challenged all of Moore's talents and did directly challenge Lawson's was the political and social turbulence of the 1960s. The times were changing, as the song of the day loudly proclaimed, and many Americans, particularly older people, strongly disapproved of civil rights demonstrations, student protests, new sexual mores, opposition to the war in Vietnam, and social welfare programs that blossomed with President Lyndon Johnson's Great Society. Some Americans, especially young ones, thought their churches had special obligations to be on the front lines, promoting social change through political action. In many main line Protestant congregations liberal clergy attempted to lead a sometimes reluctant flock toward racial integration or opposition to the war in Vietnam. Some commentators proclaimed the death of God, the emergence of a post-Christian era, or the dawning of the Age of Aquarius. With optimism and hope mingled despair and disillusionment, however, as crisis after crisis rumbled through the churches and all of America in the 1960s.[25]

Eli Lilly did not approve of the changing times. He tried to understand. A friend sent a copy of one of the most popular tracts of the day, Charles A. Reich's *The Greening of America*, which asserted that the youth of America, in beads, bell bottoms, and long hair, were effecting a revolution that "promises a higher reason, a more human community, and a new and liberated individual."[26] Lilly read Reich's prognosis for the coming revolution and wrote back: "To sum up the book, I would say that there are quite a number of starry-eyed ideas set in the matrix of rot with never a hint of how such heights of virtue are to be attained."[27] There were other, more concrete changes he did not approve. To Indiana University President Herman B Wells, Lilly wrote in 1968 to "tell you confidentially . . . that the recent action of the Board of Trustees of mixing sexes in dormitories has robbed me of pride and interest in Indiana University."[28] Ruth Lilly was more bitter and outspoken about these kinds of changes. Eli's reactions tended more toward disappointment than bitterness. Often he remained silent or tried to make the best of a controversial situation, a position perhaps derived from learning to cope with his own daughter's troubled youth.[29] When a close friend wrote to complain about the evils of the decade, particularly as caused by long-haired young Americans, Lilly replied: "The only thought worth having these days is that the present generation has always thought that the younger ones were going to spoil everything and it isn't spoiled yet—altogether!"[30]

The social and political tempest that blew through the 1960s whistled loudly at the doors of Christ Church. As it threatened to change radically the institution he so loved, Lilly reacted defensively and then angrily. Peter Lawson, the new thirty-four-year-old dean and rector, became the lightning rod of the storm. The new dean was bright and articulate but did not have Moore's stature or tact. And he had no experience leading a congregation like Christ Church. Yet he was determined to effect change, to ride the winds of the 1960s to a better world. Lilly spoke at the reception welcoming Lawson to his new position in early 1964. In his remarks the seventy-eight-year-old vestryman sounded a familiar tune for his Christ Church audience: "The best policy is to select fine leaders and back them through thick and thin."[31] But Lilly and Lawson were not kindred spirits, and although they had lunch several times Lawson found it difficult to get Lilly to say what was on his mind.[32] By mid-1964 there were signs of serious friction as Lawson's activist inclinations began to disturb some in the congregation. John G. Rauch, Sr., a member of Christ Church and Lilly's friend and personal attorney, met with Lawson in May to warn him that "he had to choose whether he would confine his activities to religious, theological, and philosophical objectives or to enter the political arena and engage in debate and agitations . . . such as public housing; juvenile delinquency; crime; racial integration."[33]

Lawson continued his political interests into the 1964 presidential campaign. The decisive event occurred at the Episcopal Church's St. Louis convention in October. Malcolm Boyd and other activist priests attracted great attention by circulating a petition condemning Republican presidential candidate Barry Goldwater as a racist. Lawson did not sign their document, but in St. Louis and back home in Indianapolis the young clergyman made known his strong opposition to Goldwater. Lilly, who strongly favored Goldwater, was furious and complained to Bishop Craine, who tried unsuccessfully to calm the waters.[34]

In December 1964 Lilly decided to have a frank talk with Lawson. So intense was his preparation for their meeting that he gathered his objections and wrote them out in essay form. He began his paper for the proposed talk by saying that "I have lost more sleep over this than ever before over any subject." Lilly estimated that a survey of the attitudes of the congregation would "show 30% on the left, 40% in the middle, and 30% on the right" with "as many dedicated Christians on the right as on the left." Yet "the image of Christ Church . . . is that our main interest is socialistic politics and not Religion." Citing the Biblical injunction to "'Render unto Caesar,' etc.," Lilly advised that "a minister who indulges in politics is bound to offend and lose quite a segment of his congregation. . . . I love Christ Church," he wrote. "Ruth and I would hate to leave . . . [but] we cannot very much longer attend and continue to support Christ Church with its present socialistic-political policy."[35]

In addition to a general unhappiness with Lawson's involvement in politics, Lilly's discontent by 1964 focused on two specific issues—public housing and racial integration. He outlined his concerns on small notecards he prepared to use to make his case before an unidentified audience, perhaps the Christ Church vestry or authorities of the diocese. Lilly began his notes with a general complaint about socialism in American politics and about the support the Episcopal Church had given as it "swung to the left of all other denominations." He then spoke of progress in housing and integration, pointing to the Talbot Fund and the resulting good work at Christ Church. But he labeled irresponsible the "statement by a clergyman of this diocese to the effect that the housing condition here is the worst in the land and endorsing federal housing." His notes also guided him through a discussion of racial integration, beginning with his assertion that "every Christian must support it." He outlined with pride the record of integration at Eli Lilly and Company during the 1950s and the support by the Lilly

Endowment for the United Negro College Fund and other programs to aid black Americans. But he expressed anxiety about the growing numbers of blacks attending Christ Church, encouraged first by Moore and then by Lawson. "I have not seen an objectional Negro in C[hrist] C[hurch]," Lilly admitted. "However we all know of numberless instances where neighborhoods and schools have been gradually infiltrated and taken over." Christ Church, Lilly warned, "is the most vulnerable point that the diocese has in the integration process. If we do not wish C[hrist] C[hurch] to become a negro church we will have to do some very careful planning." Lilly reiterated his understanding of racial equality: "Negroes should be treated the same as any other people—not more favored." Consequently, he advised, "all recruitment efforts should be stopped."[36]

Dean Lawson did not share these more traditional views of race, housing, or the ministry of Christ Church. He had great respect for Lilly and hoped that the two men could agree to disagree and that Lilly would continue to back him. That the older man could not do. In 1965 Eli Lilly took one of the most extreme steps of his life. He resigned from the vestry of Christ Church and as a proctor of the diocese. He did not formally surrender his membership in the church, but the pew in which he had sat for decades was empty as he and Ruth began attending services at Trinity Episcopal Church. And he stopped his financial contributions, writing Craine that "until Christ Church changes from a Socialist to a primarily religious organization, I will not give one cent directly or indirectly for its support." The Lilly Endowment, which had been contributing $25,000 a year to Christ Church, also ceased support. Lawson soon found it necessary to cut back staff and programs, including Cathedral House. By 1965 Christ Church faced a budget deficit.[37]

Lawson, as he later recalled, "was dancing on a tight rope."[38] He had won support of many younger, more liberal members of the congregation, but many others were alienated. The split was deep, and now the most prominent member of the congregation and the source of much of the parish's financial well-being had departed in anger. Lawson tried to patch up his difference with Lilly, writing him that "behind all my foolishness there lies a very personal and sonlike love and affection for you." Lilly refused to reply to Lawson's letter.[39] The courageous young dean continued speaking on controversial issues, including civil rights and later a sermon on the Vietnam War that sparked anger among some in the congregation.[40] Bishop Craine wrote to Moore in Washington, lamenting that "I have no choice other than to have him removed from his present position," asking

Moore to help in obtaining a place for Lawson. Rauch wrote Moore with a similar request, pleading, "For God's sake help us get rid of him!" Moore replied that he would offer help only if Lawson asked and added, "I am afraid I would agree with much Peter has done!"[41]

Lawson walked his tight rope at Christ Church until June 1971, when he announced his resignation. Lilly received the news with relief, delivered to him by Bishop Craine, who had stayed in close touch through correspondence and lunch meetings. During the summer and fall of 1971, the two men talked often, both recognizing that the wounds at Christ Church were not immediately healed with Lawson's departure. Lilly was particularly worried "about persuading any new rector to take over the wreck on the circle until the situation can be made to look more inviting."[42]

Craine took a step to make the situation more inviting when in November 1971 he appointed a Cathedral Select Committee to study and define the role of Christ Church in the Indianapolis Diocese. The committee reported that two major interest groups existed. One group preferred development "along more traditional parish lines" with limited involvement in the community. The other believed that Christ Church "should live on the cutting edge of Christian witness to the community" and that it "ought to be innovative in its ministry and fearless in its witness . . . in spite of conservative public opinion." The committee condemned the "present state of divisive factionalism" and urged the congregation "to understand and accept the diversity of its membership as a very positive strength." Christ Church, the committee suggested, could serve both the parish needs and the larger community needs if a more tolerant and democratic spirit prevailed.[43]

Lilly joined in the spirit of reconciliation by resuming financial contributions and attendance at Christ Church soon after Lawson's resignation. He was pleased by the appointment of a new dean and rector, Roger Scott Gray, in 1972, and in 1973, in addition to his customary annual contribution of $10,000, he gave Gray a check for $70,000 for building repairs. "Things seem to be getting along first rate on the Circle," he wrote a friend.[44] To the Lilly Endowment head he wrote: "during the incumbency of our late 'hippie dean' we didn't give anything. I am wondering if the Endowment wouldn't consider reinstating Christ Church in order to help keep it on the circle."[45]

Christ Church was once more closer to what Lilly hoped it would be. He developed a good relationship with Roger Gray, and they visited often in his last years. Gray later remembered vividly one of his early conversations with Lilly. After Ruth's funeral service Lilly invited the new dean back to the house on Sunset Lane. "Mr. Dean, do you know what your job is?" Lilly asked, as they sat down in his library. When Gray expressed uncertainty Lilly told him the terms of his will, which would provide 10 percent of his assets to Christ Church. He never told Gray how Christ Church should use the bequest, but remained content that Gray and future deans, vestrymen, and members would decide best. Lilly's only major stipulation was that Christ Church must remain always on the Circle.[46]

Christ Church did change, but not in the rapid or radical way that the 1960s promised. Membership did become more pluralistic, especially as more blacks sat in pews and moved into positions of leadership. At Christ Church in 1977 the nation's first woman Episcopal priest was ordained. And with money that Eli Lilly gave, particularly in the Talbot Fund and in his bequest of 309,904 shares of stock in Eli Lilly and Company in 1977, the church expanded its missions and welfare work in Indianapolis and as far away as South Africa. A decade after his death the church's endowment funds, which by then were valued at about $37 million, supported aid for the homeless, summer camps for inner-city children, alcohol and drug abuse programs, and many other extensions of the ideas Lilly, Moore, and Craine had discussed in the 1950s. And Christ Church stood firm—as a vital parish church, as a community of Indianapolis Episcopalians with a sense of stewardship, and as the little church on the Circle.[47]

Chapter 10

The Later Years, 1948-1977

When Eli Lilly left the presidency of the pharmaceutical company in 1948, he entered a period of his life that offered the potential of more time for personal leisure and relaxation. Leisure to him, however, was never simply quiet evening walks or idle gossip. Indeed, in the years from 1948 until near his death in 1977 his level of activity hardly declined and perhaps even intensified. It certainly expanded in range and scope, as he extended earlier interests and developed new passions. Like many people with active minds, he read widely. His attraction to the past continued in the 1950s and 1960s with archaeological and historical pursuits that centered on Angel Mounds, Walam Olum, the Indiana Historical Society, Shakertown, Conner Prairie, Historic Landmarks Foundation, and his own writing. He enlarged his quest for methods to develop moral character, and he spent many hours in a variety of philanthropic pursuits, contributing personally and through the Lilly Endowment.

Eli Lilly never retired. When he referred in correspondence to "my retirement," he placed quotation marks around the words.[1] Lilly was modest, unassuming, and quiet, yet under his placid exterior was an inquiring mind and an abundant physical energy that never went willingly into retirement. He believed in hard work, all his life. He believed in obligations, duties, responsibilities—all of which increased significantly after 1948. His sense of purpose and outlook on life often brought strains and burdens. Many people sought access to his wealth, and he sometimes felt weighed down by "the strenuous life of too many begging letters."[2] The organizations, boards, and committees he served were sometimes rent by divisiveness in which he found himself in the middle of conflict and hurt feelings, a situation he very much abhorred. Usually in such circumstances he tried to take a moderate, compromise position, as in a squabble over Clowes Hall, where he proposed to "lie low in the bottom of the boat as ballast,

which I hope will be of some use to everybody."[3] In a few instances, as in
the storm over Christ Church in the 1960s, Lilly was in the unhappy center
of the controversy. Meetings and correspondence of all sorts often required
his presence in Indianapolis. As summer turned to fall in 1957, he and
Ruth returned early from a respite at their beloved Lake Wawasee in order
"to plunge into a lot of activities that we would like to avoid—but they
seem necessary. We would so like to have watched the leaves turn at
Wawasee."[4]

Despite his active life Lilly did set aside time to enjoy some of the
prerogatives of a wealthy senior citizen. He found time to travel. There were
trips with Glenn and Ida Black to New Orleans on the steamboat *Delta
Queen* in 1949, to Mesa Verde and the Southwest in 1963, and often to
archaeological sites and to Williamsburg. Sometimes also the Lillys joined
Howard and Dorothy Peckham in Williamsburg. Often Eli and Ruth traveled alone on short trips to Shakertown, Kentucky, on longer trips to
southern California in 1950, 1954, and 1957, to the Canadian Rockies in
1953, to Yellowstone in 1967, and in 1952 to Mexico, where the pyramids
of San Juan Teotihuacan "fairly knocked our eyes out."[5] They made two
trips to Europe in these later years, first through England in summer 1954
and then to Italy, Switzerland, and France in 1957. Lilly kept detailed
diaries of the itinerary on each.[6]

No place was as appealing as the family cottage on Lake Wawasee.
There each summer he and Ruth escaped the heat of the city and the
immediate burdens of their responsibilities. Lilly was an entirely different
person there, one associate on McCarty Street recalled. His enthusiasms
burst out in guiding visitors over the lake on his pontoon boat and telling
them stories of early residents and events, or in displaying a new ice-
making machine, checking his wind gauge to see if he could sail his large
Dutch scow, waking late-morning sleepers by playing the Wawasee Waltz
on his hand-cranked Victrola, or simply enjoying easy conversation at
cocktail time on the big front porch or in his downstairs study, which he
called the hilarium. And there was time at Wawasee for the solitary life of
the mind, for reading and writing in the several fields that caught his
intellectual curiosity and commitment.[7]

There was more time in the later years for smaller amusements, too.
Lilly loved words. He continued his efforts at improving his writing, adding
new words and phrases to his "Shining Phrase" collection.[8] His letters to
friends, always brief, began to contain the sparkle of his father's correspondence, referring, for example, to the industrial south side location of

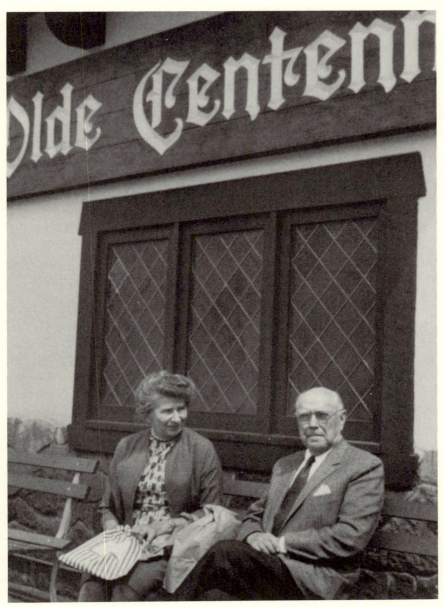

Eli and Ruth Lilly, ca. 1965.   *Eli Lilly and Company Archives*

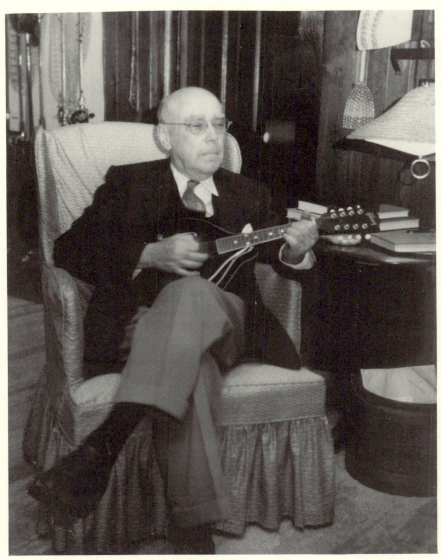

Eli Lilly playing the mandolin at his Wawasee
cottage, ca. 1959.

Eli Lilly and Company Archives

the pharmaceutical company as "the verdant valley of the Pogue," an allusion to a very small stream that flowed through the area.[9] He began to write poetry as verbal gifts, thank-you notes, and commentaries on everyday events. His trip to the Grand Tetons, for example, led to his commentary on modern dress among American tourists in a poem he titled "An Allergy Wrote in an American Resort," one stanza of which read:

> *Here nature's beauty is more solid than rock,*
> *While vacationer's styles are worse by the clock.*
> *You should just hear Ruthie's audible snorts*
> *At the women's tight britches and beach-boy shorts!*[10]

And, of course, he had more time to indulge his passion for reading, sometimes reading aloud with Ruth. He continued his interest in music, attending operas with the Blacks at Indiana University and listening to radio and to recordings of opera and of nineteenth-century American popular songs.[11] He developed a woodworking hobby, sawing, hammering, and painting in his basement shop at Sunset Lane and in a new garage shop at Wawasee. He stored his wood at the Wawasee shop in alphabetical order, from ash to walnut, and Ruth told visitors that he could find a paint can at midnight, blindfolded. He made a footstool, book display stand, dining table, and other items. A masterpiece of which he was especially proud was a Chinese tea table, which took form when he discovered some old pieces that the Indianapolis Children's Museum was planning to throw away. Lilly took them home and, he told Black, "painted up three very fancy phoenixes in Chinese red after gluing them together, and am now operating on a frame containing a bunch of twisted dragons, waves, and clouds to make a tea table."[12]

Lilly's tastes in amusement were simple and often inexpensive. He did indulge himself in some of the trappings of wealth. He bought a 1959 Rolls Royce Silver Wraith, for example, though in the first dozen years he owned it the odometer turned only 33,434 miles.[13] When Ruth wasn't along, he usually rode in the front seat with his driver so they could swap stories. He also owned a 1959 Ford Thunderbird, but his favorite cars were a small Nash Metropolitan and a Nash Rambler because "they never break down."[14]

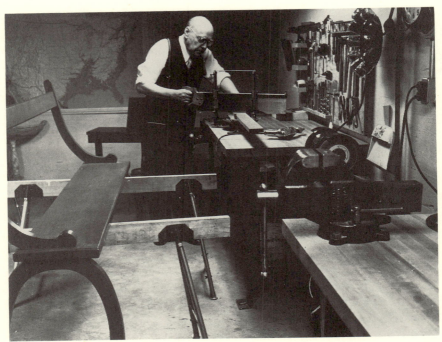

Eli Lilly in his basement workshop, Sunset Lane, 1957.   *Eli Lilly and Company Archives*

Like many wealthy men, Lilly also developed an interest in collecting art, though never the intense interest his brother showed in book, coin, miniature soldier, and other collecting. Eli Lilly bought in 1940 a Gilbert Stuart portrait of George Washington, which hung in his living room at Sunset Lane.[15] Later he acquired two paintings of Maxfield Parrish, whose art, he believed, "seems to sing of a golden age before Pandora opened her fateful chest, or to look forward to a bright supernatural future when all wrongs are righted."[16] His primary attention focused on Chinese art. At the end of World War II, Lilly expressed an interest in the subject to George H. A. Clowes, his pharmaceutical company associate who was also a serious art collector. Clowes asked around and learned that C. T. Loo of New York City was the best dealer in the field. Lilly visited Loo's shop and bought a couple of Song vases. In early 1947 he began serious collecting and purchased a dozen items from the New York dealer, including several bronze vessels, pottery vases, and hanging scrolls, for a total price of $21,000. Lilly was particularly interested in Song-type landscape paintings, but after Loo brought a collection of Song pottery to Indianapolis to show him Lilly could not resist buying it. Despite his effort to bargain with Loo, Lilly ended up giving the Chinese antique dealer his full price of just over $54,000. Loo made other profitable trips to Indianapolis and so did other dealers from New York and also from San Francisco and Los Angeles during the late 1940s and early 1950s.[17] In less than a decade Lilly had amassed "one of the finest comprehensive collections of Chinese art built by an individual in this country."[18]

Lilly had advisors in his purchases of Chinese bronzes, jade, ceramics, and paintings. In addition to Clowes, another researcher at the company also assisted. Pharmacologist Ko Kuei Chen served as Lilly's intermediary with several art dealers. Even more important was Wilbur Peat, director of Indianapolis's John Herron Art Museum. Peat was born in China, the son of missionaries, and combined an interest in Chinese art with an equally intense interest in pioneer Hoosier painters and architects. Peat and Lilly got along very well. Lilly never bought anything without first getting Peat's advice. Peat and the institution he headed benefited handsomely from the arrangement.[19] Lilly kept a small part of his Chinese collection at his home, but most he sent on loan to the Herron Art Museum. His intention, he told Loo, was to keep it there on loan until he and Ruth died, when it would become the museum's property—unless "we should be financially embarrassed before our departure."[20] Such an unhappy prospect dimmed considerably as the years passed, as did Lilly's interest in Chinese art. In 1960 he presented the entire collection to the museum.[21]

Lilly's ten-year period of active interest in Chinese art led to a related pursuit. In 1949 he purchased 115 acres of woodland along White River, adjacent to his Conner Farm holdings in Hamilton County. On the property was an abandoned summer home, situated high on a bluff overlooking the river. Lilly decided to transform the interior in Chinese style. He had the ceilings exquisitely painted with Chinese symbols and the rooms fitted with appropriate furniture and accessories. Lilly himself made two tables and painted a four-leaf screen. Chen presented several scrolls and portraits of Song emperors and helped select a name, "The House of Sylvan Harmonies," which he translated as "Shen Ho Shi." Lilly usually referred to the remodeled cottage simply as the Chinese house. He and Ruth used it as a weekend retreat and a place to entertain friends. It was the site, for example, of the sixtieth reunion of Lilly's 1891 kindergarten class. Long, wide porches overlooking the river were especially delightful but could not match the surprise and pleasure of visitors who walked into this Hoosier summer home and found such a dramatic interior.[22]

A Chinese house and art collection were hobbies for Eli Lilly. He once turned down an opportunity to purchase a group of paintings because the financial arrangement was too complicated. "I am looking for amusement rather than work and responsibility," he wrote Loo.[23] Yet Lilly's Chinese interest became more than a weekend hobby. He began after World War II to read about China and Chinese art, and, as in his other serious reading, to underline and take notes. This quest for knowledge derived in part from Lilly's general curiosity about the past, extending from ancient Greece to the prehistoric peoples of Angel Mounds and the Walam Olum to the pioneers of nineteenth-century Indiana. But it related to other interests as well, especially to his growing concern about values and the conflicts of the modern world. One of the first books he read was F. S. C. Northrop's *The Meeting of East and West*, which contained the message, Lilly later recalled, that "both the East and West must learn to appreciate the ways and thoughts of the other if disastrous clashes were to be avoided in the future."[24] Very much on Lilly's mind was the recently ended world war and the continuing conflict in China. His developing notions of Chinese culture as subjective, reflective, and mystical became part of his larger interest in moral character and the human condition, mingling with his reading of Sorokin, Ligon, and others. In a draft he sent Wilbur Peat for an introduction to a booklet on Song pottery, Lilly urged the need to "look beyond the mere perfection of the article and fully realize the universal response to beauty inherent in the Chinese people." In such character traits as "abiding serenity of spirit and gentle sympathy," he wrote, "we westerners fall far short of the Orientals." Materialistic westerners must strive "to attain, personally and nationally, a high appreciation of the beautiful tranquility of spirit and compassion."[25] Similar thoughts appeared in the pharmaceutical company magazine, where Lilly urged employees to "exercise more of the aesthetic values taught by the sages of the Orient: namely, compassion, sensitivity to all things beautiful, and equanimity, the calm joy of the spirit."[26]

Lilly's interest in Chinese art combined with his civic responsibility to make him a major benefactor of the Indianapolis Museum of Art, the successor to the Herron Museum. The major turning point in the institution's history came during the 1960s, with a search for a new building and location. Lilly was involved from the start, but the great incentive for change came after the death of J. K. Lilly, Jr., in 1966, when his son and daughter agreed to donate his home, Oldfields, and the forty-two acres surrounding it for the new museum. To this gift Eli Lilly added $1.7 million worth of pharmaceutical company stock, and he participated in the challenge to raise the many more millions of dollars the new museum would require. The chief fund raiser was Kurt F. Pantzer, an Indianapolis attorney and major collector of the work of the English painter J. M. W. Turner. Pantzer kept Lilly fully informed of the effort, particularly the wooing of Indianapolis businessman Herman C. Krannert. It was a difficult process because the relationship of Krannert and Lilly was not at all comfortable, in part because each was sensitive about treading on the philanthropic territory of the other. Krannert eventually pledged $3 million, and the Lilly Endowment added another $2 million. Another major gift came from the family of George Clowes. The two major portions of the new museum building were named the Clowes Pavilion and the Krannert Pavilion. Lilly not only refused to allow his name on the building but begged off speaking at the opening ceremony in the fall of 1970, "since," he wrote Krannert, "I know nothing about art or speaking either. I hope to enjoy the proceedings from the back row."[27]

Lilly was proud of the Indianapolis Museum of Art. Often he would take out-of-town guests there, bragging that now there was something to show visitors other than the 500-mile racetrack.[28] And he provided handsomely for the museum in his will. But compared to some other enthusiasms his attachment to the art museum was lukewarm and tentative, reflecting his sense of civic obligation rather than a driving personal interest. He worried in the late 1960s that the board of trustees, of which he was vice-chairman, had taken too large a financial risk in the massive building program, and he warned them "not to expect me personally or the Lilly Endowment to pull the project out of the hole."[29] As he had feared, however, the operating costs of the new museum were huge, and the Endowment did have to pull the institution out of the hole. Lilly approved such a course of rescue action in 1971, because the museum was "a great asset to the city and from a civic standpoint, the good citizens of Indianapolis cannot afford to let it fall on its face." The Endowment would play the part of good citizen, but Lilly was reassured by the fact that the new president of the museum board was Henry F. DeBoest, a pharmaceutical company executive he very much liked and trusted. Consequently, Lilly concluded, the Endowment could risk continuing "our policy of hand-to-mouth support" because DeBoest will "tip us off each time the sheriff approaches so that we can bail them out from time to time to prevent the sheriff's entrance."[30]

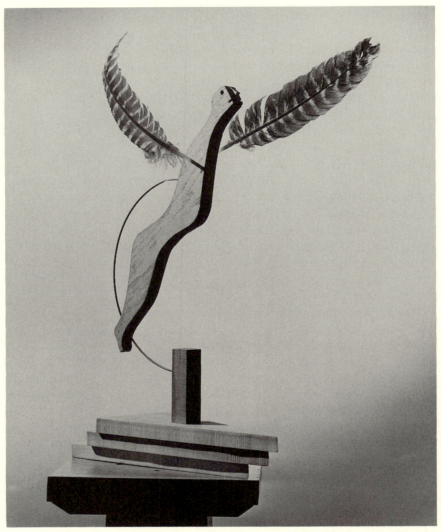

Eli Lilly's "Winged Victory of Sammy's Place,"   *Eli Lilly and Company Archives*
1972.

Lilly was cautious about the museum in part because, he wrote in 1971, "my dislike for extreme modern art is such that I have little enthusiasm for the whole business."[31] He thought contemporary artists and their admirers took themselves too seriously. To make his point he created a piece of modern art with some scraps from his wood shop and wax, wire, and feathers. He called it "Winged Victory of Sammy's Place," and with cooperation from Henry DeBoest and museum director Carl J. Weinhardt, Jr., the piece was exhibited at a contemporary show at the museum in 1972. On seeing his masterpiece in the show's catalog, Lilly wrote Weinhardt, with tongue firmly in cheek, that the photograph "was taken from the best position to get all the grace and composition that it possesses."[32]

Lilly's interest in art tended less to modern abstractions than to craftsmanship and beauty of the kind he admired in the Chinese porcelains he had collected. He visited the new museum often in the early 1970s, always spending time in the Oriental galleries, admiring the collection and reminiscing about how he and Peat had acquired specific pieces. He and Ruth also collected rare jeweled watches, which at her death went to the museum. When Weinhardt and his assistants came to Sunset Lane to pack the watches, Lilly and the museum director talked at length about the technical ingenuity and fine craftsmanship that the watches represented. Lilly then showed Weinhardt his collection of Paul Revere silver, also a superb example of craftsmanship. When Weinhardt expressed surprise and delight that such treasures existed in Indiana, Lilly said, "Well, they probably should go to the museum too." The assistants finished packing the watches and then moved to the silver, which, Weinhardt later recalled, was probably even more valuable than the watches.[33]

Most of his activities and obligations in his later years attracted Lilly not simply out of a sense of duty but because he was actively and personally engaged. In many instances this engagement and absorption provided a sense of accomplishment and a pride of achievement. Such was the case with his "retirement" years at Eli Lilly and Company.

His close, day-to-day responsibility at the pharmaceutical company ended in 1948, but he remained very much involved in fundamental decision making. He became chairman of the board in 1948, when his brother assumed the presidency. In 1953 he became honorary chairman of the board, and his brother became chairman. The death of J. K. Lilly, Jr., in 1966 brought Eli back to the chairmanship until 1969, when he moved

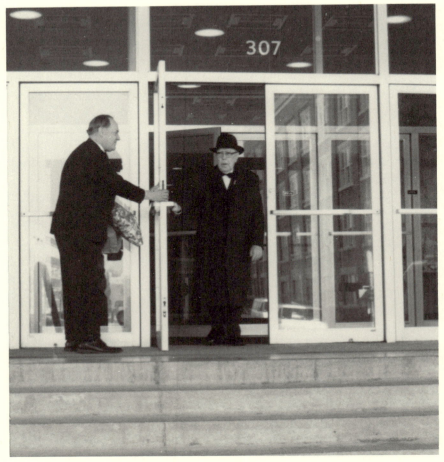

Eli Lilly leaving his office on his ninetieth birth-   *Eli Lilly and Company Archives*
day, 1 April 1975. Holding the door is his chauf-
feur, Peter Flokowitsch.

again to the honorary position. Lilly came to the office on a regular Monday, Wednesday, Friday schedule. He arrived punctually at 9:10 A.M. and left at 3:00 P.M., usually wearing one of his wide-brimmed Borsalino hats which he tipped to women he passed. Once in his office he would answer his mail and welcome visitors with and without appointments. Often he would walk through the halls on an errand of one sort or another, partly as an excuse to visit with fellow employees. At lunchtime he went to the company cafeteria, carrying his tray through the line. To many employees he was known with genuine affection as "Mr. Eli."[34]

Through these later years Lilly kept in close touch with active management, particularly with Eugene N. Beesley, the man he and his brother chose as president in 1953. The Lilly brothers were closely involved in the company reorganization of the early 1950s and in the selection and development of new managers in these transitional years.[35] President Beesley did not make a major decision without consulting Eli and, until 1966, J. K. Lilly, Jr., sometimes meeting in their offices, sometimes through memoranda, and sometimes in visits to Wawasee. Eli Lilly participated actively in decisions about such general matters as the proportion of budget expenditures to devote to research, discounts to wholesalers, bonuses for scientific researchers, and, in 1960, a new organization plan. And he participated in such specific challenges as attracting Jonas Salk's cooperation in producing polio vaccine and, as late as 1974, in a decision to acquire a new product line. Perhaps above all he remained eager that the large, complex company retain the corporate culture and particularly the employee morale that he associated with the decades when the Lilly triumvirate were in day-to-day leadership. He listened to employee concerns and faithfully attended twenty-five year banquets and retirement luncheons, serving, he said, as a cheerleader on the sidelines.[36]

Lilly took great pride in the company his grandfather had founded. In the early 1960s he and his brother decided that a full company history ought to be written. They engaged R. C. Buley, a Pulitzer Prize-winning historian at Indiana University, to write the history, assisted by Gene E. McCormick, who took primary responsibility for the project after Buley's death in 1968. In conversation and memoranda the researchers and Lilly exchanged information about the company's past. Like many successful businessmen, Lilly regretted that the company had not kept fuller records of the earlier years of the business. The project led to collection of additional family and company materials and a large number of oral history interviews. As Buley and later McCormick finished chapter drafts, Lilly read and critiqued them. He did not force his interpretation of events on the historians, nor did he want his own role exaggerated. Indeed, the pressure McCormick felt most acutely derived from Lilly's clear wish to keep his own achievements submerged in the larger story. Although the history was never completed or published, the typescript drafts and the materials gathered constitute very good sources about many aspects of the history of Eli Lilly and Company.[37]

There was good reason for Lilly's pride in the pharmaceutical company, for it was clearly among the most successful businesses in America. He was proud that the institution continued to hold to many of the traditions established during the active leadership of the Lilly family. Research remained fundamental to the business, as it had been since the Lillys hired Clowes in 1919. A survey of basic research in American industry in 1955 ranked Eli Lilly and Company twelfth among all industrial corporations.[38] Major drugs developed during Eli Lilly's active involvement, particularly insulin and penicillin, continued as sales leaders, even as new pharmaceuticals appeared. The attention to employee well-being continued, too, as did the impression that "Lillys" was one of the best places to work, whether for a high-school graduate looking for a job on a production line or a research chemist wanting to find a cure for cancer. There were changes, brought by growth, by competition, and by increasing government regulation. And there was diversification into agricultural and other products. But much remained the same.[39]

Eli Lilly never sought honors, but they came to him and the company. A survey of 423 business executives by the University of Michigan in 1967 ranked him among the twenty-five greatest living American businessmen.[40] In 1958 the American Pharmaceutical Association awarded him its highest tribute, the Remington Honor Medal. Letters of appreciation poured in. At the banquet ceremony in New York City the Indianapolis company's competitors turned out in large numbers to honor one of the most respected men in the business. In response to a request from the dinner organizers for choice of music, Lilly suggested that "arias of Italian opera, Victor Herbert, and Stephen Foster would fill the bill." Lilly's acceptance speech was sprinkled with quotations from his "Shining Phrase Book" and marked by tributes to his father and other associates in the business.[41]

Lilly's Remington address also touched on the subject of government regulation. Like many American businessmen, he had been grumbling about government since the New Deal, but in the late 1950s and early 1960s the issue became increasingly worrisome. In his 1958 Remington speech Lilly expressed his hope that the pharmaceutical industry "will continue to demonstrate beyond all socialistic propaganda to the contrary, that free enterprise in all areas of the health field will best insure the quality of medical care that the citizens of this great country have come to expect as their natural right."[42] Contrary to Lilly's wishes, however, many Americans were beginning to believe that health care was an issue of large public interest, one that required greater government regulation.

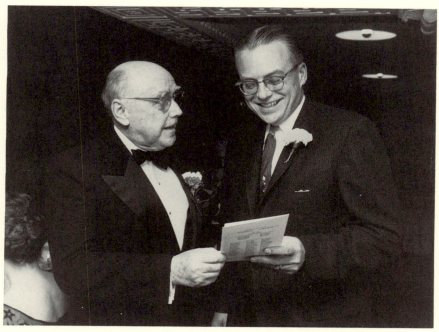

Eli Lilly and Eugene Beesley, president of Eli Lilly   *Eli Lilly and Company Archives*
and Company, at Remington Medal award dinner,
1958.

Even one of Eli Lilly and Company's great triumphs of the 1950s produced government entanglement. Following Jonas Salk's discovery of a polio vaccine in 1953, the Indianapolis company won a major role in mass production of the new vaccine. It was a difficult and laborious process, one that Lilly watched closely in 1954 and 1955, perhaps remembering the hard and glorious days of the insulin work in the early 1920s. Eventually the Lilly label appeared on more than half the Salk vaccine used, vaccine that helped produce a decrease in the number of paralytic cases of polio in the United States from 18,308 in 1954 to only several dozen by the late 1960s. The achievement brought public acclaim and substantial sales increases, but it also brought the attention of the federal government.[43] In 1958 the government charged the Indianapolis company and four others with price fixing in selling polio vaccine. Lilly was irate. To a friend he wrote that "we are hot under the collar here because of the government's accusation of our having connived with our competitors to fix prices on

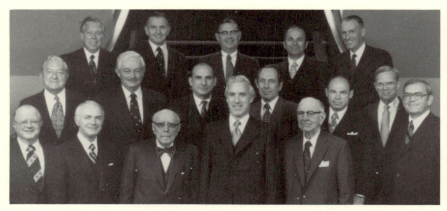

Eli Lilly and Company Board of Directors, 1976. *Eli Lilly and Company Archives*
Top row, left to right, Earl B. Herr, Robert S.
MacNeill, A. Malcolm McVie, Mel Perelman,
Eugene F. Ratliff; middle row, left to right, Albert
L. Williams, Burton E. Beck, C. Harvey Bradley,
Jr., Raymond E. Crandall, Eugene L. Step,
William McC. Martin, Jr.; bottom row, left to
right, Harold M. Wisely, Thomas H. Lake, Eli
Lilly, Richard D. Wood, Nicholas H. Noyes,
Cornelius W. Pettinga.

polio vaccine. It is a most absurd charge and we feel pretty small reward for the risks and efforts that we have put forth."[44] Long litigation followed. Defended by New York lawyer and 1948 Republican presidential candidate Thomas E. Dewey, the five drug companies eventually were exonerated, as the federal court held that the government prosecutors failed to substantiate their accusations.[45]

By the late 1950s there was more than a price fixing case to worry Lilly, Beesley, and other company executives. After years of basking in high profits and public respect, the pharmaceutical industry found itself the target of intense criticism in the press and Congress. Critics attacked the quality, safety, and cost of ethical drugs. Senator Estes Kefauver led the charge, using what many in the pharmaceutical industry thought were unfair and sensational methods to gain public support for tighter regulation. Kefauver's case gained powerful cogency when Americans learned that a new drug, thalidomide, had caused European women to give birth to babies without hands or feet. In 1962 Congress passed the Kefauver-Harris bill, which tightened earlier regulatory legislation, particularly in seeking to ensure safe and effective drugs.[46]

Lilly looked scornfully on this meddlesome activity in Washington. "It takes about fifty percent of the time of our top brass to fight our own government," he grumbled in 1961.[47] In addition to opening a regular legislative office in the capital, the Indianapolis company also began a more concerted public relations campaign, one in which Lilly was closely involved. Included were slogans such as, "For four generations we've been making medicines as if people's lives depended on them." And there were advertisements designed to present the industry's point of view. These ads, Lilly wrote a friend in 1963, would "help inform the public that brother Kefauver did not know what he was talking about. Before Kefauver, only six percent of the people of the United States thought the drug companies were making too much money. The ornery Kefauver put it up to sixty percent, so we have a disagreeable job ahead of us."[48]

Beesley and other executives at Eli Lilly and Company learned, as managers at all successful American corporations had to learn, how to function within the new regulatory climate of the 1960s. Lilly by this time was moving closer to the sidelines than the center of the playing field and did not have to compete actively under the new rules. He was affected nonetheless, particularly in his political attitudes.

Politics was never one of Eli Lilly's passions. He contributed small sums to Republican campaigns and only occasionally lobbied a politician on a special issue, such as preservation of his beloved Angel Mounds.[49] In the late 1940s he joined his brother and others in contributing to Indiana Senator Homer E. Capehart's study of social welfare in England. The results, Lilly concluded, showed that the British were sinking "into the muck and quicksand of socialism." He was particularly distressed "to see them trying out state medicine and other nefarious practices at our expense!" But, he concluded, "if their failure will prevent our pitching headlong into the same quagmire, it will be well worth the present cost (to us)."[50] Lilly had a lifelong animus against Franklin D. Roosevelt and the New Deal, noting in 1952 that "I would vote for anybody against that New Deal crowd, especially Kefauver."[51] His conservatism was not all-inclusive, however, for he rejected unequivocally Indiana's vigorously anticommunist senator of the 1950s, William Jenner. On an ocean voyage to Europe in 1957 Lilly rejoiced in meeting a passenger whose "dislike for Senator Jenner put us on common ground."[52] Nor did he like conservative Republican Robert Taft, thinking him an isolationist who could not win election to the presidency. Rather, Lilly was a strong supporter of Dwight Eisenhower in 1952 and later, a man whose qualities he listed as: "Great administrator! Great Personality! *Can* get the votes!"[53]

During the early 1960s, when politicians were harassing his company, Lilly showed a stronger interest in politics. He read and underlined *The Businessman's Guide to Practical Politics,* published in 1959.[54] More important, he read, doubtless at his brother's urging, Barry Goldwater's *The Conscience of a Conservative.*[55] Goldwater's call for a return to free enterprise and a reduction in government regulation and taxation was the sound of Gideon's trumpet to Lilly's ear. Lilly believed fervently that "competition unlimited is what has put the U.S. way ahead of other nations whose cartels protected the weak & reduced ambition all around."[56] And he was convinced that free enterprise in the economic sphere was closely connected to personal liberty in the political sphere, a cause his brother and the Lilly Endowment embraced in the early 1960s. Goldwater's dismal failure in the 1964 presidential election showed that the American people did not share this brand of conservatism. Even Hoosiers rejected the Arizona Republican, casting their first majority vote for a Democratic presidential candidate since 1936. Lilly was disheartened by the election results. "We are now among the socialist nations," he lamented. "Ruth and I have said a number of times we are glad we are as old as we are."[57] The Goldwater bust left Lilly disenchanted with politics. He refused a request from Gerald R. Ford in 1967 to contribute to the Republican party treasury: "When the Republicans cease to be a 'me too' party to the left, I shall be glad to help once more."[58] Lilly did resume small contributions to Republicans later, but without the enthusiasm he had shown for Goldwater.

After 1964 Lilly's favorite politician was a Democrat. Roger D. Branigin was elected governor of Indiana in his party's landslide victory in 1964. A folksy raconteur, Branigin represented the wing of the state's Democratic party that had never been fully comfortable with the New Deal nor with President Lyndon Johnson's Great Society. Lilly thought him "the best governor we have had for my lifetime at least" and took to describing himself as "a Goldwater American who is also a Branigin Hoosier."[59] The two men got along very well, sharing a love of history and a joy in telling stories and jokes. Lilly supported Branigin's causes, ranging from Franklin

College, his alma mater, to his campaign against Robert F. Kennedy in Indiana's 1968 primary. In 1973 he put Branigin on the board of the Lilly Endowment.[60]

In politics and in many other areas more important to him Lilly faced the challenges of aging. "Old age ain't no place for Sissies," he often told visitors. One friend put the saying on a pillow, which Lilly fondly kept in his library. And to acknowledge greetings on his ninetieth birthday, he composed one of his short poems:

> *A recent saying that seems sage*
> *States sissies are not for old age*
> *But kind words from friends*
> *Make full amends*
> *And certify we haven't turned the last page.*[61]

Changing times brought new ways he did not understand or approve, from the new social activism at Christ Church to modern art at the Indianapolis museum and modern music at the Indianapolis Symphony. Much popular entertainment he found distasteful. At Butler University's Clowes Hall, where Lilly served on the advisory board and to which he made large contributions, the popular musicals were far different from those he so loved from turn-of-the-century America. The breaking point came in 1973, with a performance of *Grease*, a Broadway musical about teenage love set to rock-and-roll music. Lilly resigned in protest, writing Dr. Clowes's son that he was simply "out of patience with the present tendency of many of the performances being so full of four-letter words, innuendo and vulgar situations."[62]

A more personal challenge of aging came with the loss of friends. "Most of our dear old friends are in the churchyards," Lilly wrote in 1973.[63] Only a few of the Rowdy Revelers, his Wawasee fishing group, were still alive to reminisce about the annual spring visit to the lake. Archaeology friend Glenn Black died in 1964. History friend Howard Peckham remained

active, "representing the only live friend I have left," Lilly wrote in 1971.[64]
Lilly could make humor of the situation, telling the story of Clemens
Vonnegut, one of the city's nineteenth-century settlers who also outlived
most of his contemporaries. At the service for one of the last of his friends
at Flanner and Buchanan, the local funeral home, Vonnegut remained
seated after the conclusion of the proceedings. To an attendant who finally
inquired if he was feeling well, Vonnegut replied, as Lilly told the story,
"Oh, yes, I was just wondering whether it's worth the trouble to go home
or not."[65]

Not only did Lilly outlive the men of his generation, but he also found
it difficult in later years to make new friends. Peckham was one of the few
people left who addressed him by his first name. To nearly everyone else
he was Mr. Lilly or Mr. Eli. His age, wealth, and status were barriers many
people could not overcome. And Lilly himself could not always be sure if
others were interested in him or his money. He did make a few new friends
in these later years. The unpretentious sincerity of Landrum and Frances
Bolling made them comfortable and trusting, and they visited often.[66] But
many others found closeness difficult. Wabash College president Byron K.
Trippet was one of many later acquaintances who never got to know him
well: "I often wondered if anyone was really close to him. One of America's
richest men, his modesty, his preference for anonymity, his shrewdness
about people and business, his dry sense of humor—all of these attributes,
it seemed to me, kept him at arm's length from others."[67]

Death took family as well as friends. His brother died in 1966. His
daughter, Evelyn Lilly Lutz, died in 1970 at age fifty-one. Evie found some
stability and contentment in her last years. Her struggles with alcoholism
in the 1940s led to sometime membership in Alcoholics Anonymous, but
she battled the disease all her life. Following two unhappy marriages, she
wed Herbert Lutz in 1953. Her father attended the ceremony at the couple's
farm in Pennsylvania. "Whitey" Lutz was little more settled vocationally
or emotionally than Evie, and he was not always faithful to her, but the
marriage was a happy one. They eventually settled on the island of St.
Thomas in the Caribbean, where they built a theater and set up a charitable
fund to provide medical care. Eli came to trust her sufficiently by 1958 to
give her company stock outright rather than in trust. Evie and Whitey
visited occasionally at Sunset Lane, but she never felt entirely comfortable
there, even though her father and stepmother did all they could to provide
that comfort. There is every indication nonetheless that father and daughter
loved each other. In her last letters she addressed him as "Old Beeswax"

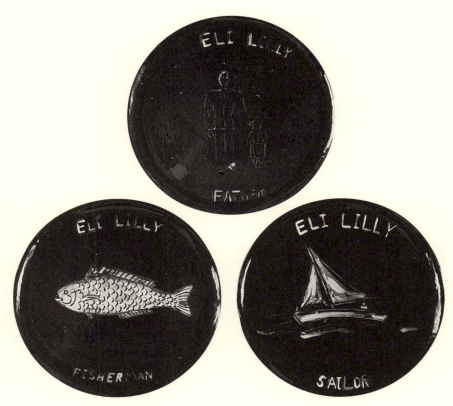

Three of the plates Evie Lilly made for her father,   *Eli Lilly and Company Archives*
depicting major interests of his life.

and "Dearest love." In one of her avocational interests she made him a set
of pottery dinner plates. Each plate had his name at the top, a description
of one of his interests at the bottom, and a drawing of that interest in the
center. The activities Evie chose to depict were farmer, horseman, fisher-
man, pharmacologist, Indian authority, sailor, and father. Evie died of throat
cancer on 5 April 1970. At her request, she was buried at the Moravian
Church in Lititz, Pennsylvania. Her father attended the service, and at the
conclusion turned to Evie's mother, whom he had not seen in years. They
did not speak, but Lilly kissed Evelyn Fortune Lilly Bartlett on the cheek
before walking away from the grave of their daughter. He was now truly
the "last of the Mohicans."[68]

Evie left one final unhappiness for her father. In early 1968 she and Whitey adopted Whitey's infant granddaughter, Sarah. Evie intended to tell her father, but kept postponing it. Lilly learned of the adoption only after Evie's death. He was furious. The brunt of his anger was directed at John Rauch, Sr., his personal attorney and the father and law partner of John Rauch, Jr. The younger Rauch was Evie's attorney and the lawyer who had handled the adoption and then, after Evie's death, became the trust guardian of young Sarah. Lilly firmly believed that the senior Rauch had an obligation to tell him of the adoption. Rauch had been his attorney for decades and was a personal friend, closely associated with Lilly at Christ Church, the Indiana Historical Society, and the Indianapolis Museum of Art. Lilly felt betrayed. In early July 1970 he fired Rauch, as extreme a personal act as Lilly had taken since his divorce. He then went to Byron P. Hollett's law office, without an appointment, and called him out of a bank directors' meeting to ask if he would become his personal attorney. Hollett had no idea what was happening except that Lilly was clearly very upset.[69]

Part of Lilly's anger had to do with large sums of money in family trusts for Evie, trusts established by her father and grandfather that now might go to a child he did not know. Lilly held no bitterness toward Sarah or Herbert Lutz. As he explained to the senior Rauch, "my gratitude and affection for Herbert Lutz himself and for his loving care of Evie are very strong. For his son and daughter-in-law and little Sarah our feelings are very warm, and we hope that Old Father Time will strengthen these bonds."[70] But Lilly's belief that he had been deceived made it impossible for him to assent to this unknown child inheriting large sums of family money. The trusts stipulated that Evie's issue would be the beneficiary. Evie had no children born to her. The sticky legal point centered on whether the word "issue" included adopted children. Hollett might have argued that it did not at the time the trusts were created and that this meaning should prevail. The trusts therefore should revert to Eli Lilly. Lilly recoiled at any publicity over the dispute, however, and insisted that Hollett settle the matter in a quiet manner. Eventually, the lawyers and the court agreed to a Solomonic settlement that divided Evie's trusts in half, with one half going to Sarah and the other to Lilly. Lilly eventually received 600,000 shares of company stock from the settlement, which he immediately gave away—to Earlham College, Wabash College, and the Children's Museum.[71]

Evie's ability to make her father unhappy thus extended beyond the grave. Why Evie adopted the child and why she never told her father of the adoption is unclear. In this intensely personal and sad affair Lilly kept

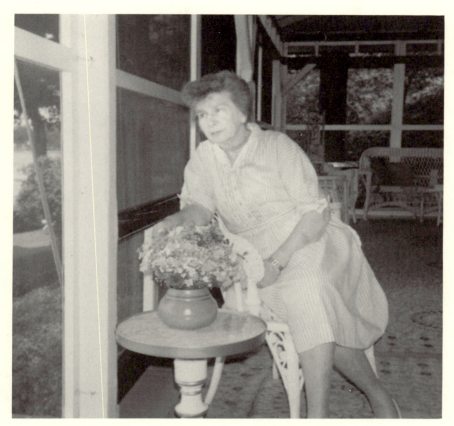

Ruth Lilly on the porch of the Wawasee cottage,   *Eli Lilly and Company Archives*
ca. 1965.

his thoughts to himself. He could not hide his anger for the senior Rauch, however, nor could he hide from Hollett his disappointment with Evie for not confiding in him.[72] He had tried so hard to be a good father. His failure with Evie was perhaps the greatest disappointment of his life.

A year after Evie's death doctors found an ominous spot on Ruth Lilly's lung. Earlier, breast cancer had led to mastectomies. Now, in early 1971, doctors began a severe course of cobalt treatments that slowed but did not stop the cancer. In December 1972 Eli wrote a friend that Ruth was "gallantly holding her own, but we are a good deal like the ancient Greeks who, in connection with agriculture, prayed to the gods for success but kept their hands to the plowtail." Ruth died on 14 March 1973 at the age of eighty-one. She had been his wife for more than forty-five years, his best friend and closest confidante. He adored her. After her death there were no more Christmas trees at Sunset Lane, no more magical summer evenings on the front porch at Wawasee. On her tombstone he placed her birth date and, rather than death date, the symbol for infinity.[73]

Through most of his life Lilly's health was excellent, with only minor problems. Into his mid-eighties his step was sure and firm, his hands steady, his mind alert. He complained of lumbago in the 1930s. In mid-1947 he had an emergency appendectomy and minor surgery again in late 1965. Gradually he granted aging its due and made concessions. In 1956 he wrote the Rowdy Revelers, following their fortieth annual fishing trip, that perhaps it was time to "call it a day, with many happy and priceless memories." Three years later he sold the last of his sailboats, noting that for the first time in sixty-four years he was without a sailboat.[74] His most troubling health problems were a deterioration of hearing and then sight. By the mid-1960s he was wearing a hearing aid, without which, he wrote, "I can't hear thunder."[75] When presented the Alexander Graham Bell Award in 1966 for his service to the deaf, Lilly played "Amaryllis," one of the songs from his childhood, on his hearing aid, whistling the notes the instrument could not play. The local newspaper reported that "his virtuosity brought down the house."[76] After his driver Peter Flokowitsch was treated for throat cancer, Lilly told him that "now, we're the perfect couple. You can't talk and I can't hear."[77] Loss of reading vision also caused problems during his last four or five years of life, especially after Ruth's death. His secretary, Anita Martin, would read to him, as would friends like Frances Bolling. Lilly became especially excited about books recorded on tape. "They are my life saver and I have listened to about 30 or 40 in the last year," he wrote an old Rowdy Reveler in 1974. "One of the best things about it, they don't cost a cent at any time! Our blind school provides the machine and the records or cassettes come postpaid in your mailbox."[78]

Eli Lilly was lonely in his last years. He missed Ruth terribly. His intense energy and quiet enthusiasm were no longer as apparent. Yet he did not retreat from life, nor did he become crabby and abrasive. Callers came to Sunset Lane, where he continued his practice of greeting them at the door and walking with them to their car at the end of a visit. He went to small dinner parties, to church services, to meetings, and three days a week to the pill factory. Friends planned special occasions for him. One was a dinner party, where the Dean of the Indiana University Music School played the piano, and Lilly and a few friends joined eagerly in requesting

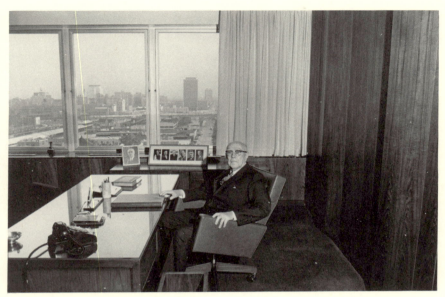

Eli Lilly in his office, looking over downtown
Indianapolis, 1968. To his right are photographs
of his father and the other six men, he always
told visitors, who "taught me the business."

Eli Lilly and Company Archives

folk songs and popular tunes of the late nineteenth century. Often he would
visit Conner Prairie, and sometimes the art museum. He attended the
ceremonies for the new Ruth Allison Lilly Theater at the Indianapolis
Children's Museum and enjoyed immensely listening to Robert Merrill's
selection of songs on that occasion. He and Merrill had met on an ocean
crossing in the 1950s and exchanged vitamins for record albums in the
years after. There were also memories to provide company. In 1975 he
wrote insulin scientist Charles Best that "I often think of the stirring and
delightful times we have had together and take great pleasure in living
them over."[79] Sometimes he would reminisce to his secretary, Anita Martin,
explaining changes in the city as he stood looking out the large window
in his twelfth-floor office. He doted on two small dogs he and Ruth had
acquired. The little affenpinschers were "cuter than punch," he admitted,
especially because "I like dogs the nearer they approach zero in size."[80]
The spring after Ruth's death he retreated to Wawasee: "The dogs and I
and the Talking Books start out for the lake tomorrow morning to see how
long we can stick it out."[81] He made a few more short visits to his beloved

Lake Wawasee but after a brief stay in the summer of 1975 doubted he would "ever go again because the place is not what it used to be without Ruthie."[82]

_____

Having no illusions of immortality, Eli Lilly prepared for death with the care and thoughtfulness that characterized his other projects. His brother had refused to draw a will that would specify disposal of his home and many of his collections. During Joe's last year Eli tried to talk with him about the subject, but without success. Thus, much to Eli's frustration, there were huge taxes due on his brother's estate, which necessitated selling some of the family's pharmaceutical company stock. There was also, Eli regretted, "the unfortunate publicity about stamps and coins and the death taxes upon them [which] would have been avoided" with a properly drawn will. [83]

Eli Lilly carefully planned the disposition of his property. Before he died he settled all arrangements for his real estate holdings. The apple orchard north of Indianapolis, which his father had given him and his brother, went to Park School in 1965.[84] The Wawasee cottage he committed to the three oldest children of J. K. Lilly III, to be claimed on his and Ruth's death. He wrote them in 1968 to explain this intended bequest. As with most of his giving, he attached no strings to the Wawasee property, "for my experience has taught me that it is futile and often pernicious for one generation, which has passed on, to leave behind restrictions which often prove to be fallacious." He did tell the young Lillys, however, that even though he was the sole owner of the cottage he had "always considered it to be a family estate," descended from their great-great-grandfather. He hoped they would "keep it in the family."[85] To nurture that wish, he began carefully to encourage visits during the summers. As he explained in 1973, he was "trying to vaccinate the young people to the old cottage and seem to be succeeding very well."[86]

Lilly also planned a future for his Sunset Lane home. In 1971 he committed the property and most of its contents to Indiana University, to be used, after his death, as the Indianapolis residence of the university president. His father's home next door he also gave to the university for use by the head of the Indianapolis campus. In late 1971, as these arrangements were being concluded, Lilly made a thoughtful addition to the gift. University chancellor Herman B Wells came away from a visit with Lilly carrying a personal check for $1 million, given as an endowment to maintain the homes.[87]

Lilly's assets in company stock, cash, and bonds were considerably larger than his real estate holdings. By the end of 1959 these included 392,310 shares of Eli Lilly and Company stock, worth $31.5 million, about $1 million in cash, and $2.5 million in tax-free bonds.[88] His strategy for disposing of these assets, which continued to grow in the 1960s and 1970s, was to keep his estate "as simple as possible."[89] Thus, he planned to give it all to about a dozen recipients on the basis of designated percentages of the total value of the estate. Lilly carefully insisted that Ruth and Evie should receive the same amount, which he set in 1968 at 5 percent of the total. The rest would be divided among Lilly's favorite institutions. In January 1968, for example, he decided this would mean 10 percent each to the Indiana Historical Society, the Indianapolis Art Association, the Indianapolis Children's Museum, Earlham College, Wabash College, the Philadelphia College of Pharmacy, and Butler University for support of Clowes Hall. Six other institutions would receive 5 percent of the estate: Park School, Orchard School, Historic Landmarks Foundation, Trinity Episcopal Church, St. Paul's Episcopal Church, and Tudor Hall School. Lilly paid close attention to "this percentage business," as he called it, working out different arrangements on scratch paper and changing the numbers and the institutions to suit changing circumstances. Most important, perhaps, was the absence of Christ Church and the Episcopal Diocese of Indianapolis from the list during the late 1960s and their addition later.[90]

Fund raisers of all sorts sought access to Lilly's wealth in his last years. He was "hounded to make investments, gifts, contributions, etc., etc., etc."[91] His will provided a means of easing the pressure in a few instances. Approached for additional contributions to Clowes Hall, for example, he replied that "I would prefer not to give anything at the present time unless there is dire trouble, because my will is all on a percentage basis and I can't give any large sums without robbing all the rest on the list."[92] He could also respond to impatient fund seekers by pointing to his age: "My will calls for certain things to be done for Butler University, and you may not have long to wait because I am almost 83 years old," he wrote in 1967.[93] Only a few people knew the nature of Lilly's will. He did discuss it with Bolling, McLaughlin, Roger Gray, and possibly a few others, but not in much detail. Weinhardt at the art museum knew nothing about Lilly's plans for his institution.[94]

Ruth's death gave Lilly additional determination in turning away fund raisers. He explained the situation to Bishop John Craine in 1975: "My will is now frozen as regards such things as a result of an agreement with Ruth just before she left us that I would not change a thing in regard to the 23 favorite projects of ours."[95] Lilly incorporated his agreement with Ruth into his will by setting aside 20 percent of his holdings of Eli Lilly and Company stock for distribution on a percentage basis to Ruth's eleven special interests. At his death this 20 percent of his stock holdings amounted to 774,760 shares, worth nearly $33.8 million. The shares were distributed as follows: Ruth's favorite institution, the Children's Museum of Indianapolis, received 14 percent; 11 percent went to Save the Children Federation and to each of three struggling Southern schools she had supported, The Berry Schools, Mt. Berry, Georgia, The Piney Woods Country Life School, Piney Woods, Mississippi, and Alice Lloyd College, Pippa Passes, Kentucky; and 7 percent each for the Day Nursery Association of Indianapolis, the American Committee for Keep, Cooperative for Relief Everywhere, Fellowship in Prayer, Episcopal Diocese of Indianapolis, and the Washington Cathedral.[96]

The remaining 80 percent of Lilly's 3,873,800 shares of pharmaceutical company stock he distributed to his most favored thirteen institutions. Receiving 10 percent each (309,904 shares with a value at Lilly's death of about $13.5 million) were the Indianapolis Museum of Art, Butler University, Earlham College, Wabash College, Philadelphia College of Pharmacy, the Indiana Historical Society, the Children's Museum of Indianapolis, and Christ Church. The five institutions that received 4 percent or 123,961 shares were Orchard School Foundation, Park-Tudor Foundation, Trinity Episcopal Church, St. Paul's Episcopal Church, and Historic Landmarks Foundation of Indiana. Lilly's will also provided for small personal gifts to a few friends, relatives, and household staff.[97]

As with his gift of Wawasee to another generation of the Lilly family, Eli Lilly made few restrictions in his will. He stipulated that his bequests to the Indianapolis Museum of Art, Philadelphia College of Pharmacy, and Wabash College were not to be used to construct buildings. He wanted Clowes Hall to have first call on the bequest to Butler, and Conner Prairie first rights to the Earlham bequest. The only other restriction was on Christ Church, which did not receive its bequest directly. Lilly's will set up trusts at three Indianapolis banks, the income from which would go to the church only so long as it remained on the Circle.[98] Beyond these, there were no other restrictions, reflecting Lilly's belief that such constraints were unwise and unnecessary.

The institutions to which he bequeathed his money were those closest to him personally. They reflected his interests in history, historic preservation, education, and religion. In many instances he had played an important and personal role in shaping the institution and knew well the people in responsible positions. His bequests were the last of a series of gifts that had included not only his money but his active engagement. To the end, he gave his money not simply to dispose of it and not simply out of a sense of civic obligation, but because he believed—sometimes passionately—in the institutions and causes that were the objects of his philanthropy. Uniting nearly all was their location in Indianapolis and Indiana, marking Lilly's permanent affection for a particular place.

The value of Lilly's estate at his death was about $165,775,000.[99] During his long life he had given away many more millions of dollars, as had the Lilly Endowment. But Lilly was never much impressed with the size of his fortune or his philanthropy. Money was important to him. He watched it carefully and did not waste it. But it was not the currency with which he kept score in the game of life.

In his last year there were several special occasions—a birthday party at the Morris-Butler house, the dedication of the new building of the Indiana Historical Society, and a luncheon of his closest associates at Conner Prairie.[100] Perhaps most important was the centennial of Eli Lilly and Company. Lilly participated in planning the occasion, making clear that "I would hate to hear this rock and roll business like we had at our last 25-year dinner." Instead, he suggested Strauss waltzes, Gilbert and Sullivan, Victor Herbert ("any number of his"), Stephen Foster, Tchaikovsky, Verdi, and, most specifically, "There's a Tavern in the Town."[101] As his health deteriorated the centennial of the company became increasingly important. "I have just gotten through my 90th birthday by the skin of my teeth," he wrote an old friend after suffering a mild stroke in April 1975, "and my main thought in life is to last another year to celebrate the 100th

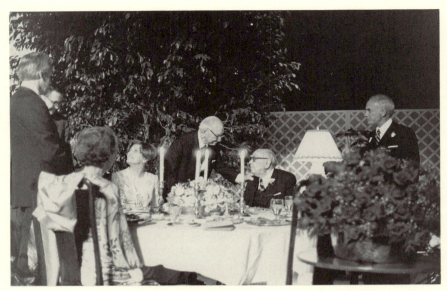

Head table at Eli Lilly and Company's 100th   *Eli Lilly and Company Archives*
anniversary dinner, 1976. Left to right: Richard
D. Wood, A. Malcolm McVie, Mrs. Thomas H.
Lake (seated, back to camera), Anita Martin,
Nicholas H. Noyes, Eli Lilly, Thomas H. Lake.

anniversary of the company on the 10th of May, 1976."[102] Lilly survived
to attend the anniversary affair, a gala occasion for which the Indianapolis
Convention Center was decorated to look like Pearl Street in 1876. He
arrived without fanfare in the middle of the celebration, but as the crowd
noticed he was there a quiet descended and soon tears glistened in the
eyes of more than a few employees.[103]

By mid-1976 Lilly was using a wheelchair much of the time. He tired
easily, but his mind remained clear. He dressed every day in suit and tie,
and on those days he felt too tired to come to the office his secretary went
to Sunset Lane to take care of correspondence and read to him. In mid-
December his doctors discovered he had liver cancer. Lilly refused to use
the word "cancer," referring to it as "my old enemy," the disease that had
killed his grandfather, father, wife, and daughter. In early January 1977 he
insisted on making the traditional New Year's call on Indianapolis pharmaceutical wholesalers, a custom begun by his grandfather. It was his last
duty for the company he had joined in 1907.[104]

Lilly entered University Hospital in mid-January. He died the after-noon of 24 January 1977, with Anita Martin and Roger Gray, the dean and rector of Christ Church, nearby. It was a cold winter day, fitting Lilly's observation that he was born during one of the coldest winters of the nineteenth century and would die during one of the coldest of the twentieth century. Three years earlier Lilly had instructed his attorney, Byron P. Hollett, and Anita Martin of the procedures to follow at his death. They informed the people he had listed, selected a casket according to his instructions, arranged for the funeral service at the Gothic Chapel in Crown Hill Cemetery and burial in the family lot immediately after, followed a few days later by a memorial service in Christ Church. He wanted flowers like those at Ruth's funeral. And he wanted placed in his casket a blue velvet pillow from his library that had been made from Ruth's wedding dress. In his instructions to Hollett and Martin, Lilly insisted also that "the regular Episcopal Service from the Prayer Book (dated 1928) be used," and added, "I do not want any eulogies or remarks made at the service." He advised Hollett and Martin to be sure there was security for his house so that his domestic staff could attend the funeral if they wished, told them to give his clothing to the Episcopal Church, and reminded them that Topsy and Tiger, his affenpinscher dogs, were to go to live with Anita Martin in the country.[105]

Notes

Abbreviations used in the notes of this book are: Eli Lilly = EL; J. K. Lilly, Sr. = JKL, Sr.; J. K. Lilly, Jr. = JKL, Jr. The Eli Lilly Papers are abbreviated ELP. Unless otherwise noted, all unpublished sources cited in the following notes (including ELP and record groups, such as XBLl) are from Eli Lilly and Company Archives, Lilly Center, Indianapolis.

Preface

1. EL to C. W. Hackensmith, 21 Apr. 1972, Hackensmith Folder, ELP.
2. Quoted in Leon Edel, *Henry James: A Life* (New York: Harper & Row, 1985), 432.

Chapter 1

1. EL to Russell C. Hill, 12 Jan. 1973, American Institute for Character Education Folder, ELP.
2. JKL, Sr., to EL, 1 Apr. 1940, EL Miscellaneous Papers, Lilly Family Papers, XBLl.
3. Birth announcement, Photo Album 1, Eli Lilly Room, Lilly Center. After his grandfather's death Lilly did not use the Jr. Eli's father studied the Lilly genealogy and located the family's first Eli in Sweden in 1470. The first American Eli Lilly migrated to Maryland from England in 1789. He was the great-great-grandfather of the subject of this biography. J. K. Lilly, Sr., "The Name Lilly," *Lilly Review* 2 (May 1942): 21; (Aug. 1942): 17.
4. John W. Rowell, *Yankee Artillerymen: Through the Civil War with Eli Lilly's Indiana Battery* (Knoxville: University of Tennessee Press, 1975), 8.
5. Ibid., 3-124; John W. Rowell, *Yankee Cavalrymen: Through the Civil War with the Ninth Pennsylvania Cavalry* (Knoxville: University of Tennessee Press, 1971); R. C. Buley, "A History of Eli Lilly and Company," typescript, 1966, chapter 2, pp. 8-65.
6. EL to Jackson G. Henderson, 24 Dec. 1969, H Miscellaneous Folder, ELP; EL, "Reminiscences," typescript, 1966-69, XBLl. This very important document is unpaged.
7. Sidney Speed to EL, 6 July 1918, XBLl; Rowell, *Yankee Artillerymen*, 269-71, 273; Gene E. McCormick, "A History of Eli Lilly and Company," typescript, 1974, chapter 10, pp. 194-96.
8. EL, "Reminiscences."
9. Jacob Piatt Dunn, *Greater Indianapolis: The History, the Industries, the Institutions, and the People of a City of Homes,* 2 vols. (Chicago: Lewis Publishing Co., 1910), 2:689. See also Buley, "History of Eli Lilly and Company," chapters 3, 4, 5; Roscoe Collins Clark,

Threescore Years and Ten: A Narrative of the First Seventy Years of Eli Lilly and Company 1876-1946 (Indianapolis: Eli Lilly and Co., 1946), 7-40.

10. JKL, Sr., "Reminiscences," 6-8, 33-36, typescript, 1940, XBLl. Quotation on page 35. See also Buley, "History of Eli Lilly and Company," chapter 3, pp. 8-13, 44-46, 60-64. Colonel Lilly and his second wife, Maria, had one child, a daughter born in 1871, who died in 1884.

11. JKL, Sr., "Reminiscences," 64; Buley, "History of Eli Lilly and Company," chapter 4, p. 4.

12. EL, "Reminiscences." One of the reasons Lilly got along so well with a new secretary late in his life was that they both discovered on their first meeting that as children they were deathly afraid of owls. Anita Martin, interview with author, 5 May 1988.

13. EL, "Reminiscences"; Eli Lilly, *History of the Little Church on the Circle: Christ Church Parish Indianapolis 1837-1955* (Indianapolis: Christ Church, 1957), 236. Sometime in the 1970s Lilly came to his office and dictated to his secretary the names of the families living on Tennessee Street. He then checked his memory against a city directory. In most cases he was correct. Martin, interview with author. See also Charlotte Cathcart, *Indianapolis from Our Old Corner* (Indianapolis: Indiana Historical Society, 1965), 68, 70, 72-73.

14. Booth Tarkington, "The Middle West," *Harper's Monthly* 106 (Dec. 1902): 79. Tarkington did not identify Indianapolis by name in this article, but it is surely his hometown that provided the primary source of his sketch, as it did for much of his fiction.

15. Meredith Nicholson, "Indianapolis: A City of Homes," *Atlantic Monthly* 93 (1904): 840.

16. Anna McKenzie, comp., *Red Book of Indianapolis 1895-6* (Dallas, Tex.: Holland Brothers Publishing Co., 1895), 7. See also Cathcart, *Indianapolis from Our Old Corner,* 55.

17. Lilly, *History of the Little Church on the Circle,* 246-47.

18. Hester Anne Hale, *Indianapolis: The First Century* (Indianapolis: Marion County/Indianapolis Historical Society, 1987), 40-56, 84-89, 94-114; Indianapolis Board of Trade, *Indianapolis: The Great Manufacturing Center of America* (n.p., 1894).

19. Booth Tarkington, *The Magnificent Ambersons* (Garden City, N.Y.: Doubleday, Page & Co., 1918), 386.

20. Nicholson, "Indianapolis: A City of Homes," 839.

21. Robert G. Barrows, "Hurryin' Hoosiers and the American 'Pattern,'" *Social Science History* 5 (1981): 197-222; Robert G. Barrows, "Beyond the Tenement: Patterns of American Urban Housing, 1870-1930," *Journal of Urban History* 9 (1983): 395-420; Hale, *Indianapolis,* 125. For Hoosier moderation see James H. Madison, *The Indiana Way: A State History* (Bloomington and Indianapolis: Indiana University Press and Indiana Historical Society, 1986); and Peter T. Harstad, "Indiana and the Art of Adjustment," in *Heartland: Comparative Histories of the Midwestern States,* ed. James H. Madison (Bloomington and Indianapolis: Indiana University Press, 1988), 158-85.

22. Eli Lilly, *Early Wawasee Days: Traditions, Tales, and Memories Concerning That Delectable Spot* (Indianapolis: Studio Press, Inc., 1960), 51-54. Quotation on page 54.

23. EL, "Reminiscences"; Lilly, *Early Wawasee Days,* 75. Eli's brother, J. K. Lilly, Jr., shared this enthusiasm for "The Gunboat Series" and in the 1930s collected three hundred copies

of Castlemon's books and had a bibliography of his writings prepared. David A. Randall, *Dukedom Large Enough* (New York: Random House, 1969), 45-46, 349-50.

24. EL, "Reminiscences."

25. Last Will and Testament of [Colonel] Eli Lilly, 12 May 1898, Folder 3, Box A, 1, Legal Records, Vault; EL, "Reminiscences"; McCormick, "History of Eli Lilly and Company," chapter 8, pp. 90-104. Decades later Lilly would write his father that hearing a song such as "The Daring Young Man on the Flying Trapeze" "took me back to Tennessee Street." EL to JKL, Sr., 12 Aug. 1935, JKL, Sr., Letters, Vault.

26. Cathcart, *Indianapolis from Our Old Corner*, 23-26; JKL, Sr., "Reminiscences," 28; Robert G. Barrows, "A Demographic Analysis of Indianapolis, 1870-1920" (Ph.D. dissertation, Indiana University, 1977), 97; Gene E. McCormick, interview with author, 2 May 1988; Richard O. Ristine, interview with author, 27 Apr. 1988.

27. EL, "Reminiscences."

28. EL, undated notes for talk, ca. 1957, p. 2, Speeches Folder, ELP.

29. EL to Gene E. McCormick, 26 Feb. 1969, Lilly Company History Folder, ibid. See also Howard Peckham, interview with author, 2 Aug. 1985.

30. McCormick, "History of Eli Lilly and Company," chapter 10; McCormick, interview with author; Martin, interview with author; James B. Griffin, interview with author, 26 Dec. 1986; EL, "Reminiscences."

31. EL to Margaret Ridgely, 4 Mar. 1906, EL Miscellaneous Papers, Lilly Family Papers, XBLl; Ridgely to EL, 24 Dec. 1927, ibid.; EL, "Reminiscences"; Lilly, *History of the Little Church on the Circle*, 282.

32. EL, "Reminiscences"; *Indianapolis News*, 24 Nov. 1962.

33. EL, "Reminiscences."

34. Ibid. See also EL, undated notes for talk, ca. 1957, p. 1, Speeches Folder, ELP; Laura Sheerin Gaus, *Shortridge High School 1864-1981: In Retrospect* (Indianapolis: Indiana Historical Society, 1985), 61-74. In 1947 Lilly referred to Charity Dye and her quotation of Van Dyke in the pharmaceutical company publication *SuperVision* 2 (July 1947): 1.

35. Gaus, *Shortridge High School*, 73; *Shortridge Annual, 1903*; EL, "Reminiscences."

36. EL, Astronomy Scrapbook, Miscellaneous Cabinet 2; EL, Astronomy Scrapbooks, Album 1, Eli Lilly Room; Simon Newcomb, *Popular Astronomy* (New York: Harper & Brothers, 1878). Lilly's copy of the book is in the Eli Lilly Room, Lilly Center.

37. EL, "Confidential: First Marriage, a Confession of Failure" [1968], p. 1, Memoirs, Miscellaneous Cabinet 1.

38. EL, "Confidential: First Marriage, a Confession of Failure," 1; Evelyn Fortune Lilly Bartlett, interview with author, 15, 16 Jan. 1986; Madeline Fortune Elder, interview with author, 11 Dec. 1985.

39. EL, "Remarks at 25-Year Banquet," 3 May 1972, p. 2, XBLl. Lilly told this story on other occasions as did Charles J. Lynn, who added, "As the years have passed, the business has 'smelled' sweeter and sweeter for all." Charles J. Lynn to Eugene N. Beesley, 1 June 1957, XBLl.

40. John S. Wright, "Reminiscences of Thirty Four Years in the Lilly Laboratories," typescript, 15 Dec. 1926, XCAa.

41. EL, "Remarks at 25-Year Banquet," 3. See also EL, undated notes for talk, ca. 1957, p. 1, Speeches Folder, ELP.

42. EL, undated notes for talk, ca. 1957, p. 1, Speeches Folder, ELP.

43. Joseph W. England, ed., *The First Century of the Philadelphia College of Pharmacy 1821-1921* (Philadelphia: Philadelphia College of Pharmacy and Science, 1922), 159-60, 183; Glenn Sonnedecker, *Kremers and Urdang's History of Pharmacy,* 4th ed. rev. (Philadelphia: J. B. Lippincott Co., 1976), 193, 269, 284, 482; EL, "Reminiscences."

44. *The Graduate 1907: Philadelphia College of Pharmacy* (Philadelphia: Philadelphia College of Pharmacy and Science, 1907), 66; EL, "Reminiscences"; Peckham, interview with author; Bartlett, interview with author.

45. Bartlett, interview with author; JKL, Sr., to EL, 16 Dec. 1904, Lilly Letters, Vault; EL to Margaret Ridgely, 4 Mar. 1906, EL Miscellaneous Papers, Lilly Family Papers, XBLl.

46. "Red Lilly" refers to the trademark adopted by the company in 1900, a duplicate in red of Colonel Lilly's signature, accompanied by the motto, "If It Bears a Red Lilly It's Right." Buley, "History of Eli Lilly and Company," chapter 6, p. 16.

47. JKL, Sr., to EL, 29 Mar. 1906, Lilly Letters, Vault.

Chapter 2

1. JKL, Sr., to EL and Evelyn Lilly, 3 Sept. 1907, Lilly Letters, Vault. See also *Indianapolis Star,* 29 Aug. 1907.

2. Copies of these and other books inscribed from William Fortune are in the Eli Lilly Room, Lilly Center.

3. Evelyn Fortune Lilly Bartlett, interview with author, 15, 16 Jan. 1986.

4. Ibid.

5. Ibid.

6. Ibid.; EL, "Confidential: First Marriage, a Confession of Failure" [1968], p. 1, Memoirs, Miscellaneous Cabinet 1.

7. *Budget* 5 (15 May 1909). See also Jonathan Liebenau, *Medical Science and Medical Industry: The Formation of the American Pharmaceutical Industry* (Baltimore: Johns Hopkins University Press, 1987), 46; J. Worth Estes, "The Pharmacology of Nineteenth-Century Patent Medicines," *Pharmacy in History* 30 (1988): 3-18; James Harvey Young, *The Toadstool Millionaires: A Social History of Patent Medicines in America before Federal Regulation* (Princeton, N.J.: Princeton University Press, 1961).

8. R. M. Reahard, "Forty-Three Years in Retrospect," *SuperVision* 3 (Oct. 1948): 4.

9. EL, undated notes for talk, ca. 1957, p. 1, Speeches Folder, ELP.

10. Reahard, "Forty-Three Years in Retrospect," 4.

11. EL, Economic Department Notebook, June-Aug. 1907, XBLl; JKL, Sr., "History of Eli Lilly and Company," XCAa.

12. EL, Economic Department Notebook, 24 May 1909, Mar. 1908, 11 Jan. 1909, 24, 27 Aug. 1907, Dec. 1908; *Budget* 5 (30 Apr. 1908): 4; *Budget* 8 (30 Apr. 1909): 2.

13. EL, Economic Department Notebook, 12 Jan. 1909, 28 Mar. 1908; *Budget* 5 (30 Apr.

1908): 2; Eli Lilly, "A Great Industry Adopts an Insurance Man's Short Cut," *System* 49 (1926): 73.

14. EL, Economic Department Notebook, 21 Nov. 1907.

15. *Laboratory Notes* 2 (21 Dec. 1907); 3 (22 Jan. 1908).

16. JKL, Sr., to EL, 10 Aug. [1909], Lilly Letters, Vault. This letter has an added penciled date of 1907, but internal evidence strongly suggests 1909 rather than 1907.

17. JKL, Sr., to EL, 10 Mar. 1911, Lilly Letters, Vault.

18. JKL, Sr., "History of Eli Lilly and Company," 35, 36, 41.

19. Ibid., 36, 46, 49; R. C. Buley, "A History of Eli Lilly and Company," typescript, 1967, chapter 6, pp. 43-47; Harmon W. Marsh, "Glue Jackets for Disagreeable Medicines: How Gelatin Capsules Are Manufactured," *Scientific American* 117 (15 Sept. 1917): 194.

20. Eli Lilly, "We Find Out How to Speed-Up Production 50%," *System* 48 (1925): 545.

21. EL, memorandum, 1971, attached to the copy of Frederick Winslow Taylor's *The Principles of Scientific Management* (New York: Harper, 1919) in the Eli Lilly Room. Lilly noted that he had read the earlier, 1911, printing of the book. His memory of his reading is in Gene E. McCormick, note of interview with EL, 3 Feb. 1967, Scientific Management Folder, Drawer 1, Cabinet 8, Company History Files.

22. Daniel Nelson, *Frederick W. Taylor and the Rise of Scientific Management* (Madison: University of Wisconsin Press, 1980); Daniel Nelson, "Scientific Management, Systematic Management, and Labor, 1880-1915," *Business History Review* 48 (1974): 479-500; Samuel Haber, *Efficiency and Uplift: Scientific Management in the Progressive Era 1890-1920* (Chicago: University of Chicago Press, 1964); David Montgomery, *The Fall of the House of Labor: The Workplace, the State, and American Labor Activism, 1865-1925* (New York: Cambridge University Press, 1987), 216-56. No significant evidence of worker reaction to scientific management at Eli Lilly and Company has been located.

23. JKL, Sr., to EL and Evelyn Lilly, 19 Mar. 1911, Lilly Letters, Vault.

24. EL to Miss Reibel, 3 Sept. 1912, Scientific Management Folder, Drawer 1, Cabinet 8, Company History Files; Emerson Company, "Investigation Report of Eli Lilly & Company," 8 Nov. 1913, pp. 206-7, XIRq.

25. Emerson Company, "Investigation Report of Eli Lilly & Company," 36, 265-66.

26. Haber, *Efficiency and Uplift,* 52-57; Nelson, *Frederick W. Taylor,* 127, 130, 153; Daniel A. Wren, *The Evolution of Management Thought,* 2d ed. (New York: John Wiley & Sons, 1979), 181-85.

27. Emerson Company, "Investigation Report of Eli Lilly & Company." Quotations are on pages 6, 321, 4.

28. JKL, Jr., to JKL, Sr., 27 Feb. 1914, Lilly Letters, Vault.

29. Emerson Company, "Final Report of the Efficiency Work in the Plant of the Eli Lilly & Company," 27 June 1914, XIRq. Quotation on page 147. See also McCormick, memorandum of interview with EL, 8 Apr. 1966, Scientific Management Folder, Drawer 1, Cabinet 8, Company History Files.

30. EL, "Remarks at 25-Year Banquet," 3 May 1972, p. 4, XBLl; Emerson Company, "Investigation Report of Eli Lilly & Company," 37-38; Buley, "History of Eli Lilly and Company," chapter 6, pp. 100-101.

31. Lilly, "We Find Out How to Speed-Up Production 50%," 546; EL to McCormick, 24 Feb. 1969, Lilly Company History Folder, ELP; Buley, "History of Eli Lilly and Company," chapter 6, p. 101.

32. EL to S. O. Sharp, 8 Jan. 1914, Memorandums-Misc., 1912-29, XPDc. This ring binder of production-related memoranda provides good evidence of Lilly's close involvement in production matters and the struggle for systematization and quantification of production.

33. JKL, Sr., to EL and JKL, Jr., n.d. [1916], 9 Apr. 1916, Lilly Letters, Vault; Nicholas H. Noyes, "Essay of the Past," 1951, Noyes Folder, Drawer 4, Cabinet 2, Company History Files.

34. Buley, "History of Eli Lilly and Company," chapter 6, pp. 95-100; JKL, Jr., "Report on the Subject of Employment," 7 Oct. 1916, XIRa; JKL, Jr., to Charles J. Lynn, 9 Oct. 1916, XIRa; "Efficiency Division, 1912-1925," [ca. 1925], XIRa.

35. The clearest indication of the familial relationship is in Lilly Letters, Vault. See, for examples, JKL, Sr., to EL, 19 Dec. 1915, 26 Jan. 1917.

36. See, for example, JKL, Sr., to EL, 19 Jan. 1917, ibid.

37. JKL, Sr., "Possible Economies and Advantages from Amalgamation," n.d., attached to JKL, Sr., to Charles J. Lynn et al., 2 May 1946. The undated document is in J. K. Lilly's hand and from internal evidence was probably written in 1918-19.

38. Alfred D. Chandler, Jr., and Stephen Salsbury, *Pierre S. Du Pont and the Making of the Modern Corporation* (New York: Harper & Row, 1971), 37, 593-99; David A. Hounshell, *From the American System to Mass Production, 1800-1932: The Development of Manufacturing Technology in the United States* (Baltimore: Johns Hopkins University Press, 1984), 277; Charles W. Cheape, *Family Firm to Modern Multinational: Norton Company, a New England Enterprise* (Cambridge, Mass.: Harvard University Press, 1985), 99-113, 152-60.

39. JKL, Sr., "History of Eli Lilly and Company," 39.

40. Ibid., 39-40.

41. Ibid., 38-40, 42; Buley, "History of Eli Lilly and Company," chapter 6, pp. 29, 53-58.

42. JKL, Sr., to EL and JKL, Jr., 9 Apr. 1916, Lilly Letters, Vault.

43. JKL, Sr., to EL, 29 Jan. 1919, ibid.

44. McCormick, notes of interview with EL, 29 Nov. 1967, Chapter 6 Folder, Drawer 1, Cabinet 8, Company History Files.

45. EL, "Remarks at 25-Year Banquet," 3.

46. EL, "Response at Dinner on the Fiftieth Anniversary with Eli Lilly and Company," 1 June 1957, XBLl.

47. McCormick, notes of interview with EL, 29 Nov. 1967.

48. Lynn to Eugene N. Beesley, 1 June 1957, 50th Anniversary File, XBLl; McCormick, notes of interview with EL, 29 Nov. 1967; E. J. Kahn, Jr., *All in a Century: The First 100 Years of Eli Lilly and Company* ([Indianapolis: Eli Lilly & Co., 1976]), 52; Emerson Company, "Investigation Report of Eli Lilly & Company," 146.

49. EL, "Too Much Conservatism," 13 Oct. 1919, XBLl.

50. EL to Beesley, 22 Jan. 1968, Beesley Folder, XBLl.

51. JKL, Sr., to EL, 16 Oct. 1919, XBLl. See also McCormick, notes of interview with EL, 29 Nov. 1967.

52. EL to Beesley, 22 Jan. 1968, XBLl.

53. Eli Lilly and Company, *The First One Hundred Years* (n.p., n.d.), 8. In commenting on two different efforts to write the history of the company, Lilly was very modest in any references to his own contributions. Only in considering his work in production in these early years did he ask that the writers "please give us a little credit along those lines." EL to McCormick, 24 Feb. 1969, Lilly Company History Folder, ELP. See also EL to John F. Modrall, 26 Nov. 1962, M Miscellaneous Folder, ELP.

Chapter 3

1. JKL, Sr., to EL and JKL, Jr., 4 Feb. 1917, Lilly Letters, Vault.

2. JKL, Sr., "History of Eli Lilly and Company," 57-61, XCAc; Benjamin D. Hitz, ed., *A History of Base Hospital 32* (Indianapolis, 1922); Alma S. Woolley, "A Hoosier Nurse in France: The World War I Diary of Maude Frances Essig," *Indiana Magazine of History* 82 (1986): 37-68.

3. Jonathan M. Liebenau, "Scientific Ambitions: The Pharmaceutical Industry, 1900-1920," *Pharmacy in History* 27 (1985): 3-11. For the general evolution of big business see Alfred D. Chandler, Jr., *The Visible Hand: The Managerial Revolution in American Business* (Cambridge, Mass.: Harvard University Press, 1977).

4. JKL, Sr., "A Plan for Promoting the Affairs of Eli Lilly & Company during the Years 1920-21-22-23," 26 Oct. 1919, XCAe. Quotations are on pages 8, 11.

5. EL to JKL, Sr., 12 Feb. 1920, XCAe; JKL, Sr., to Board of Directors, 20 Feb. 1920, XCAc.

6. Eli Lilly, "We Find Out How to Speed-Up Production 50%," *System* 48 (1925): 598.

7. EL, Economic Department Notebook, 15 June 1907, XBLl; Emerson Company, "Investigation Report of Eli Lilly & Company," 8 Nov. 1913, pp. 148-49, XIRq; Everett K. Todd, interview with Gene E. McCormick, 7, 9 Feb. 1968, p. 11, Drawer 1, Cabinet 3, Company History Files.

8. Theodore R. Olive, "Applying Mass Production Methods in a Pharmaceutical Plant," *Chemical & Metallurgical Engineering* 35 (1928): 81. See also Gene E. McCormick, "A History of Eli Lilly and Company," typescript, 1971, chapter 7, pp. 121-26.

9. Olive, "Applying Mass Production Methods in a Pharmaceutical Plant," 79-83; JKL, Sr., "History of Eli Lilly and Company," 73, 78; *Budget* 22 (Mar. 1925): 2.

10. *Budget* 21 (Apr. 1924): 3. See also JKL, Jr., "Planning Department," 15 Dec. 1919, XPDv.

11. JKL, Sr., to EL, 12 Jan., 15 Mar. 1920, Lilly Letters, Vault; EL to S. O. Sharp, 17 Sept. 1921, Memorandums—Misc., 1912-29, XPDc; John C. Siegesmund, interview with McCormick, 10 Dec. 1968, p. 34, Drawer 1, Cabinet 3, Company History Files; Earl Beck, "Installing Wage Incentive Systems That Work," *Factory* 32 (1924): 826, 943; Earl Beck to EL, 18 Jan., 28 May 1924, Earl Beck File, XIRi; *Lilly Balance* 1 (Dec. 1919): 6; EL to Wils Fox, 22 Mar. 1926, Efficiency Division, XIRa.

12. Earl Beck, "Close Control Cuts Maintenance Costs," *Management* (July 1931): 69; JKL,

Sr., to EL, 26 July 1922, 1 Aug. 1923, Lilly Letters, Vault; George Meihaus to EL, 2 Oct. 1922, Planning Department, 1920-22, XPDv; Eli Lilly, "Every Product a Salesman," *Factory and Industrial Management* 83 (1932): 97-99.

13. George Meihaus to Mr. Taylor, 14 Nov. 1928, Manufacturing Tickets—Followup, 1928, Planning Department, XPDv; Methods and Standards Department Manual, typescript, no page numbers, 1929, XIRe. See also Earl Beck, "Executive Control Affects All Operations," *Management* (Apr. 1931): 28-39.

14. W. J. Rice to EL, 13 Oct. 1921, Memorandums, Production Department, 1920-24, XPDc; EL to Sharp, 6 Sept., 3 Oct. 1923, Memorandums—Misc., 1912-29, XPDc.

15. Todd, interview with McCormick, 23; Lester H. Hoopes, interview with McCormick, 11 Oct. 1967, pp. 3-4, Drawer 4, Cabinet 2, Company History Files.

16. JKL, Sr., to R. A. Whidden, 18 Mar. 1925, JKL, Sr., Letters, XCAc; EL, interview with McCormick, 22 July 1969, Facilities Improvement Folder, Drawer 4, Cabinet 5, Company History Files.

17. John C. Siegesmund, interview with McCormick, 10 Dec. 1968, pp. 16-17, Drawer 1, Cabinet 3, Company History Files.

18. JKL, Sr., "History of Eli Lilly and Company," 69.

19. Quoted in James Harvey Young, "Public Policy and Drug Innovation," *Pharmacy in History* 24 (1982): 5. See also John K. Crellin, "Folklore and Medicines—Medical Interfaces: A Kaleidoscope and Challenge," in *Folklore and Folk Medicines,* ed. John Scarborough (Madison, Wisc.: American Institute of the History of Pharmacy, 1987), 112-13.

20. Liebenau, "Scientific Ambitions: The Pharmaceutical Industry, 1900-1920," 9-10; Harry F. Dowling, *Medicines for Man: The Development, Regulation, and Use of Prescription Drugs* (New York: Alfred A. Knopf, 1970), 18.

21. Glenn Sonnedecker, "The Rise of Drug Manufacture in America," *Emory University Quarterly* 21 (1965): 80-83; Jonathan Liebenau, *Medical Science and Medical Industry: The Formation of the American Pharmaceutical Industry* (Baltimore: Johns Hopkins University Press, 1987), 36-44.

22. John Parascandola, "Industrial Research Comes of Age: The American Pharmaceutical Industry, 1920-1940," *Pharmacy in History* 27 (1985): 12-21; Liebenau, *Medical Science and Medical Industry,* 109-24.

23. JKL, Sr., "History of Eli Lilly and Company," 36.

24. JKL, Sr., "A Plan for Promoting the Affairs of Eli Lilly & Company," 11.

25. JKL, Sr., to Board of Directors, 20 Feb. 1920, XCAc.

26. EL to JKL, Sr., 12 Feb. 1920, XCAe.

27. George H. A. Clowes, Jr., "George Henry Alexander Clowes, PhD, DSc, LLD (1877-1958): A Man of Science for All Seasons," *Journal of Surgical Oncology* 18 (1981): 197-217; EL "Notes on Research," 23 Jan. 1969, Drawer 1, Cabinet 5, Company History Files.

28. G. H. A. Clowes to G. W. McCoy, 9 Oct. 1919, G. H. A. Clowes Correspondence, XRDc.

29. *Budget* 16 (2 June 1919): 35.

30. G. H. A. Clowes, "Preliminary Report of Research Department for Year Ending October 20th, 1921," XRDe.

31. Quoted in R. C. Buley, "A History of Eli Lilly and Company," typescript, 1967, chapter 6, p. 164.

32. Kenneth Hartman, interview with McCormick, 10 Dec. 1971, p. 85, Drawer 2, Cabinet 3, Company History Files.

33. Clowes, "George Henry Alexander Clowes," 210, 214; EL, "Notes on Research"; JKL, Sr., to EL, 20 Sept. 1929, Lilly Letters, Vault.

34. JKL, Sr., to EL and JKL, Jr., 30 Jan. 1920, Lilly Letters, Vault.

35. Michael Bliss, *The Discovery of Insulin* (Chicago: University of Chicago Press, 1982), 104-6; G. H. A. Clowes, "Banting Memorial Address," 7 June 1947, p. 5, typescript, Insulin Folder, Drawer 2, Cabinet 8, Company History Files. An abbreviated version of the insulin story is Michael Bliss, "Resurrections in Toronto: Fact and Myth in the Discovery of Insulin," *Bulletin of the American Academy of Arts and Sciences* 38 (Dec. 1984): 15-36. My account relies heavily on Bliss's excellent book, which is essential and very interesting reading. For more on the human side of the Toronto story see Michael Bliss, *Banting: A Biography* (Toronto: McClelland and Stewart, 1984).

36. Bliss, *Discovery of Insulin,* 20-44.

37. Ibid.; EL, "Notes on Research."

38. Bliss, *Discovery of Insulin,* 137-39; John Patrick Swann, "Insulin: A Case Study in the Emergence of Collaborative Pharmacomedical Research, Part I," *Pharmacy in History* 28 (1986): 4-7.

39. EL to Charles H. Best, 3 Feb. 1975, Best File, ELP; Best to Richard D. Wood, 25 Jan. 1977, XBLl; Best, interview with McCormick, 24 Sept. 1968, Drawer 3, Cabinet 2, Company History Files.

40. EL to J. J. R. Macleod, 17 June, 10 July 1922, Insulin—Section 6 Folder, Drawer 3, Cabinet 5, Company History Files; Robert H. Rhodehamel, interview with author, 18 July 1986. Robert H. Rhodehamel recalls not seeing his father, Harley, for days and days during this early insulin work.

41. JKL, Sr., to EL, 25 July 1922, Lilly Letters, Vault. See also JKL, Sr., to EL, 29 July, 3 Aug. 1922, ibid.

42. Bliss, *Discovery of Insulin,* 171-72; Swann, "Insulin, Part I," 8-10; Clowes to Macleod, 5 Sept. 1922, Insulin Folder, Drawer 2, Cabinet 8, Company History Files; McCormick, "History of Eli Lilly and Company," chapter 7, pp. 54-58.

43. JKL, Sr., to EL [May 1923], Lilly Letters, Vault.

44. EL to John F. Modrall, 26 Nov. 1962, "M" Miscellaneous File, ELP. For the company-sponsored account of insulin, see Roscoe Collins Clark, *Threescore Years and Ten: A Narrative of the First Seventy Years of Eli Lilly and Company, 1876-1946* (Indianapolis: Eli Lilly & Co., 1946), 56-61.

45. EL, "Notes on Research."

46. JKL, Sr., to EL, 23 Jan. 1923, Lilly Letters, Vault.

47. Bliss, *Discovery of Insulin,* 174, 178-81; John Patrick Swann, "Insulin: A Case Study in the Emergence of Collaborative Pharmacomedical Research, Part II," *Pharmacy in History* 28 (1986): 65-66; Minutes of the Meeting of the Special Committee on Insulin, 2 Apr. 1923, University of Toronto, Insulin Folder, Drawer 2, Cabinet 8, Company History Files.

48. Clowes to Macleod, 14 Apr. 1923, Unitage-Insulin Folder, Drawer 3, Cabinet 5, Company History Files. See also Clowes to Macleod, 7, 14 Mar. 1923, Insulin Folder, Drawer 2, Cabinet 8, ibid.

49. Minutes of the Meeting of the Special Advisory Committee on Insulin, 2 Apr., 8 May, 13 June 1923, University of Toronto, Insulin Folder, Drawer 2, Cabinet 8, ibid.; EL, "Notes on Research"; Swann, "Insulin, Part II," 70-71; Bliss, *Discovery of Insulin,* 180-81.

50. EL to F. Lorne Hutchison, 12 Apr. 1924, Insulin Folder, Drawer 3, Cabinet 5, Company History Files.

51. Swann, "Insulin, Part II," 73.

52. JKL, Sr., "A History of Eli Lilly and Company," 69. See also JKL, Sr., to R. J. Bynum, 12 Feb. 1924, Edward Zink Folder, ELP. J. K. Lilly, Sr., estimated the company's after-tax profits at $1,338,000 for 1923.

53. Minutes of the Special Advisory Committee on Insulin, 18 Sept. 1923, University of Toronto, Insulin Folder, Drawer 2, Cabinet 8, Company History Files; Swann, "Insulin, Part II," 71.

54. Swann, "Insulin, Part II," 72; Bliss, *Discovery of Insulin,* 151-65, 188, 243-44. Elizabeth Hughes was the daughter of Charles Evans Hughes, the 1916 Republican presidential candidate and later chief justice of the Supreme Court.

55. JKL, Sr., to John Uri Lloyd, 13 Aug. 1924, Insulin Folder, Drawer 3, Cabinet 5, Company History Files.

56. JKL, Sr., to Ernest Stauffen, 26 May 1925, Lilly Letters, Vault.

57. Austin H. Brown, "Address before Twenty-Five Year Group," typescript, 10 May 1949, Drawer 1, Cabinet 5, Company History Files. See also Rhodehamel, interview with author. Inadequate data on individual American pharmaceutical companies make it impossible to rank them by size, but it is likely that Eli Lilly and Company was second, behind Parke-Davis, at the end of the 1920s. McCormick, "History of Eli Lilly and Company," chapter 7, p. 298.

58. Eli Lilly and Company, *The First One Hundred Years* (n.p., n.d.), 9.

59. JKL, Sr., to EL, 2 July 1924, Lilly Letters, Vault; Parascandola, "Industrial Research Comes of Age," 12-21.

60. John P. Swann, *Academic Scientists and the Pharmaceutical Industry: Cooperative Research in Twentieth-Century America* (Baltimore: Johns Hopkins University Press, 1988), 24-56; Parascandola, "Industrial Research Comes of Age," 17-20; Williams Haynes, *American Chemical Industry,* 6 vols. (New York: D. Van Nostrand, 1945-54), 3:394; Roger L. Geiger, *To Advance Knowledge: The Growth of American Research Universities, 1900-1940* (New York: Oxford University Press, 1986), 94-101, 174-77; David A. Hounshell and John Kenly Smith, Jr., *Science and Corporate Strategy: Du Pont R & D, 1902-1980* (Cambridge, England: Cambridge University Press, 1988), 290-94.

61. EL to JKL, Sr., 8 July 1930, Scientific Fellowships Folder, Drawer 4, Cabinet 5, Company History Files.

62. EL to JKL, Sr., 14 Aug. 1929, ibid. See also EL, "Notes on Research."

63. JKL, Sr., to EL, 20 Sept. 1929, Lilly Letters, Vault.

64. K. K. Chen, interview with McCormick, 6, 16 Feb. 1968, pp. 37-38, 40, Drawer 4,

Cabinet 2, Company History Files; Leon G. Zerfas, interview with McCormick, 22, 25 Oct. 1968, pp. 19-20, Drawer 2, Cabinet 2, ibid.

65. EL to Clowes, 20 Sept. 1924, XCAc. See also McCormick, "History of Eli Lilly and Company," chapter 7, pp. 188-90.

66. Zerfas, interview with McCormick, 22. See also Robert H. Rhodehamel interview with author; McCormick, "History of Eli Lilly and Company," chapter 7, pp. 195-99.

67. Chen, interview with McCormick, 34.

68. Zerfas, interview with McCormick, 22.

69. J. P. Scott to George D. Beal, 16 Dec. 1938, C38(a)I, Lilly and Co., Kremers Reference Files, School of Pharmacy, University of Wisconsin, Madison.

70. McCormick, "History of Eli Lilly and Company," chapter 7, pp. 79-82, 153-56, 157-58, 179-84; Chen, interview with McCormick, 1-5; K. K. Chen, "Two Pharmacological Traditions: Notes from Experience," *Annual Review of Pharmacology and Toxicology* 21 (1981): 1-6; E. J. Kahn, *All in a Century: The First 100 Years of Eli Lilly and Company* ([Indianapolis: Eli Lilly & Co., 1976]), 104.

71. JKL, Sr., to EL, 5 Apr. 1927, Lilly Letters, Vault; EL, "Notes on Research"; Zerfas, interview with McCormick, 15-16; McCormick, "History of Eli Lilly and Company," chapter 7, pp. 160-78; Francis M. Rackemann, *The Inquisitive Physician: The Life and Times of George Richards Minot* (Cambridge, Mass.: Harvard University Press, 1956), 141-60; Swann, *Academic Scientists and the Pharmaceutical Industry,* 150-69. Swann's book provides excellent detail and analysis of the liver extract cooperation. I am grateful to him for sharing copies of his dissertation before the book was published.

72. Eli Lilly and Company, *Sales Bulletin* 30 (Feb. 1929): 1. See also Eli Lilly and Company, *The Lilly Research Laboratories* (Indianapolis, 1933, 1942).

73. Swann, *Academic Scientists and the Pharmaceutical Industry,* 150-69; EL to George H. Whipple, 8 Sept. 1930, Liver Extract No. 55 Folder, Drawer 4, Cabinet 5, Company History Files; EL, "Notes on Research"; McCormick, "History of Eli Lilly and Company," chapter 7, p. 71.

Chapter 4

1. Robert H. Rhodehamel, interview with author, 18 July 1986.

2. EL, undated notes for talk, 1957, p. 2, Speeches Folder, ELP. See also Louis J. Nickel, interview with Gene E. McCormick, 19 Jan. 1972, p. 40, Drawer 2, Cabinet 3, Company History Files; Gene E. McCormick, "A History of Eli Lilly and Company," typescript, 1971, chapter 7, p. 118.

3. JKL, Sr., to EL, 25 Aug. 1924, Lilly Letters, Vault.

4. EL, "Reminiscences," typescript, 1966-69, XLBl; "Record of Fish Caught, 1916-31, by Rowdy Revelers," XBLl. Lilly sent invitations in 1923 to Bowman Elder, Garvin Brown, Charles Latham, George L. Denny, William Stafford, R. B. Failey, Anton Vonnegut, Russell Fortune, Nicholas H. Noyes, Fred Appel, J. K. Lilly, Jr., and Sylvester Johnson, Jr. EL to Bowman Elder, 26 Mar. 1923, XBLl.

5. Evelyn Fortune Bartlett, interview with author, 15, 16 Jan. 1986.

6. Ibid.; Madeline Fortune Elder, interview with author, 11 Dec. 1985.

7. EL, "Confidential: First Marriage, a Confession of Failure," [1968], pp. 1-2, Memoirs, Miscellaneous Cabinet 1.

8. Bartlett, inverview with author; JKL, Sr., to EL, 8, 15 Feb. 1922, Lilly Letters, Vault.

9. EL, "Confidential: First Marriage, a Confession of Failure," 2. Lilly incorrectly remembered the date of the trip. It is verified as the summer of 1922 in JKL, Sr., to EL, 14 Aug. 1922, Lilly Letters, Vault.

10. Bartlett, interview with author; JKL, Sr., to EL [May 1923], Lilly Letters, Vault.

11. Gene E. McCormick, interview with author, 2 May 1988; EL and Evelyn Fortune Lilly, "Memorandum of Settlement," 15 May 1926, Miscellaneous Folder, EL Legal Records, Vault.

12. Bartlett, interview with author. Because of the prominence of the Lilly and Fortune families the divorce "really shook up the town" and forced many to take sides in a private matter that became public. Allen Clowes, interview with author, 11 Nov. 1988.

13. JKL, Sr., to EL, 8 Mar. 1926, Lilly Letters, Vault.

14. Ibid.

15. *Evelyn F. Lilly* v. *Eli Lilly,* 3 July 1926, Marion County Clerk of Courts Office, City-County Building, Indianapolis; EL and Evelyn Fortune Lilly, "Memorandum of Settlement."

16. EL to Evie Lilly, 11 July 1926, XBLl.

17. Ibid., 25 July 1926. Dante was the nickname for Evie's nurse, Miss Johnson.

18. Ibid., 19 Sept. 1926, 8, 15 Dec. 1929; JKL, Sr., to EL, 26 Mar. 1928, 20 Sept. 1929, Lilly Letters, Vault.

19. Howard H. Peckham to author, 28 June 1986, in author's possession; EL, "Reminiscences"; E. J. Kahn, Jr., *All in a Century: The First 100 Years of Eli Lilly and Company* ([Indianapolis: Eli Lilly & Co., 1976]); EL, "Confidential: First Marriage, a Confession of Failure," 2.

20. Gene E. McCormick, "A History of Eli Lilly and Company," typescript, 1972, chapter 8, pp. 72-80.

21. JKL, Sr., to EL, 7 Jan. 1927, Lilly Letters, Vault. See also Bartlett, interview with author.

22. JKL, Sr., "A Stockholder's Complaint," 14 Aug. 1929, Corporate Affairs Folder, Drawer 1, Cabinet 8, Company History Files.

23. Bartlett, interview with author. See also *Indianapolis Star,* 8, 15 Apr. 1934; Evelyn Bartlett Scrapbooks, Bonnet House, Fort Lauderdale, Florida; and Carl J. Weinhardt, Jr., "Bonnet House," *Connoisseur* 215 (Jan. 1985): 98-103. The Bartlett Collection at the Art Institute of Chicago is among the most important collections of modern art in America.

24. EL, "Confidential: First Marriage, a Confession of Failure," 3.

25. Ibid.; Marriage License, Miscellaneous Folder, EL Legal Records, Vault; EL, "Reminiscences"; JKL, Sr., to EL, 31 Dec. 1927, Lilly Letters, Vault.

26. EL, Confidential: First Marriage, a Confession of Failure," 1; Howard and Dorothy Peckham, interview with author, 2 Aug. 1985.

27. EL, Diary, 26 Nov. 1955, XBLl; Howard and Dorothy Peckham, interview with author; Gene E. McCormick, "A History of Eli Lilly and Company," typescript, 1974, chapter 10, p. 174; EL, "Reminiscences"; Glenn Black to Carl E. Guthe, 15 Nov. 1933, Glenn A. Black Papers, Glenn A. Black Laboratory of Archaeology, Indiana University, Bloomington.

28. EL to Black, 28 June 1934, 17 Feb. 1941, 3 Aug. 1942, 9 July 1943, 6 Aug. 1947, Black Papers, Black Laboratory; EL to JKL, Sr., 10 Aug. 1936, JKL, Sr., Papers, Vault.

29. EL, "Wawasee Fever (with apologies to John Masefield)," Poems Folder, ELP.

30. EL to E. Y. Guernsey, 19 Apr. 1937, Guernsey Folder, EL Papers, Black Laboratory.

31. EL, "An Allergy: Wrote on a Hoosier Lakeside," Poems Folder, ELP.

32. EL, "Reminiscences." See also Robert B. Parrott to EL, 16 Mar. 1943, XBLl; EL to Rowdy Revelers, 12 Mar. 1943, XBLl; *Indianapolis Times,* 1 May 1949.

33. JKL, Sr., to EL, 19 Oct. 1929, Lilly Letters, Vault; EL, interview with McCormick, 26 Jan. 1972, Residences Folder, EL Drawer, Cabinet 4, Company History Files; B. W. Duck to EL, 1 Aug. 1970, Homes Folder, ELP.

34. JKL, Sr., to EL, 31 July 1930, Lilly Letters, Vault. The senior Lilly's spelling of chauffeur is indicative of his delight in making play with words, not his spelling. See also Patricia Curry, *Lilly House* (Bloomington: Indiana University Publications, n.d.).

35. *Indianapolis Star,* 15 July 1971; Grant Wood to Albert Bailey, 23 July 1934, XPLl; EL to Mrs. John Pusey, 7 Oct. 1966, XPLl.

36. EL, "Plan for Developing Proper Outlook on Life," [1934], XBLl.

37. Black to EL, 12 Sept. 1934, Black Papers, Black Laboratory; EL to Black, 13 Sept. 1934, ibid.

38. H. A. Overstreet, *About Ourselves: Psychology for Normal People* (New York: W. W. Norton & Co., 1927), 7.

39. *New York Times Book Review,* 18 Mar. 1928, p. 28.

40. EL, "Plan for Developing Proper Outlook on Life"; Benjamin Franklin, *The Autobiography of Benjamin Franklin* (New York: Washington Square Press, 1955), especially 104-6.

41. EL to Carl Voegelin, 14 Apr. 1937, Voegelin Folder, EL Papers, Black Laboratory.

42. Many of the most influential books in Lilly's personal library are in the Eli Lilly Room, Lilly Center. Most of his books remain in the Sunset Lane house, some with his paper slips and other markers.

43. EL to Black, 28 Jan. 1932, Black Papers, Black Laboratory.

44. Byron P. Hollett, interview with author, 24 Sept. 1985.

45. EL, "Remington Honor Medal Acceptance Address," 10 Dec. 1958, Remington Medalist Scrapbook, XBLl.

46. JKL, Sr., to EL, 28 Mar. 1928, Lilly Letters, Vault; JKL, Sr., to EL, 1 Apr. 1933, 1 Apr. 1940, EL Miscellaneous Papers, Lilly Family Papers, XBLl.

47. EL to JKL, Sr., [Feb. 1945], 26 Feb. 1946, EL and JKL, Sr., Correspondence, ELP.

48. JKL, Sr., "Reminiscences," 50-54, typescript, 1940, XBLl; McCormick, "History of Eli Lilly and Company," chapter 8, pp. 41-69, 140, 147-48; J. K. Lilly, Sr., "The Name Lilly," *Lilly Review* 2 (Apr. 1942): 13; (May 1942): 21-22; (June 1942): 14; (Aug. 1942): 17. For a useful overview of J. K. Lilly, Sr.'s, life, see Gene E. McCormick, "Josiah Kirby Lilly, Sr., the Man (1861-1948)," *Pharmacy in History* 12 (1970): 57-67; and Irene D. Neu, "Josiah Kirby Lilly," John A. Garraty and Edward T. James, eds., *Dictionary of American Biography: (Supplement Four, 1946-1950)* (New York: Charles Scribner's Sons, 1974), 499-500.

49. JKL, Sr., to EL and JKL, Jr., 26 Dec. 1947, JKL, Sr., Personal Papers; EL to Douglass Hayes, 3 May 1954, Hayes Folder, ELP.

50. McCormick, "History of Eli Lilly and Company," chapter 8, pp. 89-90, 100-104.

51. JKL, Sr., "Reminiscences," 104. See also JKL, Sr., to John Uri Lloyd, 15 Dec. 1930, Lilly Letters, Vault.

52. McCormick, "History of Eli Lilly and Company," chapter 8, pp. 130-32; *Indianapolis Star,* 20 Apr. 1934.

53. McCormick, "History of Eli Lilly and Company," chapter 8, pp. 134-39, 183.

54. Otto N. Frenzel to EL, 20 May 1957, 50th Anniversary Letters, XBLl.

55. EL, "Shining Phrase Book," XBLl, 59; EL, "Remington Honor Medal Acceptance Address." The Remington Medal was even more meaningful because his father had received it in 1942.

56. EL, "Confidential: First Marriage, a Confession of Failure," 2; John G. Rauch, Jr., interview with author, 4 May 1988; Elder, interview with author; J. K. Lilly III, interview with author, 4 Sept. 1986; EL to Guernsey, 4 May 1936, 28 Aug. 1933, Guernsey Folder, EL Papers, Black Laboratory; EL, "Reminiscences."

57. EL to Black, 25 June 1937, Black Papers, Black Laboratory. See also *Indianapolis Times,* 21, 24 June 1937; *Indianapolis News,* 19, 23, 24, 25 June 1937; *Indianapolis Star,* 20, 23, 24 June 1937; J. K. Lilly III, interview with author; Hollett, interview with author; Rauch, Jr., interview with author; Clowes, interview with author.

58. EL to Evie Lilly, 29 Sept. 1939, Evelyn Lutz Folder, ELP.

59. Declaration of Family Accord, 6 May 1970, Miscellaneous Legal Records, Vault; EL to Rauch, Sr., 17 Nov. 1948, Folder 1, Box A, 1, Legal Records, Vault; EL to Rauch, Sr., 14 Feb. 1966, Rauch Folder, ELP.

60. J. K. Lilly III, interview with author; Elder, interview with author; EL to JKL, Sr., 13 Jan., 20 Mar. 1939, JKL, Sr., Papers, Vault.

61. EL to Guernsey, 26 Nov. 1940, Guernsey Folder, EL Papers, Black Laboratory.

62. Bartlett, interview with author; J. K. Lilly III, interview with author.

63. EL to Rauch, Sr., 17 Nov. 1948, Folder 1, Box A, 1, Legal Records, Vault; EL to Black, 13 May 1948, Black Papers, Black Laboratory.

64. EL to Ruth Lilly, 19 Nov. 1948, Folder 1, Box A, 1, Legal Records, Vault.

65. EL to JKL, Jr., 19 Nov. 1948, ibid.; EL, Will, 24 Nov. 1948, ibid. It is nearly certain that Ruth and Joe Lilly never saw these letters, for they remained with the will in Rauch's office until the 1970s.

66. *Indianapolis Times,* 30 Dec. 1939.

67. EL to Tom D. Spies, 28 Dec. 1942, XCAx.

68. Black to EL, 25 Sept. 1934, 30 Dec. 1935, Black Papers, Black Laboratory; EL to Maxfield Parrish, 18 June 1962, XBLl; EL to Stith Thompson, 24 Feb. 1941, F Miscellaneous Folder, ELP.

69. Work Projects Administration, *Indiana: A Guide to the Hoosier State* (New York: Oxford University Press, 1941), 206, 209.

70. Ibid., 206-11; Judith E. Endelman, *The Jewish Community of Indianapolis: 1849 to the Present* (Bloomington: Indiana University Press, 1984), 113-17; EL to JKL, Sr., 29 Jan. 1945, EL and JKL, Sr., Correspondence, ELP; Booth Tarkington, *Image of Josephine* (Garden City, N.Y.: Doubleday, Doran & Co., 1945). The woman was Caroline Fesler, whose taste for modern art neither Tarkington nor Lilly shared.

71. EL, undated notes for talk, 4; EL to Sloane Graff, 11 Apr. 1952, Graff Folder, ELP; EL, "On the Brink of Destruction and Slavery," Poems, Songs, and Other Writings Folder, ELP. Many historians, including the author, believe the New Deal was a major force in preserving and extending freedom and enterprise.

72. EL, Federal Income Tax Records, ELP; EL to Rauch, Sr., 30 Dec. 1959, Rauch Folder, ELP.

73. *Indianapolis News*, 4, 5 May 1934; EL to Guernsey, 4 May 1934, Guernsey Folder, EL Papers, Black Laboratory; EL, interview with McCormick, 26 Feb. 1968, Philanthropic-Personal Folder, EL Drawer, Cabinet 4, Company History Files. The newspaper reports did not identify Lilly by name, but only as a "high official in the Eli Lilly & Co." But Guernsey and presumably many others in Indianapolis immediately identified Lilly as the object of the plot. Guernsey to EL, 4 May 1934, Guernsey Folder, EL Papers, Black Laboratory.

Chapter 5

1. *Lilly Review* 2 (May 1942): 14.

2. JKL, Sr., to EL and JKL, Jr., 17 Apr. 1934, JKL, Sr., Letters to Sons, XBLk. With this transfer J. K. Lilly, Sr.'s, holdings were 120,000 shares. The Lillys listed the value of the stock on 3 Aug. 1934 at $55.81 a share. EL, Gift Tax Form, 1934, Income Tax Records, ELP.

3. EL to Glenn Black, 29 Aug. 1945, Glenn A. Black Papers, Glenn A. Black Laboratory of Archaeology, Indiana University, Bloomington.

4. Eli Lilly and Company, Consolidated Operating Results, 30 Mar. 1977.

5. EL to JKL, Sr., et al., 20 June 1932, Research Organization, 1932-44, Drawer 1, Cabinet 6, Company History Files.

6. *Lilly Research Laboratories: Dedication* (Indianapolis: Eli Lilly & Co., 1934), xi-xii, 94, 121-28.

7. Ibid., passim; John P. Swann, *Academic Scientists and the Pharmaceutical Industry: Cooperative Research in Twentieth-Century America* (Baltimore: Johns Hopkins University Press, 1988), 41-43; John Parascandola, "Industrial Research Comes of Age: The American Pharmaceutical Industry, 1920-1940," *Pharmacy in History* 27 (1985): 12-21.

8. George B. Walden, Sr., interview with Gene E. McCormick, 5 Nov. 1968, p. 25, Drawer 1, Cabinet 3, Company History Files; Swann, *Academic Scientists and the Pharmaceutical Industry,* 50-54; EL to G. H. A. Clowes, 5 Feb. 1936, XCAc. The quotation is from EL to Research Committee, 21 May 1942, Research Committee, +XRDj.

9. EL, "Notes on Research," 23 Jan. 1969, Drawer 1, Cabinet 5, Company History Files; Clowes to EL, 1 Dec. 1944, Clowes Folder, ELP. Quotation is on page 26. Lilly reacted to this memorandum from Clowes with handwritten marginal comments.

10. JKL, Jr., to EL, 16 July 1940, Research Organization, 1932-44, Drawer 1, Cabinet 5, Company History Files. See also Raymond Rice, interview with McCormick, 19 Aug. 1977, Research Organization, 1932-44, Drawer 1, Cabinet 6, Company History Files; Robert H. Rhodehamel, interview with author, 8 Dec. 1986.

11. J. P. Scott to George D. Beal, 16 Dec. 1938, C38(a)I, Lilly & Co., Kremers Reference Files, School of Pharmacy, University of Wisconsin, Madison.

12. Clowes to EL, 1 Dec. 1944, Clowes Folder, ELP; Rice, interview with McCormick.

13. EL, "History of Eli Lilly and Company, 1876-1950," typescript, 105-6, 135. In 1932 Eli Lilly took over this annual compilation and report begun by his father in 1908.

14. EL, "The Progress of Eli Lilly and Company: Past, Present and Future," 18 Feb. 1946, typescript, 5-9, XCAi; EL, "The President's Column," *SuperVision* 2 (Feb. 1947): 1.

15. EL, "History of Eli Lilly and Company," 112. See also EL to McCormick, 26 Feb. 1969, Lilly Company History Folder, ELP; J. L. Rosenstein to McCormick, 24 Nov. 1969, Herman H. Young Foundation Folder, Drawer 1, Cabinet 9, Company History Files.

16. J. L. Rosenstein, *Psychology of Human Relations for Executives* (New York: McGraw-Hill, 1936).

17. EL to McCormick, 26 Feb. 1969, Lilly Company History Folder, ELP; EL to Earl Beck, 22 May 1934, Paternalism Folder, Drawer 1, Cabinet 9, Company History Files.

18. EL to McCormick, 26 Feb. 1969, Lilly Company History Folder, ELP.

19. Beck to EL, 15 Dec. 1936, Efficiency Division Reports, XIRa.

20. *Catalog of Employees' Hobby Show 1936,* Employee Activities Folder, Drawer 3, Cabinet 6, Company History Files.

21. Beck to EL, 31 Dec. 1937, Efficiency Division Reports, XIRa.

22. Ibid.; Everett K. Todd, interview with McCormick, 7, 9 Feb. 1968, Drawer 1, Cabinet 3, Company History Files; Robert H. Rhodehamel, interview with author, 18 July 1986; Gene E. McCormick, "A History of Eli Lilly and Company," typescript, 1971, chapter 7, pp. 117-18.

23. Eli Lilly, "A Plan for Accomplishing More Effective Research," *Proceedings of the Indiana Academy of Science* 48 (1938): 10.

24. Daniel A. Wren, *The Evolution of Management Thought,* 2d ed. (New York: John Wiley & Sons, 1979), 297-323; Sanford M. Jacoby, "Employee Attitude Testing at Sears, Roebuck and Company, 1938-1960," *Business History Review* 60 (1986): 602-7; Sanford M. Jacoby, *Employing Bureaucracy: Managers, Unions, and the Transformation of Work in American Industry, 1900-1945* (New York: Columbia University Press, 1985), 241-74.

25. F. J. Roethlisberger, "Some Impressions Regarding the Social Organization of Eli Lilly and Company," typescript, Feb. 1941, XIRe. Roethlisberger's ideas at the time of his visit to Indianapolis are contained in F. J. Roethlisberger, *Management and Morale* (Cambridge, Mass.: Harvard University Press, 1941). See also F. J. Roethlisberger, *The Elusive Phenomena: An Autobiographical Account of My Work in the Field of Organizational Behavior at the Harvard Business School* (Cambridge, Mass.: Graduate School of Business Administration, Harvard University, 1977). In late 1941 Lilly sent three executives to visit the Western Electric Hawthorne Works, where Mayo and Roethlisberger had done so much of their pioneering work. Beck to EL, 19 Dec. 1941, Efficiency Division Reports, XIRa.

26. Emma Lou Thornbrough, "Breaking Racial Barriers to Public Accommodations in Indiana, 1935-1963," *Indiana Magazine of History* 83 (1987): 302, 316-18; Emma Lou Thornbrough, "Segregation in Indiana during the Klan Era of the 1920's," *Mississippi Valley Historical Review* 47 (1961): 594-618; Kenneth T. Jackson, *The Ku Klux Klan in the City, 1915-1930* (New York: Oxford University Press, 1967), 144-60; Work Projects Adminis-

tration, *Indiana: A Guide to the Hoosier State* (New York: Oxford University Press, 1941), 206.

27. E. H. Adriance to M. D. Snead, 23 Aug. 1934, Want List Folder, Drawer 1, Cabinet 9, Company History Files; Adriance to George Horton, 8 Sept. 1934, ibid.

28. EL to Beck, 30 Dec. 1935, Industrial Relations Folder, Drawer 3, Cabinet 6, ibid.

29. Beck to EL, 24 Sept. 1946; EL to Beck, 25 Sept. 1946; Beck to EL, 11 Mar. 1947; Beck to JKL, Jr., 30 Nov. 1948; E. N. Beesley to Beck, 4 Jan. 1949; JKL, Jr., to Beck, 9 Dec. 1948; H. G. Brannen to Division Directors, 19 Feb. 1951; all in ibid.

30. *Indianapolis Recorder,* 4 Jan. 1958.

31. Judith E. Endelman, *The Jewish Community of Indianapolis: 1849 to the Present* (Bloomington: Indiana University Press, 1984), 118, 172; Dale F. Ruedig, interview with McCormick, 24-25 Nov. 1969, p. 83, Drawer 2, Cabinet 3, Company History Files; James Ronald Newlin, "Women at Lilly: The Role of Female Labor in an American Industry, 1910-1950," typescript, 1980, Drawer 1, Cabinet 9, Company History Files; EL to JKL, Jr., 30 Apr., 1 June 1934, Women at Work Folder, Drawer 1, Cabinet 9, Company History Files.

32. JKL, Sr., to John Uri Lloyd, 1 Oct. 1924, Insulin Folder, Drawer 2, Cabinet 8, Company History Files.

33. EL, "History of Eli Lilly and Company," 114.

34. Ibid., 116-17. See also *Lilly Review* 7 (Sept. 1947): 12; Margaret W. Smith, interview with McCormick, 21 Dec. 1971, Drawer 1, Cabinet 3, Company History Files.

35. C. Rufus Rorem and Robert P. Fischelis, *The Costs of Medicine: The Manufacture and Distribution of Drugs and Medicines in the United States and the Service of Pharmacy in Medical Care* (Chicago: University of Chicago Press, 1932), 234.

36. Charles O. Jackson, *Food and Drug Legislation in the New Deal* (Princeton, N.J.: Princeton University Press, 1970), esp. 81, 151-74, 215-17; David F. Cavers, "The Evolution of the Contemporary System of Drug Regulation under the 1938 Act," in *Safeguarding the Public: Historical Aspects of Medicinal Drug Control,* ed. John B. Blake (Baltimore: Johns Hopkins Press, 1970), 158-70; EL, "History of Eli Lilly and Company," 126. Lilly was grateful for the national legislation because it drove out "a plethora of drastic laws by individual states." EL, "History of Eli Lilly and Company," 121.

37. EL, "History of Eli Lilly and Company," 124. See also Ellis W. Hawley, *The New Deal and the Problem of Monopoly: A Study in Economic Ambivalence* (Princeton, N.J.: Princeton University Press, 1966), 420-55.

38. *United States* v. *Eli Lilly and Company et al.,* case no. 67571 (criminal), District Court of the United States for the District of Columbia, 31 Mar. 1941, pp. 5, 6. See also *New York Times,* 8 Feb., 1, 26 Apr. 1941; *Business Week,* 20 July 1940, p. 44, 5 Apr. 1941, p. 8.

39. JKL, Jr., to JKL, Sr., 14 Mar. 1941, JKL, Sr., Personal Papers. See also EL, "History of Eli Lilly and Company," 143, 152.

40. Smith, interview with McCormick; EL to Black, 14 June 1941, Black Papers, Black Laboratory; EL, "History of Eli Lilly and Company," 152. See also Joseph Cornwall Palamountain, Jr., *The Politics of Distribution* (Cambridge, Mass.: Harvard University Press, 1955), 90-106.

41. JKL, Sr., to EL, 27 June 1941, Antitrust Folder, 1941, Drawer 2, Cabinet 6, Company History Files.

42. James H. Madison, *Indiana through Tradition and Change: A History of the Hoosier State and Its People, 1920-1945* (Indianapolis: Indiana Historical Society, 1982), 370-407.

43. JKL, Sr., to Hazel Allison, 4 Apr. 1943, Allison Family Folder, ELP.

44. JKL, Jr., to JKL, Sr., and EL, 18 Nov. 1941, JKL, Sr., Personal Papers.

45. EL, "Progress of Eli Lilly and Company"; Robert H. Rhodehamel, interview with author, 18 July 1986; EL to Black, 18 Feb. 1943, Black Papers, Black Laboratory.

46. EL, "Progress of Eli Lilly and Company," 5. Lilly reported that annual labor turnover increased from 6 percent in the depths of the Great Depression to 49 percent in 1944.

47. C. F. Eveleigh to JKL, Jr., 3 Oct. 1947, Efficiency of Production Departments, XCAo; JKL, Jr., to EL, 6 Oct. 1947, ibid.; Eli Lilly and Company, "Consolidated Operating Results," 30 Mar. 1977; H. W. Rhodehamel to Scott, 6 Sept. 1945, Research Folder, Drawer 3, Cabinet 6, Company History Files; EL to Sloane Graff, 17 Dec. 1943, Graff Folder, ELP.

48. EL to Graff, 13 Nov. 1942, Graff Folder, ELP; EL, "Progress of Eli Lilly and Company," 1-2.

49. EL to JKL, Sr., 5 Mar. 1945, EL and JKL, Sr., Correspondence Folder, ELP.

50. EL, "Progress of Eli Lilly and Company," 2.

51. EL to Clowes, 22 Oct. 1943, Clowes Correspondence, XRDc. See also Clowes to Vincent du Vigneaud, 9 Apr. 1943, ibid.

52. Clowes to EL, 26 Nov. 1943, ibid. See also EL to Clowes, 2 Dec. 1943, ibid.

53. Clowes to EL, 6 Dec. 1943, 10 Mar. 1944; Clowes to Charles H. Best, 5 Dec. 1945; George B. Walden to Clowes, 21 Feb. 1947; Clowes to Russell M. Wilder, 29 May 1947, all in ibid.

54. Clowes to EL, 10 Mar. 1944, ibid.; David P. Adams, "The Penicillin Mystique and the Popular Press (1935-1950)," *Pharmacy in History* 26 (1984): 134-42.

55. Arnold Thackray, "University-Industry Connections and Chemical Research: An Historical Perspective," National Science Board, *University-Industry Research Relationships* (Washington, D.C.: U.S. Government Printing Office, 1983), 225-26; Otto K. Behrens, "Biosynthesis of Penicillins," in *The Chemistry of Penicillin,* eds. Hans T. Clarke, John R. Johnson, and Robert Robinson (Princeton, N.J.: Princeton University Press, 1949), 657-79.

56. J. M. McGuire, "The Antibiotics—Past, Present, and Future," *Proceedings of the Indiana Academy of Science* 71 (1961): 249-51. McGuire was an Eli Lilly and Company scientist closely involved in penicillin work in the 1940s. See also W. H. Helfand et al., "Wartime Industrial Development of Penicillin in the United States," in *The History of Antibiotics: A Symposium,* ed. John Parascandola (Madison, Wisc.: American Institute of the History of Pharmacy, 1980), 31-36; Harry F. Dowling, *Fighting Infection: Conquests of the Twentieth Century* (Cambridge, Mass.: Harvard University Press, 1977), 125-57; David Wilson, *In Search of Penicillin* (New York: Alfred A. Knopf, 1976), 187-98; John C. Siegesmund, interview with McCormick, 10 Dec. 1968, Drawer 1, Cabinet 3, Company History Files.

57. McGuire, "The Antibiotics," 250; Helfand et al., "Wartime Industrial Development of Penicillin," 36-38.

58. McGuire, "The Antibiotics," 252-53; Helfand et al., "Wartime Industrial Development of Penicillin," 46; "Antibiotics," *Research Today* [Lilly Research Laboratories] 2 (Spring 1945): 19-30; Research Committee Minutes, 598, 13 May 1943, Research Committee,

+ XRDj; Clowes to EL, 6 Dec. 1943, Clowes Correspondence, XRDc; George B. Walden, Sr., interview with McCormick, 5 Nov. 1968, Penicillin Folder, Drawer 2, Cabinet 6, Company History Files; John A. Leighty, interview with McCormick, 23 July 1968, Penicillin Folder, Drawer 2, Cabinet 6, Company History Files.

59. Clowes to EL, 1 Dec. 1944, Clowes Folder, ELP; Walden, interview with McCormick, 5 Nov. 1968, Drawer 1, Cabinet 3, Company History Files; Helfand et al., "Wartime Industrial Development of Penicillin," 46-51; John C. Sheehan, *The Enchanted Ring: The Untold Story of Penicillin* (Cambridge, Mass.: MIT Press, 1982), 75-92; John Patrick Swann, "The Search for Synthetic Penicillin during World War II," *British Journal for the History of Science* 16 (1983): 154-90.

60. U.S., Congress, House, Committee on Appropriations, *Hearings on the National War Agencies Appropriation Bill for 1945,* 78th Cong., 2d sess., 1944, p. 430. See also EL to JKL, Sr., 15 Jan. 1946, EL and JKL, Sr., Correspondence Folder, ELP.

61. H. W. Rhodehamel to Scott, 6 Sept. 1945, Research Folder, Drawer 3, Cabinet 6, Company History Files.

62. Louis Lasagna, "1938-1968: The FDA, the Drug Industry, the Medical Profession, and the Public," in *Safeguarding the Public: Historical Aspects of Medicinal Drug Control,* ed. John B. Blake (Baltimore: Johns Hopkins University Press, 1970), 171; Eli Lilly and Company, Consolidated Operating Results, 30 Mar. 1977; EL to McCormick, 21 Aug. 1967, Facilities Improvement Folder, Drawer 4, Cabinet 5, Company History Files.

63. JKL, Jr., to JKL, Sr., 21 Jan. 1947, JKL, Sr., Personal Papers, reporting a conversation with EL. See also ibid., 29 July 1946.

64. EL to JKL, Sr., 6 Aug. 1946, EL and JKL, Sr., Correspondence, ELP; EL, "The Progress of Eli Lilly and Company"; *SuperVision* 1 (June 1946): 1; *SuperVision* 3 (Jan. 1948): 4; John C. Siegesmund, interview with McCormick, 10 Dec. 1968, Drawer 1, Cabinet 3, Company History Files.

65. JKL, Sr., to EL, 29 July 1947, EL and JKL, Sr., Correspondence, ELP.

66. Charles J. Lynn to William Fortune, 7 Sept. 1923, Folder 23, William Fortune Papers, Indiana Historical Society Library. See also William R. Spurlock, interview with McCormick, 9 Aug. 1968, Drawer 1, Cabinet 3, Company History Files; E. J. Kahn, Jr., *All in a Century: The First 100 Years of Eli Lilly and Company* ([Indianapolis: Eli Lilly & Co., 1976]), 52.

67. EL, "History of Eli Lilly and Company," 131. See also Report of Melvin T. Copeland, 23 Apr. 1937, pp. 31-32, XMMe; *Lilly Review* 7 (Jan. 1947): 3; Roscoe Collins Clark, *Threescore Years and Ten: A Narrative of the First Seventy Years of Eli Lilly and Company, 1876-1946* (Indianapolis: Eli Lilly & Co., 1946), 112-15.

68. JKL, Jr., "History of Eli Lilly and Company," 188; EL, "Progress of Eli Lilly and Company," 3; *SuperVision* 2 (July 1947): 9.

69. Research Committee Minutes, #33, 12 Jan. 1945, Research Committee, + XRDj.

70. J. P. Scott, "Planning of Our Post War Research Contacts," 19 Sept. 1944, Research Committee, + XRDj; Research Committee Report #83, 7 Jan. 1948, and Research Committee Report #91, 6 July 1948, Research Folder, Drawer 3, Cabinet 6, Company History Files; Research Committee Minutes, #47, 18 Jan. 1946, Research Committee, + XRDj.

71. EL, "Progress of Eli Lilly and Company," 4.

72. *SuperVision* 2 (July 1947): 9.

73. EL, "Progress of Eli Lilly and Company," 6.

74. R. C. Clark to JKL, Jr., 21 Mar. 1944, Public Relations Folder, Drawer 3, Cabinet 6, Company History Files; EL to Beck, 29 Feb. 1944, EL Miscellaneous Papers, Lilly Family Papers, XBLl; Rhodehamel, interview with author, 18 July 1986.

75. Roethlisberger, "Some Impressions Regarding the Social Organization of Eli Lilly and Company," 2.

76. Beck to EL, 12 June 1944, Organization Structure Proposal, 1944-48, XCAo. See also Beck to N. H. Noyes, 2 Mar. 1944, ibid.; Beesley to Beck, 25 Jan. 1944, ibid.

77. Beck to EL, 12 June 1944, Organization Structure Proposal, 1944-48, XCAo; Clark, *Threescore Years and Ten,* 76-77, 120-24.

78. E. H. Adriance and B. E. Beck, "Decentralizing the Staff Personnel Function," *Personnel* 24, no. 2 (1947): 3.

79. Rhodehamel, interviews with author.

80. JKL, Sr., to EL and JKL, Jr., 1 Sept. 1946, JKL, Sr., Personal Papers.

81. EL, "Progress of Eli Lilly and Company," 4.

82. EL to Beck, 13 Mar. 1947, Decentralization Folder, Drawer 3, Cabinet 6, Company History Files.

83. Beck, Progress Report of Plant Studies Committee, 9 Aug. 1948, Plant Studies Committee, 1947-48, XEMp. Quotation on page 1.

84. Ibid., 4.

85. Roethlisberger, "Some Impressions Regarding the Social Organization of Eli Lilly and Company," 2.

86. EL, "Progress of Eli Lilly and Company," passim. See also Rhodehamel, interview with author, 8 Dec. 1986.

87. EL, "Progress of Eli Lilly and Company," passim.

88. *SuperVision* 1 (Jan. 1946): 1. The need for big businesses to develop supervisors with good listening and communication skills was a fundamental tenet of the industrial relations literature of the 1930s and 1940s. Wren, *Evolution of Management Thought,* 318-20.

89. Direct quotations are from "The President's Column" in *SuperVision,* page 1, for the issues of Jan. 1946, Mar. 1948, and Aug. 1946.

90. Direct quotations are from *SuperVision,* page 1, issues of Jan. 1947 and Nov. 1946.

91. For speakers in the industrial relations lecture series see *SuperVision,* passim.

92. Alfred D. Chandler, Jr., *The Visible Hand: The Managerial Revolution in American Business* (Cambridge, Mass.: Harvard University Press, 1977), 451-53, 490-92.

93. JKL, Sr., to EL and JKL, Jr., 21 June 1922, JKL, Sr.'s, Objective Plan, Drawer 4, Cabinet 5, Company History Files; JKL, Sr., to Maria Lilly, 27 Feb. 1926, JKL, Sr., Miscellaneous Papers, Lilly Family Papers, XBLl; JKL, Sr., to EL and JKL, Jr., 1 Sept. 1946, JKL, Sr., Personal Papers. See also JKL, Sr., to EL and JKL, Jr., 8 Jan. 1925, unindexed material.

94. JKL, Sr., to Charles Lynn et al., 2 May 1946, Wheeler Folder, Drawer 3, Cabinet 6, Company History Files. The memorandum from W. M. Wheeler has not survived, though his proposals were apparently adopted by the board of directors. The identification of family with company pervades JKL, Sr., "Reminiscences," typescript, 1940, XBLl.

95. EL to J.K. Lilly III, 6 May 1941, J. K. Lilly III Folder, ELP; EL to JKL, Sr., 26 Feb. 1946, EL and JKL, Sr., Correspondence, ibid.

96. J. K. Lilly III, interview with author, 4 Sept. 1986.

97. EL to J. K. Lilly III, 20 Sept. 1946, J. K. Lilly III Folder, ELP.

98. Melvin T. Copeland, Report, June 1925, XMMe. The ever watchful company treasurer, Nicholas H. Noyes, strongly objected to the costs of Copeland's consulting visits. In the 1930s the company paid him $500 a day plus expenses. Noyes fumed: "I have never heard of any college professor, no matter how much of an expert or how competent, who charged over $200 a day for his time, and most of them charge $100 a day." Noyes to JKL, Jr., 15 May 1934, Melvin T. Copeland Correspondence, XMMc.

99. Copeland, Report, 29 Apr. 1947, p. 8, 14 Nov. 1944, pp. 16, 17.

100. Beesley to Beck, 25 Jan. 1944, Organization Structure, 1944-48, XCAo; Kahn, *All in a Century,* 149-50.

101. Melvin T. Copeland, Report, 20 June 1934, XMMe; "America's Best-Managed Companies," *American Business* 17 (Feb. 1947): 20-22; "Our Best Managed Companies," *American Business* 17 (June 1947): 18-19. Respondents to the poll were described as leading bankers, business editors, and security dealers.

Chapter 6

1. EL to Evie Lilly, 15 Dec. 1929, XBLl. An earlier version of part of this chapter appeared as James H. Madison, "Eli Lilly: Archaeologist," Glenn A. Black Laboratory of Archaeology, *Research Reports* No. 8 (1988).

2. EL to Glenn Black, 29 Jan. 1947, Black Papers, Glenn A. Black Laboratory of Archaeology, Indiana University, Bloomington.

3. EL to E. Y. Guernsey, 1 June, 3 May 1933, Guernsey Folder, EL Papers, Black Laboratory.

4. Ibid., 3 Nov. 1930.

5. EL to A. L. Addis, 17 Feb. 1931, Addis Folder, ibid. See also EL, Gift to Indiana Historical Society, 22 Dec. 1933, EL Folder, Box 3, Indiana Historical Society Business Office Files, Indiana Historical Society Library.

6. EL to Thomas Hendricks, 20 Aug. 1930, Hendricks Folder, EL Papers, Black Laboratory.

7. EL to B. H. Hall, 4 May 1932, Hall Folder, ibid.

8. EL to W. A. McGuire, 13 Feb. 1932, McGuire Folder, ibid.

9. Ronald L. Michael, "Indiana Archaeology: 1800-1930," *Indiana Archaeology Bulletin* 1 (1976): 65-85; Glenn A. Black, ". . . that what is past may not be forever lost. . . ." *Indiana History Bulletin* 38 (1961): 52-55; Robert Silverberg, *Mound Builders of Ancient America: The Archaeology of a Myth* (Greenwich, Conn.: New York Graphic Society, 1968).

10. Lana Ruegamer, *A History of the Indiana Historical Society, 1830-1980* (Indianapolis: Indiana Historical Society, 1980), 135-36, 261-69; James H. Kellar, *An Introduction to the Prehistory of Indiana* (Indianapolis: Indiana Historical Society, 1983), 13-16. Among the contributors to the archaeology section work was J. K. Lilly, Sr. He gave $200 in 1926 and $100 in 1927. There is no contribution recorded for Eli Lilly in these early years. Christopher B. Coleman to JKL, Sr., 18 July 1928, Archaeology Folder, Indiana Historical Bureau Correspondence, Archives Division, Indiana Commission on Public Records, Indiana State Library and Historical Building, Indianapolis.

11. Coleman to EL, 20 Nov. 1933, Archaeology Folder, 1928-36, Indiana Historical Society Library; Ruegamer, *History of the Indiana Historical Society,* 269-70; Glenn A. Black, "Report of Trip of Glenn A. Black and Dr. Warren K. Moorehead," 20 May 1931, Black Folder, EL Papers, Black Laboratory; Black to EL, 17 Nov. 1958, Miscellaneous Folder, EL Legal Records, Vault; EL to Warren K. Moorehead, 18 May 1931, Moorehead Folder, EL Papers, Black Laboratory.

12. EL to E. R. Burmaster, 27 Aug. 1931, Burmaster Folder, EL Papers, Black Laboratory.

13. Ibid., 31 Dec. 1931. See also Eli Lilly, "A Cedar Point 'Glacial Kame' Burial," *Proceedings of the Indiana Academy of Science* 51 (1941): 31-33.

14. EL to Black, 3 July 1931, Black Papers, Black Laboratory. See also EL to John J. Davis, 13 Feb. 1931, Black Papers, Black Laboratory; John C. Householder, interview with author, 5 Dec. 1986.

15. Eli Lilly, "Bibliography on Indiana Archaeology," *Indiana History Bulletin* 9 (1932): 445-79; EL, "Reminiscences," typescript, 1966-69, XBLl.

16. EL to Moorehead, 17 Aug. 1931, Moorehead Folder, EL Papers, Black Laboratory.

17. James H. Kellar, "Glenn A. Black," in untitled dedication booklet for the Glenn A. Black Laboratory of Archaeology, 21 Apr. 1971, Indiana University Publications; Ruegamer, *History of the Indiana Historical Society,* 257-59, 270-72; EL to Black, 15 Sept. 1931, Black Papers, Black Laboratory.

18. EL to Black, 17 Aug. 1931, Black Papers, Black Laboratory. See also EL to Black, 24 June 1931, Black Folder, EL Papers, Black Laboratory.

19. EL to Moorehead, 15 Aug. 1931, Moorehead Folder, EL Papers, Black Laboratory.

20. H. C. Shetrone to William R. Teel, 28 Sept. 1931, Teel Folder, ibid.

21. Shetrone to EL, 19 May 1932, Shetrone Folder, ibid.; Black to Shetrone, 27 Dec. 1935, Black Papers, Black Laboratory.

22. EL to Black, 6 Nov. 1931, Black Folder, EL Papers, Black Laboratory. See also Black to EL, 23 Oct. 1931, Black Papers, Black Laboratory.

23. EL to Black, 29 Oct. 1931, Black to EL, 30 Oct. 1931, EL to Black, 2 Nov. 1931, all in Black Papers, Black Laboratory.

24. EL to Black, 9 Mar. 1932, ibid.

25. Teel to Black, 11, 13 July 1932, ibid.

26. EL to Black, 28 June 1934, ibid.

27. EL to Coleman, 1 June 1933, Archaeology Folder, 1928-36, Indiana Historical Society Library. See also Ruegamer, *History of the Indiana Historial Society,* 281. Lilly's contributions to the Society were sometimes personal, sometimes made through the Lilly Endowment. Of the $1,172,321 that the Lilly Endowment gave the Society in the years 1939-68, $663,251 was directed to archaeology. Endowments Grants to Indiana Historical Society, 1919-68, n.d., Indiana Historical Society Folder, EL Drawer, Cabinet 4, Company History Files.

28. EL to James B. Griffin, 24 Dec. 1936, Griffin Folder, EL Papers, Black Laboratory.

29. EL to Black, 6 Sept. 1934, Black Papers, Black Laboratory; EL to Griffin, 12 Jan. 1937, Griffin Folder, EL Papers, Black Laboratory; Howard H. Peckham, letter to author, 22 Aug. 1985. For Franklin's model, see Benjamin Franklin, *The Autobiography of Benjamin Franklin* (New York: Washington Square Press, 1955), 19-20.

30. Eli Lilly, *Prehistoric Antiquities of Indiana: A Description of the More Notable Earthworks, Mounds, Implements and Ceremonial Objects Left in Indiana by Our Predecessors, Together with Some Information As to Their Origin and Antiquity, and the Prehistory of Indiana* (Indianapolis: Indiana Historical Society, 1937), v; Frederica De Laguna, review, *American Journal of Archaeology* 43 (1939): 552-53; Warren King Moorehead, review, *Mississippi Valley Historical Review* 25 (1938-39): 86-87; EL to Nellie Armstrong, 4, 15, 16 June 1937, EL Folder, Publication Files, Indiana Historical Society; *Indianapolis Times,* 12 Feb. 1938.

31. Lilly, *Prehistoric Antiquities of Indiana,* 22, 36. Like most archaeologists of the 1930s, Lilly was concerned above all with chronology and taxonomy, but he was interested also in broader issues of culture. See Gordon R. Willey and Jeremy A. Sabloff, *A History of American Archaeology* (San Francisco: W. H. Freeman & Co., 1974), 88-126.

32. Black to EL, 6 Sept. 1932, Black Papers, Black Laboratory.

33. EL to Guernsey, 14 Feb. 1934, Guernsey Folder, EL Papers, Black Laboratory; EL to Shetrone, 9 Jan. 1933, Shetrone Folder, ibid.

34. EL to Shetrone, 6 Aug. 1931, Shetrone Folder, ibid.

35. EL to Moorehead, 21 Nov. 1931, Moorehead Folder, ibid.; Shetrone to EL, 26 Jan. 1932, Shetrone Folder, ibid.; EL to Black, 21 Jan. 1936, Black Papers, Black Laboratory.

36. EL to Carl Guthe, 12 Sept. 1932, Guthe Folder, EL Papers, Black Laboratory. See also E. Sapir, "Time Perspectives in Aboriginal American Culture, A Study in Method," Canada, Department of Mines, Geological Survey, *Memoir* 90 (Ottawa, 1916): 51-85.

37. EL to Edward Sapir, 16 Sept. 1932, Sapir Folder, EL Papers, Black Laboratory.

38. Sapir to EL, 18 Oct. 1932, ibid.

39. EL to Sapir, 31 Oct. 1932, ibid.

40. Sapir to Lilly, 5 Dec. 1932; Lilly to Sapir, 15 Dec. 1932; Sapir to Lilly, 23 Dec. 1932, ibid.

41. Lilly to Sapir, 29 Dec. 1932; Sapir to Lilly, 17 Jan. 1933, ibid.

42. Sapir to EL, 29 Mar., 5 Apr. 1933, ibid.

43. EL to Edgar S. Furniss, 7 Apr. 1933, ibid.

44. Carl Voegelin to EL, 14 Aug., 21 Dec. 1933, 6, 25 Jan. 1934, Voegelin Folder, ibid.; EL to Carl Voegelin, 2 Jan. 1934, Sapir Folder, ibid.

45. Carl Voegelin to EL, 5 Feb. 1934, Voegelin Folder, ibid.; EL to Voegelin, 12 Mar. 1934, ibid. See also Black to EL, 13 Feb. 1934, ibid.; Black to Guthe, 5 Mar. 1934, Black Papers, Black Laboratory.

46. Black to Guthe, 5 Mar. 1934, Black Papers, Black Laboratory; EL to Voegelin, 12 Dec. 1935, Voegelin Folder, EL Papers, Black Laboratory.

47. G. Bromley Oxnam to EL, 28 Apr. 1936, V Miscellaneous Folder, ELP.

48. EL to Fay-Cooper Cole, 12 Feb. 1937, Cole Folder, EL Papers, Black Laboratory; Guthe to EL, 23 Jan. 1933, Guthe Folder, ibid.; EL to Guthe, 19 Oct. 1936, Guthe Folder, ibid.; James B. Griffin, "Commentary on an Unusual Research Program," in untitled dedication booklet for the Glenn A. Black Laboratory of Archaeology, 21 Apr. 1971, Indiana University Publications. For Griffin's distinguished career, see Volney H. Jones, "James Bennett Griffin: Archaeologist," in *Cultural Change and Continuity: Essays in Honor of James Bennett Griffin,* ed. Charles E. Cleland (New York: Academic Press, 1976), xxxix-lxxvii.

49. EL to Teel, 16 Nov. 1936, Teel Folder, EL Papers, Black Laboratory. See also EL to Griffin, 4 Jan. 1937, Griffin Folder, ibid.; EL to Black, 9 Apr. 1934, Black Papers, Black Laboratory.

50. EL to Guthe, 31 May 1940, Black Folder, EL Papers, Black Laboratory. See also EL to Guernsey, 30 Sept. 1937, Guernsey Folder, ibid.; James B. Griffin, interview with author, 26 Dec. 1986.

51. Guthe to EL, 25 Oct. 1937, Guthe Folder, EL Papers, Black Laboratory.

52. *Walam Olum or Red Score: The Migration Legend of the Lenni Lenape or Delaware Indians: A New Translation, Interpreted by Linguistic, Historical, Archaeological, Ethnological, and Physical Anthropological Studies* (Indianapolis: Indiana Historical Society, 1954), ix-x; C. A. Weslager, *The Delaware Indians: A History* (New Brunswick, N.J.: Rutgers University Press, 1972), 77-97; William Barlow and David O. Powell, "'The Late Dr. Ward of Indiana': Rafinesque's Source of the Walam Olum," *Indiana Magazine of History* 82 (1986): 185-93; Charles Boewe, "The Walam Olum and Dr. Ward, Again," *Indiana Magazine of History* 83 (1987): 342-59.

53. *Walam Olum,* especially Lilly's chapter, titled "Speculations on the Chronology of the Walam Olum and Migration of the Lenape," 273-85.

54. For Lilly's interest in Schliemann and Troy, see Eli Lilly, ed., *Schliemann in Indianapolis* (Indianapolis: Indiana Historical Society, 1961), and below, chapter 7.

55. EL to Black, 11 Jan. 1932, Black Papers, Black Laboratory.

56. Black to EL, 27 Jan. 1932, ibid.

57. EL to Black, 12 Feb. 1932, ibid. See also Black to EL, 11 Feb. 1932, ibid.

58. EL to Guthe, 12 Sept. 1932, Guthe Folder, EL Papers, Black Laboratory.

59. Guthe to Black, 15 Feb. 1933, Black Papers, Black Laboratory. See also EL to Sapir, 16 Sept. 1932, Sapir to EL, 18 Oct. 1932, Sapir Folder, EL Papers, Black Laboratory.

60. EL to Voegelin, 14 Nov. 1938, Voegelin Folder, EL Papers, Black Laboratory. See also Eli Lilly, "Remarks Regarding the Pictographs of the Walam Olum," *Proceedings of the Indiana Academy of Science* 49 (1939): 32-33.

61. EL to Black, 10 Mar. 1941, Black Papers, Black Laboratory. See also Black to EL, 16 Jan. 1939, Black Papers, ibid.; EL to Black, 26 Sept. 1933, 12 Mar. 1941, 11 Apr. 1945, ibid.

62. EL to Voegelin, 2 Nov. 1942, Voegelin Folder, EL Papers, Black Laboratory. See also EL to Voegelin, 16 Mar. 1943, ibid.; EL to Black, 4 Sept. 1943, Black Papers, Black Laboratory.

63. EL to Black, 9 July 1943, Black Papers, Black Laboratory. See also EL to Black, 26 Oct. 1942, ibid.

64. EL to Black, 2 Oct. 1946, ibid.

65. EL to Dorothy Cross, 20 May 1946, Catherine McCann Folder, EL Papers, Black Laboratory; EL to William A. Ritchie, 4 June 1946, Ritchie Folder, ibid.; EL to Frank G. Speck, 20 May 1946, Speck Folder, ibid.

66. EL to Cross, 12 Aug. 1946, McCann Folder, ibid.

67. EL to Ritchie, 15 Sept. 1947, Ritchie Folder, ibid. Invited for the 10 Oct. meeting were Ritchie, Griffin, Neumann, Witthoft, Carl Voegelin, Black, Howard Peckham, Weer, Carpenter, and Richard S. MacNeish, a University of Michigan student who also worked on the

Delaware problem. Dorothy Cross, Catherine McCann, and Erminie Voegelin were not invited, evidence of the special challenges facing female academics in the 1940s.

68. EL to Carl Voegelin, 8 Jan. 1948, Voegelin Folder, ibid. See also EL to Carl Voegelin, 30 Jan. 1947, ibid.; EL to Ritchie, 6 Oct. 1947, Ritchie Folder, ibid.

69. EL to Carl Voegelin, 12 Dec. 1949, Voegelin Folder, ibid.

70. EL to Neumann, 27 Sept. 1951, ibid.; EL to Carl and Erminie Voegelin [27 Sept. 1951], 8 Oct. 1951, ibid.

71. EL to Black, 5 Mar. 1953, Black Papers, Black Laboratory. See also Howard H. Peckham to Paul Weer, 8 Sept. 1953, Walum Olum Correspondence, Publications Files, Indiana Historical Society.

72. Black to EL, 7 May 1952, Black Folder, ELP. Black and Griffin respected each other's abilities but did not feel kindly toward one another. It is likely that Carl Voegelin, John Witthoft, and perhaps others as well as Griffin came to think Walam Olum a fabrication. Griffin, interview with author; John Witthoft, letter to author, 23 Apr. 1987. Both Griffin and Witthoft remained very fond of Lilly and highly respectful of his contributions to their field.

73. Undated memorandum of Walam Olum payments, Walam Olum Folder, EL Papers, Indiana Historical Society Library; EL to Erminie Voegelin, 21 Sept. 1948, Voegelin Folder, EL Papers, Black Laboratory; Griffin to EL, 6 Jan. 1947, Griffin Folder, EL Papers, Black Laboratory; James H. Kellar, interview with author, 27 Aug. 1986. The quotation about Griffin is from George I. Quimby and Charles E. Cleland, "James Bennett Griffin: Appreciation and Reminiscences," Cleland, *Cultural Change and Continuity,* xxxi.

74. *Walam Olum.* See also R. R. Donnelley & Sons, Invoice, 4 Oct. 1954, Walum Olum Correspondence, Publications Files, Indiana Historical Society; Gayle Thornbrough to EL, 30 Apr. 1954, Walam Olum Folder, ELP.

75. Robert B. Woodbury, review, *American Antiquity* 21 (1955-56): 192. See also Martin Gusinde, review, *Anthropos* 52 (1957): 679-81.

76. C. A. Weslager, review, *Archaeology* 8 (1955): 283. Later, Weslager was more open to the possibility that the Walam Olum was a legitimate part of Delaware tradition. See Weslager, *Delaware Indians,* 77-97.

77. EL to Black, 7 Oct. 1954, enclosing Griffin to EL, 5 Oct. 1954, Black Papers, Black Laboratory.

78. EL to Black, 20 Dec. 1954, ibid.

79. James B. Griffin, review, *Indiana Magazine of History* 51 (1955): 59-65.

80. Griffin, "Commentary on an Unusual Research Program."

81. EL to Griffin, 27 Apr. 1971, Griffin Folder, ELP.

82. EL to Josephine Elliott, 12 July 1972, D Miscellaneous Folder, ibid. Earlier Lilly had supported a laborious search for Ward and Walam Olum in Ohio sources and in the Moravian Archives in Bethlehem, Pennsylvania. See Carl John Fliegel, comp., *Index to the Records of the Moravian Mission among the Indians of North America,* 4 vols. (Woodbridge, Conn.: Research Publications, Inc., 1970), 1:v; EL to James H. Rodabaugh, 8 May 1951, Moravian Mission Folder, Conner Prairie Settlement Collection, Earlham College Archives, Richmond, Indiana; EL to K. G. Hamilton, 6 Jan. 1955, Moravian Mission Folder, Conner Prairie Settlement Collection.

83. Elemire Zolla, *The Writer and the Shaman: A Morphology of the American Indian,* trans. by Raymond Rosenthal (New York: Harcourt Brace Jovanovich, 1973), 233.

84. Daniel Hoffman, *Brotherly Love* (New York: Vintage Books, 1981), 9-14, 159-60; Charles Boewe, "A Note on Rafinesque, the Walam Olum, the Book of Mormon, and the Mayan Glyphs," *Numen* 32, no. 1 (1985): 101-13; Boewe, "The Walam Olum and Dr. Ward, Again," 346-47; Herbert C. Kraft, *The Lenape: Archaeology, History, and Ethnography* (Newark: New Jersey Historical Society, 1986), xii, xiv, 4-7; Weslager, *Delaware Indians,* 80-81; Griffin, "A Commentary on an Unusual Research Program"; Griffin, interview with author; William N. Fenton, review, *New-York Historical Society Quarterly* 39 (1955): 338-41. Carbon-14 dating, which was developed after most of the work on Walam Olum was finished, does not support the time frame Lilly proposed for the Lenape migration. Kellar, *Introduction to the Prehistory of Indiana,* 18.

85. Carl Voegelin to EL, 26 Mar. 1935, Voegelin Folder, EL Papers, Black Laboratory.

86. Ibid., 28 Sept. 1941.

87. EL to Carl Voegelin, 26 Sept. 1941, 5, 11 Apr. 1944, 18 Dec. 1947, ibid.; EL to Black, 13 Oct. 1941, 15 May, 6 June 1944, Black Papers, Black Laboratory.

88. Carl Voegelin to EL, 14 Oct. 1947, Voegelin Folder, Black Laboratory.

89. Black to EL, 11 Oct. 1954, 7, 24 June 1955, Black Papers, Black Laboratory; Neumann to EL, 15 Apr. 1963, 10 May 1963, Neumann Folder, ELP. In 1963 Lilly was still providing financial support for Neumann's research.

90. Eli Lilly, "A Plan for Accomplishing More Effective Research," *Proceedings of the Indiana Academy of Science* 48 (1939): 8, 10, 11.

91. Voegelin to EL, 26 Mar. 1935, Voegelin Folder, Black Papers, Black Laboratory. See also Griffin to EL, 21 Sept. 1936, Griffin Folder, EL Papers, Black Laboratory.

92. Moorehead to EL, 20 May 1931, Moorehead Folder, EL Papers, Black Laboratory.

93. Lilly, *Prehistoric Antiquities of Indiana,* 44, 46-48. More detailed and precise data on Mound A are provided in Glenn A. Black, *Angel Site: An Archaeological, Historical, and Ethnological Study,* 2 vols. (Indianapolis: Indiana Historical Society, 1967), 1:46-48.

94. Black, *Angel Site,* 1:20-26; Ruegamer, *History of the Indiana Historical Society,* 283-86.

95. Black to Guthe, 12 Apr. 1938, Black Papers, Black Laboratory. See also Lilly to Guernsey, n.d., Guernsey Folder, EL Papers, Black Laboratory.

96. EL to Black, 18 Sept. 1939, Black Papers, Black Laboratory; EL to Coleman, 3 June 1937, Archaeology Folder, 1937-44, Indiana Historical Society Library.

97. Black to EL, 18 Mar. 1942, Black Papers, Black Laboratory; Black to EL, 10 May 1955, Black Folder, ELP; EL to Black, 19 Mar. 1941, Black Papers, Black Laboratory; Black, *Angel Site,* 1:229; Frances Martin, interview with author, 7 June 1986.

98. Black to EL, 23 June 1941, Black Papers, Black Laboratory; EL to Black, 19 Mar., 24 June 1941, 11 June 1945, ibid.

99. Black to EL, 28 June 1945, ibid.

100. EL to Black, 25 Nov. 1946, ibid. See also *Indianapolis News,* 25, 26 Nov. 1946.

101. EL to Curtis G. Shake, 3 May 1963, Harrison Mansion Folder, ELP; EL, "Reminiscences." See also EL to Richard O. Ristine, 12 June 1964, Political Contributions Folder, ELP; EL to Black, 22 Nov. 1963, Black Papers, Black Laboratory.

102. Black, *Angel Site,* 1:27-28; Black "Archaeological Activities, 1939-62," typescript, 8 Apr. 1963, Black Papers, Black Laboratory. One field technique in which Lilly was especially interested was the pioneering use of proton magnetometry at Angel site in the early 1960s, assisted by a grant from the National Science Foundation. See Richard B. Johnston, *Proton Magnetometry and Its Application to Archaeology: An Evaluation at Angel Site,* Indiana Historical Society Prehistory Research Series, vol. 4, no. 2 (Indianapolis: Indiana Historical Society, 1964), 45-140.

103. EL to Moorehead, 26 Aug. 1932, Moorehead Folder, EL Papers, Black Laboratory.

104. EL to Black, 27 Sept. 1934, Black Papers, Black Laboratory; Black to EL, 7 July 1946, ibid.

105. EL to Black, 6 Nov. 1945, ibid.

106. Black to EL, 11 June 1958, Black Folder, ELP. See also Black to EL, 18 Jan. 1954, Black Papers, Black Laboratory; EL to Black, 3 Feb. 1954, Black Papers, Black Laboratory. Black's unsigned "Tribute to Eli Lilly," on the occasion of his retirement from the presidency of the Indiana Historical Society, appeared in the *Indiana Magazine of History* 43 (1947): 63-66. Lilly immediately recognized Black as the author. EL to Black, 28 Mar. 1947, Black Papers, Black Laboratory.

107. Kellar, interview with author; James H. Kellar, "Glenn A. Black, 1900-1964," *American Antiquity* 31 (1965-66): 402-5; Martin, interview with author. See also Black Papers, Black Laboratory, for example, EL to Black, 18 Apr., 3 June 1958.

108. "The Trip Magnificent," Oct. 1963, Black Folder, ELP.

109. EL to Black, 8 Jan. 1946, Black Papers, Black Laboratory. Information on the trips comes from EL, "Reminiscences" and Black Papers, Black Laboratory. See, for example, EL to Black, 1 Mar. 1949, 25 Oct. 1954, 27 Jan., 20 Feb. 1960. Also helpful is Martin, interview with author.

110. EL to Thornton Black, 30 Sept. 1964, Black Folder, ELP.

111. Kellar, interview with author; EL, notes of telephone conversation with Dorothy Herron, 7 Sept. 1964, Black Folder, ELP; John G. Rauch, Sr., to EL, 15 Jan. 1965, Black Folder, ELP; EL to Ida Black, 24 May 1965, Black Folder, ELP; Ida Black to EL and Ruth Lilly, 25 May 1965, Black Folder, ELP; Howard and Dorothy Peckham, interview with author, 2 Aug. 1985.

112. Black, *Angel Site,* 1:vii-viii.

113. EL to Black, 13 Oct. 1941, Black Papers, Black Laboratory; EL to Roger D. Branigin, 27 Nov. 1968, Black Folder, ELP; Herman B Wells, interview with author, 30 Oct. 1984; Black Laboratory dedication booklet.

114. Elvin H. Hewins to EL, 10 Feb. 1972, Black Folder, ELP.

115. EL to Kellar, 12 Sept. 1972, Kellar Folder, ELP.

116. EL to James H. Kellar, 22 Jan. 1968, ibid.

117. EL to Branigin, 27 Nov. 1968, Black Folder, ibid.

118. EL to Kellar, 11 Feb. 1970, Angel Mounds Folder, ibid.; Rauch to Herman B Wells, 7 Mar. 1969, Rauch Folder, ibid.; EL to Rauch, 14 Mar. 1969, Rauch Folder, ibid.; Martin, interview with author.

119. Griffin, "Commentary on an Unusual Research Program."

Chapter 7

1. Lana Ruegamer, *A History of the Indiana Historical Society, 1830-1980* (Indianapolis: Indiana Historical Society, 1980), 5-173. Quotation is on page 162.

2. EL, "Reminiscences," typescript, 1966-69, XBLl; Ruegamer, *History of the Indiana Historical Society,* 224-26. Much of Lilly's financial support came by way of the Lilly Endowment.

3. Minutes of the Executive Committee, 31 Jan. 1946, Indiana Historical Society Papers, Indiana Historical Society Library.

4. EL to Hubert Hawkins, 27 Nov. 1961, Indiana Historical Society Folder, ELP. See also Gayle Thornbrough to Eva Rice Gobel, 29 June 1965, Charlotte Cathcart Folder, ibid.

5. EL, "Reminiscences." For McNutt's patronage see James H. Madison, *Indiana through Tradition and Change: A History of the Hoosier State and Its People, 1920-1945* (Indianapolis: Indiana Historical Society, 1982), 93-99. Lilly's friend and former brother-in-law, Bowman Elder, was one of McNutt's closest political associates.

6. EL, "Reminiscences"; Indiana Historical Society Minutes of the Executive Committee, 8 Dec. 1934.

7. Gayle Thornbrough, Dorothy L. Riker, and Paula Corpuz, eds., *The Diary of Calvin Fletcher,* 9 vols. (Indianapolis: Indiana Historical Society, 1972-83); Gayle Thornbrough, interview with author, 16 Dec. 1986.

8. Ruegamer, *History of the Indiana Historical Society,* 227-29; EL, "Reminiscences."

9. Indiana Historical Society Minutes of the Executive Committee, 28 Mar. 1940. See also ibid., 13 Dec. 1940.

10. Ibid., 11 Dec. 1943; EL to John G. Rauch, Sr., 13 May 1942, Hodges Suit Folder, ELP; EL to Volney M. Brown, 7 Feb. 1944, Hodges Suit Folder, ELP; Rauch to Christopher B. Coleman, 10 Mar. 1944, Hodges Suit Folder, ELP; EL, "Reminiscences."

11. Mary Dean Brossman to EL, 5 Mar. 1945, Hodges Suit Folder, ELP; EL to Brossman, 8 Mar. 1945, ibid.

12. EL to Howard Peckham, 10 June 1949, EL Folder, 1948-58, Box 3, Indiana Historical Society Business Office Files, Indiana Historical Society Library; Rauch to EL, 13 July 1949, Hodges Suit Folder, ELP. See also *Indianapolis News,* 9 June 1949.

13. EL to Thornbrough, 11 Mar. 1968, Indiana Historical Society Folder, ELP.

14. Minutes of the Board of Trustees, 11 Dec. 1968, Business Office, Indiana Historical Society; Thornbrough, interview with author; Robert L. Jones, "*The Diary of Calvin Fletcher:* A Review Essay," *Indiana Magazine of History* 80 (1984): 171.

15. EL to Glenn A. Black, 26 Dec. 1944, Glenn A. Black Papers, Glenn A. Black Laboratory of Archaeology, Indiana University, Bloomington. See also EL to Black, 4 Aug., 1 Sept. 1944, ibid.

16. Indiana Historical Society Minutes of Executive Committee, 31 Jan. 1946, 7 Dec. 1951; Ruegamer, *History of the Indiana Historical Society,* 181-87; EL to Peckham, 25 Nov. 1952, Indiana Historical Society Folder, ELP; Dorothy and Howard Peckham, interview with author, 2 Aug. 1985.

17. EL to Black, 29 Jan. 1945, Black Papers, Black Laboratory; Dorothy and Howard Peckham, interview with author.

18. Peckham to EL, 20 Sept. 1961, Peckham Folder, ELP. The inscribed book, Dwight D. Eisenhower, *At Ease: Stories I Tell to Friends* (Garden City, N.Y.: Doubleday, 1967), is in the Eli Lilly Room, Lilly Center.

19. Ruegamer, *History of the Indiana Historical Society,* 188-93; Peckham to EL, 21 July 1953, Indiana Historical Society Folder, ELP; Hubert Hawkins, interview with Lana Ruegamer, 7 Dec. 1979, tape, Indiana Historical Society Library.

20. Lilly's marginal comments are on Hubert Hawkins to Byron K. Trippet, 16 Feb. 1963, Indiana Historical Society Folder, ELP.

21. EL to Hawkins, 9 Dec. 1964, EL Folder, Box 3, Indiana Historical Society Business Office Files.

22. EL to Herman B Wells, 23 Aug. 1972, Indiana Historical Society Folder, ELP.

23. Ruegamer, *History of the Indiana Historical Society,* 201-5; Thornbrough, interview with author; Hubert H. Hawkins, interview with author, 13 Feb. 1987; Indiana Historical Society Board of Trustees Minutes, 3 May 1967.

24. Thornbrough, interview with author; Lilly Endowment Grants to Indiana Historical Society, 1939-68, n.d., Indiana Historical Society Folder, EL Drawer, Cabinet 4, Company History Files; EL, Deed of Gift, 8 May 1968, EL Folder, Box 3, Indiana Historical Society Business Office Files; Rauch to EL, 20 May 1968, Indiana Historical Society Folder, ELP.

25. Peckham to EL, 3 July 1968, Peckham Folder, ELP; EL to Rauch, 9 July 1968, Indiana Historical Society Folder, ibid.; Rauch to William T. Alderson, 12 July 1968, Indiana Historical Society Folder, ibid.; Rauch to Hawkins, 25 July 1968, Indiana Historical Society Folder, ibid.

26. William T. Alderson, Report on the Organization and Operations of the Indiana Historical Society, 21 Sept. 1968, Indiana Historical Society Folder, ELP. See also Ruegamer, *History of the Indiana Historical Society,* 207-9.

27. EL to John F. Wilhelm, 25 Aug. 1972, Indiana Historical Society Folder, ELP.

28. Ruegamer, *History of the Indiana Historical Society,* 211-12; EL to Hawkins, 15 Jan. 1973, EL Folder, 1965-73, Box 3, Indiana Historical Society Business Office Files; Hawkins, interview with author.

29. Ruegamer, *History of the Indiana Historical Society,* 205-7, 212, 231, 238; Indiana Historical Society Board of Trustees Minutes, 17 Jan. 1968, 19 May, 27 Oct. 1975; Alderson, Report on the Organization and Operation of the Indiana Historical Society; Thornbrough, interview with author; Hawkins, interview with author.

30. EL to Peckham, 16 Dec. 1947, EL Folder, Box 3, Indiana Historical Society Business Office Files; EL to Hawkins, 18 July 1975, ibid.

31. Hawkins to Thomas S. Emison, 15 Sept. 1964, Angel Mounds, From 1964, Folder, Indiana Historical Society Library.

32. EL to E. Y. Guernsey, 10 May 1937, Guernsey Folder, EL Papers, Black Laboratory.

33. Herman B Wells, interview with author, 30 Oct. 1984; Dorothy and Howard Peckham, interview with author; Thornbrough, interview with author; Hawkins, interview with author.

34. EL to Peckham, 13 Jan. 1947, Indiana Historical Society Folder, ELP. See also Thornbrough, interview with author.

35. EL to Gene E. McCormick, 2 Nov. 1973, Lilly Company History Folder, ELP.

36. Lilly's 5 x 8 note cards are in Miscellaneous Cabinet 1. His "Shining Phrase Book" is in XBLl.

37. William E. Wilson, *Indiana: A History* (Bloomington: Indiana University Press, 1966), 16.

38. EL, undated notes for talk, ca. 1957, Speeches Folder, ELP; EL to Black, n.d. [Aug. 1954], Black Papers, Black Laboratory; EL to Church Historical Society, 9 Jan. 1953, Little Church on the Circle Folder, ELP; Clifford L. Lord to EL, 20 Feb., 31 Mar. 1952, Little Church on the Circle Folder, ELP; 5 x 8 note file, Miscellaneous Cabinet 1; EL's edited typescript of *Little Church on the Circle,* in XBLl.

39. Eli Lilly, *History of the Little Church on the Circle; Christ Church Parish Indianapolis 1837-1955* (Indianapolis: Christ Church, 1957).

40. Ibid. Quotations are on pages 67-68, 210.

41. Ibid., esp. 284, vii, 321, 302.

42. EL, undated notes for a talk.

43. Eli Lilly, *Early Wawasee Days: Traditions, Tales, and Memories Concerning That Delectable Spot* (n.p., Indianapolis, 1960).

44. EL to Scott Edgell, 28 July, 21 Oct. 1966, Edgell Folder, ELP; Scott A. Edgell, *Sketches of Lake Wawasee* (Indianapolis: Indiana Historical Society, 1967).

45. EL, "Reminiscences." Lilly later acquired a copy of the book, in a more recent edition, now in the Eli Lilly Room, Lilly Center. C. Witt, *Tales of Troy,* Charles DeGarmo, trans. (Bloomington, Ill.: Public-School Publishing Co., 1919). See also Patricia Curry, *Lilly House* (Bloomington: Indiana University Publications, n.d.).

46. Eli Lilly, ed., *Schliemann in Indianapolis* (Indianapolis: Indiana Historical Society, 1961), v, 82. Quotation is on page 80. Schliemann remains a controversial figure. Many of the dozens of biographies of him are romantic and uncritical. Some are fictional, including Irving Stone, *The Greek Treasure: A Biographical Novel of Henry and Sophia Schliemann* (New York: Doubleday & Co., 1975). Several scholars have recently attacked the Schliemann hagiography, asserting that he deliberately falsified, distorted, and repressed archaeological evidence. See William M. Calder III and David A. Traill, eds., *Myth, Scandal, and History: The Heinrich Schliemann Controversy and a First Edition of the Mycenaean Diary* (Detroit: Wayne State University Press, 1986).

47. Robert Payne, *The Gold of Troy: The Story of Heinrich Schliemann and the Buried Cities of Ancient Greece* (New York: Funk & Wagnalls Co., 1959).

48. EL to Robert Payne, 8 May 1959, Schliemann Folder, ELP; EL to John N. Pantazides, 29 June, 29 July 1959, 29 Jan. 1960, Pantazides Folder, ibid.; EL to Black, Black Papers, Black Laboratory; Rauch to EL, 13 Oct. 1960, Schliemann Folder, ELP.

49. EL to Indiana Historical Society, 18 Sept. 1961, EL Folder, Indiana Historical Society Business Office Files; Lilly, ed., *Schliemann in Indianapolis,* passim. Quotation is on page 19.

50. EL to Pantazides, 3 Nov. 1959, Pantazides Folder, ELP. It is nearly certain that Schliemann obtained his American citizenship and Indianapolis divorce by fradulent means. See David A. Traill, "Schliemann's American Citizenship and Divorce," *Classical Journal* 77 (1981-82): 336-42.

51. Lilly, *Schliemann in Indianapolis,* 77.

52. Francis R. Walton to EL, 16 Sept. 1961, 16 May 1962, 8 June 1964, 5 May 1967, Schliemann Folder, ELP; EL to Harry M. Lyter, 8 June 1966, ibid.; Eva Rice Goble to David Randall, 5 June 1967, ibid.; Lucy Shoe Meritt, *History of the American School of Classical Studies at Athens, 1939-1980* (Princeton, N.J.: American School of Classical Studies at Athens, 1984), 230.

53. EL to John Vint, 3 Mar. 1969, Parthenon Book Folder, ELP. See also EL to Randall, 6 Oct., 6 Dec. 1965, ibid.; EL to John P. Dessauer, 14 Nov. 1966, ibid.; Theodore Bowie, interview with author, 19 June 1987.

54. Herman B Wells to EL, 2 Oct., 15 July 1969, 4 Mar. 1970, Parthenon Book Folder, ELP.

55. Anita Martin, undated note, ibid.

56. Theodore Bowie and Diether Thimme, eds., *The Carrey Drawings of the Parthenon Sculptures* (Bloomington: Indiana University Press, 1971); Elizabeth Gummey Pemberton, review, *Art Journal* 32 (1972-73): 236.

57. George L. Denny to Ralph F. Gates, 8 Jan. 1947, Deaconess Hospital Building Folder, ELP; EL to Robert D. Starrett, 15 Oct. 1958, ibid.

58. John Lauritz Larson and David G. Vanderstel, "Agent of Empire: William Conner on the Indiana Frontier, 1800-1855," *Indiana Magazine of History* 80 (1984): 301-28; EL, notes of interview about Conner Prairie, undated, Conner Farm Folder, ELP.

59. EL to Guernsey, 12 Nov. 1934, File B2a1, RG 2, Conner Prairie Archives, Noblesville, Indiana. See also EL to Charles N. Thompson, 2 Oct. 1934, File A36, Lilly Manuscripts, ibid.; EL to Laurence Vail Coleman, 17 June 1935, B2a1, RG 2, ibid.; EL to Guernsey, 2 Aug. 1934, File B2a1, RG 2, ibid.; Guernsey to EL, 1, 31 Aug. 1934, File B2a1, RG 2, ibid.; Charles B. Hosmer, Jr., *Preservation Comes of Age: From Williamsburg to the National Trust, 1926-1949,* 2 vols. (Charlottesville: University Press of Virginia, 1981), 1:66, 391-97; EL, "Reminiscences"; EL, notes of interview about Conner Prairie, undated, Conner Farm Folder, ELP.

60. EL to Robert D. McCreary, 21 Dec. 1934, File B2a1, RG 2, Conner Prairie Archives; *Noblesville Ledger,* 3 Dec. 1934; EL, "Reminiscences."

61. EL to Guernsey, 22 Oct. 1934, File B2a1, RG 2, Conner Prairie Archives. See also EL to Mary W. Durham, 10 Aug. 1934, ibid.; *Indianapolis Star,* 20 June 1937.

62. EL to McCreary, 21 Dec. 1934, File B2a1, RG 2, Conner Prairie Archives.

63. EL to Guernsey, 29 June 1934, Guernsey Folder, EL Papers, Black Laboratory. See also EL to Ray J. Hinkle, 25 Aug. 1936, B4e, RG 2, Conner Prairie Archives.

64. EL to Guernsey, 16 June 1936, Guernsey Folder, EL Papers, Black Laboratory. See also EL, "Reminiscences"; John C. Householder, interview with author, 5 Dec. 1986.

65. EL to Black, 30 Oct. 1940, Black Papers, Black Laboratory.

66. Hosmer, *Preservation Comes of Age,* 1:131-32.

67. Ibid., 2:1,044; David G. Vanderstel, "The William Conner House: Construction to Restoration," Apr. 1983, typescript, Conner Prairie Archives.

68. *The Official Show Blue Book,* 32d ed. (New York: Official Horse Show Blue Book, Inc., 1939), 168. See also EL, "Reminiscences"; and *The Conner Prairie Farm: Something of Its*

History and Present Resources in Agriculture, Including Its Stock of Horses, Cattle, Hogs, and Sheep (Chicago: Lakeside Press, 1941). This last item was lavishly done and bears throughout the marks of Lilly's special interests and his writing style.

69. EL, "Reminiscences."

70. *The Conner Prairie Farm*, 9. See also EL, "Reminiscences." Among the books from Lilly's personal library now in the Eli Lilly Room at Lilly Center, both with his underlinings, are Laurence M. Winters, *Animal Breeding*, 4th ed. (New York: J. Wiley, 1948); and Jay L. Lush, *Animal Breeding Plans* (Ames, Iowa: Collegiate Press, 1937).

71. James B. Cope, interview with author, 24 June 1987.

72. A. M. McVie to EL, 7 Feb. 1955, Conner Farm Financial Reports Folder, ELP. See also EL to Tillman Bubenzer, 2 Oct. 1951, Conner Farm Folder, ibid.; Bubenzer to EL, 16 Aug. 1955, Conner Farm Folder, ibid.

73. EL to Bubenzer, 16 June 1955, Conner Farm Folder, ibid.

74. Bubenzer to EL, 14 July 1955, ibid.

75. Ibid., 16 Aug. 1955. See also ibid., 9 Aug. 1955.

76. Ibid., 27 Dec. 1955; EL to Bubenzer, 29 Dec. 1955, ibid. The farm's losses for 1955 were $136,280. McVie to EL, 15 Feb. 1956, Conner Farm Financial Reports, ELP.

77. EL to Rauch, 30 Dec. 1959, Rauch Folder, ELP. See also Bubenzer to EL, 12 June 1957, Conner Farm Folder, ibid.

78. McVie to EL, 23 Apr. 1962, Conner Farm Financial Reports Folder, ibid.; McVie to EL, 1 Sept. 1965, ibid.; W. M. Wheeler, Jr., to EL, 12 June 1956, Conner Farm Folder, ibid.; EL to Landrum R. Bolling, 12 Dec. 1963, Conner Prairie Farm/Earlham College Folder, ELP; James B. Cope, interview with author.

79. EL to Bolling, 12 Dec. 1963, Conner Prairie/Earlham College, ELP. See also Rauch to Bolling, 21 Jan. 1964, ibid.

80. Landrum R. Bolling, interview with author, 28 Mar. 1988; James B. Cope, interview with author; Thomas E. Jones to Bolling, 16 Oct., 2 Nov. 1963, Conner Prairie Farms Folder, President's Correspondence, Earlham College Archives.

81. Harold C. Cope to Bolling, 15 Mar. 1967, Conner Prairie Farms Folder, President's Correspondence, Earlham College Archives.

82. Bolling to Harold C. Cope, 22 May 1967, ibid.

83. Harold C. Cope to EL, 19 Feb. 1968, EL Folder, ibid.; James B. Cope to EL, 15 Feb. 1971, Conner Prairie/Earlham College Folder, ELP; Benjamin L. Jessup, "Eli Lilly and Conner Prairie" (M.A. thesis, Ball State University, 1987), 99-100.

84. EL to Coleman, 17 June 1935, B2a1, RG 2, Conner Prairie Archives. See also *Indianapolis Star*, 19 May 1935. Lilly was upset because Gov. Paul McNutt's patronage appointments had thoroughly affected the state park system and brought about the resignation of its founder and head, Richard Lieber. See Madison, *Indiana through Tradition and Change*, 96, 339.

85. Work Projects Administration, *Indiana: A Guide to the Hoosier State* (New York: Oxford University Press, 1941), 331.

86. Tillman Bubenzer, "Memories of Conner Prairie Farm," typescript, June 1986, File A2g, RG 2, Conner Prairie Archives; Jessup, "Eli Lilly and Conner Prairie," 71, 101; EL to Sloane Graff, 28 May 1963, Graff Folder, ELP.

87. Rauch to Bolling, 12 Dec. 1963, Conner Prairie Farms, President's Correspondence, Earlham College Archives; EL to Bolling, 5 May 1965, Moravian Mission Folder, Conner Prairie Pioneer Settlement Collection, Earlham College Archives; EL to Bolling, 23 Dec. 1964, File C1a, RG 2, Conner Prairie Archive; Minutes of the Conner Prairie Museum Committee, 8 Sept. 1964, EL Folder, President's Correspondence, Earlham College Archives; EL, "To the Conner Pioneers, 1966," Miscellaneous Folder, Conner Prairie Pioneer Settlement Collection, Earlham College Archives; Bolling, interview with author; James B. Cope, interview with author.

88. Howard C. Cope to EL, 19 Feb. 1968, Conner Prairie/Earlham College Folder, ELP.

89. Minutes, Conner Prairie Advisory Council, 3 Dec. 1968, Conner Prairie Museum Folder, President's Correspondence, Earlham College Archives; Bolling, "Memorandum for the Earlham College Files," 2 Mar. 1969, EL Folder, President's Correspondence, ibid.

90. "Deed of Gift by Eli Lilly to Earlham College," 24 Jan. 1969, Conner Prairie/Earlham College Folder, ELP. See also Bolling to EL, 5 Dec., 11 Feb. 1969, ibid.

91. Bolling, "Memo for the Files," 5 Oct. 1969, EL Folder, President's Correspondence, Earlham College Archives. See also Bolling, "Memorandum for the Earlham College Files," 2 Mar. 1969, ibid.

92. Harold C. Cope to Earlham Board of Trustees, 12 Mar. 1970, Conner Prairie Museum Folder, ibid. See also Bolling to EL, 4 Jan., 3 Dec. 1969, EL Folder, ibid.

93. James B. Cope, interview with author; Contributions Folder, ELP; Bolling, "Receipt and Agreement," 20 July 1972, Conner Prairie Folder, President's Correspondence, Earlham College Archives.

94. Conner Prairie Pioneer Settlement, *Annual Report, 1973-1974;* ibid., *1976.*

95. Bolling, interview with author; Esther Linenberger, interview with author, 16 June 1987.

96. See Harrison Mansion Folder, ELP.

97. EL to Calvin S. Hamilton, 30 Nov. 1960, Historic Madison, Inc., Folder, ibid.

98. EL to John T. Windle, 23 Mar. 1962, 14 Dec. 1964, ibid.; Thomas Walker, "The Oral History of Historic Preservation: A Selected Survey," *Indiana Folklore and Oral History* 15 (1986): 56; John T. Windle and Robert M. Taylor, Jr., *The Early Architecture of Madison, Indiana* (Madison and Indianapolis: Historic Madison, Inc., and Indiana Historical Society, 1986).

99. Thomas D. Clark and F. Gerald Ham, *Pleasant Hill and Its Shakers,* 2d ed. (Pleasant Hill, Ky.: Pleasant Hill Press, 1983); Earl D. Wallace, interview with author, 4 Oct. 1985; EL to Wallace, 9 Dec. 1963, Shakertown Folder, ELP; Earl D. Wallace, *The Story of Shakertown at Pleasant Hill, Kentucky, Inc.: From Inception in 1961 to 1984* (Harrodsburg, Ky.: Shakertown at Pleasant Hill, Kentucky, Inc., 1984), 6-14.

100. Wallace, interview with author.

101. Ibid.; EL to Wallace, 27 Oct. 1965, 10 Oct. 1966, 31 Oct. 1968, 17 Apr. 1972, Shakertown Folder, ELP; Contributions Folder, ELP.

102. Wallace, interview with author; Wallace, *The Story of Shakertown,* 21-22.

103. Wallace, interview with author; Wallace, *The Story of Shakertown,* 23-24.

104. Wallace, interview with author.

105. H. Roll McLaughlin, interview with author, 18 June 1987; Robert C. Braun, "Reflec-

tions of Our First Twenty-Five Years," Marion County/Indianapolis Historical Society *Circular* 7 (Dec. 1986): 1-3; EL to McLaughlin, 3 Oct. 1973, Historic Landmarks Foundation Folder, ELP; EL to Jury of Fellows, American Institute of Architects, 22 Dec. 1969, Historic Landmarks Foundation Folder, ELP; EL to James Biddle, 2 Dec. 1974, McLaughlin Personal Files.

106. McLaughlin to James Hoover, 16 Feb. 1962, McLaughlin Personal Files; EL to Hoover, 27 Sept. 1961, Historic Landmarks Foundation Folder, ELP; McLaughlin, interview with author; EL to John P. Craine, 16 May, 18 June 1962, Kemper House Folder, ELP. Lilly gave the restored Kemper house to the Episcopal Diocese of Indianapolis, which in 1977 transferred it to Historic Landmarks Foundation.

107. McLaughlin, interview with author; Contributions Folder, ELP; EL to Hoover, 6 Mar. 1964, Historic Landmarks Foundation Folder, ELP.

108. McLaughlin, interview with author.

109. EL, Deed of Gift to Historic Landmarks Foundation, 3 Feb. 1969, Historic Landmarks Foundation Folder, ELP.

110. EL to McLaughlin, 24 July 1970, ibid.; McLaughlin, interview with author.

111. McLaughlin to EL, 30 June 1965, 3 Mar. 1966, Historic Landmarks Foundation Folder, ELP; EL to McLaughlin, 2 Jan. 1968, McLaughlin Personal Files.

112. EL to McLaughlin, 1 Nov. 1972, Historic Landmarks Foundation Folder, ELP.

113. McLaughlin to EL, 1, 26 Oct. 1973, ibid.; McLaughlin, interview with author.

114. Walker, "The Oral History of Historic Preservation," 66.

Chapter 8

1. Waldemar A. Nielsen, *The Big Foundations* (New York: Columbia University Press, 1972), 309-311, provides a good sketch of the characteristics of wealthy philanthropists.

2. EL to Evie Lilly, 29 Sept. 1939, Evelyn Lutz Folder, ELP.

3. JKL, Sr., "Remarks Concerning Proposed Donations by Lilly Endowment, 1948," Lilly Endowment Folder, Drawer 3, Cabinet 1, Company History Files.

4. Lilly Endowment, Inc., *Report for 1960,* 6; John S. Lynn to EL, 22 Aug. 1967, Lilly Endowment Folder, ELP.

5. Gene E. McCormick, notes of interview with Eli Lilly, 9 Apr. 1973, Philanthropies Folder, EL Drawer, Cabinet 4, Company History Files.

6. Frederic P. Williams, interview with author, 18 Jan. 1988.

7. Waldemar A. Nielsen, *The Golden Donors: A New Anatomy of Great Foundations* (New York: E. P. Dutton & Co., 1985), 16, 18.

8. Glenn A. Black to EL, 26 June 1936, Glenn A. Black Papers, Glenn A. Black Laboratory of Archæology, Indiana University, Bloomington.

9. Eli Lilly, "A Plan for Accomplishing More Effective Research," *Proceedings of the Indiana Academy of Science* 48 (1939): 10-11.

10. EL to Pierre F. Goodrich, 8 Jan. 1951, EL Folder, Sparks Papers, Wabash College Archives. The results of Goodrich's struggles on the "seas of philosophy" are evident in the

Pierre F. Goodrich Seminar Room in Wabash College's Lilly Library. Nearly all the books discussed below are from Lilly's personal library in the Eli Lilly Room, Lilly Center.

11. Pitirim A. Sorokin, "Sociology of My Mental Life," in *Pitirim A. Sorokin in Review,* ed. Philip J. Allen (Durham, N.C.: Duke University Press, 1963), 32.

12. Robin M. Williams, Jr., "Pitirim A. Sorokin: Master Sociologist and Prophet," in *Sociological Traditions from Generation to Generation: Glimpses of the American Experience,* Robert K. Merton and Matilda White Riley (Norwood, N.J.: Ablex Publishing Corp., 1980), 100.

13. Don Martindale, "Pitirim A. Sorokin: Soldier of Fortune," in *Sorokin and Sociology; Essays in Honour of Professor Pitirim A. Sorokin,* eds., G. C. Hallen and Rajeshwar Prasad (Moti Katra, India: Satish Book Enterprise, 1972), 42.

14. Sorokin, "Sociology of My Mental Life," 34.

15. Pitirim A. Sorokin, *The Crisis of Our Age: The Social and Cultural Outlook* (New York: E. P. Dutton & Co., 1941), 195, 319, 324. See also Barry V. Johnston, "Sorokin and Parsons at Harvard: Institutional Conflict and the Origin of the Hegemonic Tradition," *Journal of the History of the Behavioral Sciences* 22 (Apr. 1986): 107-127; Barry V. Johnston, "Pitirim Sorokin and the American Sociological Association: The Politics of a Professional Society," *Journal of the History of the Behavioral Sciences* 23 (Apr. 1987): 103-122; Edward A. Tiryakian, ed., *Sociological Theory, Values, and Sociocultural Change: Essays in Honor of Pitirim A. Sorokin* (New York: Free Press of Glencoe, 1963); Pitirim A. Sorokin, *A Long Journey: The Autobiography of Pitirim A. Sorokin* (New Haven, Conn.: College and University Press, 1963).

16. E. B. Best to John S. Lynn, 24 Apr. 1967, Sorokin Folder, ELP. In this three-page memorandum a Lilly Endowment staff member quoted from and summarized correspondence and reports from files relating to Sorokin. Nearly all quotations in this chapter from Sorokin's published writings are passages underlined by EL in his personal copies, now located in the Eli Lilly Room, Lilly Center.

17. EL, "The Nemesis of Materialism" [1941], Miscellaneous Writings Folder, ELP. Internal evidence strongly suggests late 1941, before Pearl Harbor, as the date of this essay. It appears that Lilly intended the essay for oral delivery, but where and to whom is not known. Sorokin is not named in the paper, but his ideas and phrases permeate it.

18. Thomas C. Cochran, *Challenges to American Values: Society, Business, and Religion* (New York: Oxford University Press, 1985), 85-90, 112-13. Quotations are on pages 86, 90.

19. Pitirim A. Sorokin, *Man and Society in Calamity* (New York: E. P. Dutton & Co., 1942), 318.

20. *SuperVision* 1 (Oct. 1946): 1.

21. Sorokin to EL, 11 Apr. 1946, Sorokin Folder, ELP; EL to Sorokin, 17 Apr. 1946, ibid. See also Sorokin, *A Long Journey,* 276.

22. Pitirim A. Sorokin, *The Reconstruction of Humanity* (Boston: Beacon Press, 1948), 3, 234.

23. Quoted in Best to Lynn, 24 Apr. 1967, Sorokin Folder, ELP.

24. Sorokin, *A Long Journey,* 278.

25. EL to JKL, Jr., 1 Nov. 1948, Sorokin Folder, ELP; EL to Sorokin, 10, 28 Dec. 1948, ibid.; EL to James B. Conant, 17 Jan. 1949, ibid.

26. Johnston, "Pitirim Sorokin and the American Sociological Association," 108; Kay Bierwiler, "Pitirim Sorokin's Research in Altruism" (Ph.D. dissertation, State University of New York at Albany, 1978), 90-150.

27. Sorokin, *A Long Journey,* 280.

28. JKL, Jr., to EL, 10 Apr. 1951, Sorokin Folder, ELP; Earl Beck to JKL, Jr., 20 Mar. 1951; G. Harold Duling to JKL, Jr., and EL, 28 Feb. 1951, Communism, 1950-51, XCAw.

29. Best to Lynn, 24 Apr. 1967, Sorokin Folder, ELP; E. H. Volkart to EL, 13 Sept. 1967, ibid.

30. EL to Sorokin, 5 July 1967, ibid.

31. Henry C. Link, *The Return to Religion* (New York: Macmillan Co., 1937), 103. Link did send Lilly an autographed copy of his book *The Rediscovery of Morals: With Special Reference to Race and Class Conflict* (New York: E. P. Dutton & Co., 1947), which Lilly heavily marked. Lilly also had his secretary type extensive passages from the book on 5 x 8 cards, which are in Miscellaneous Cabinet 1. Lilly cited the 1947 book in *SuperVision* 2 (June 1947): 1.

32. Frances Eward, *Exploring Christian Potential: A Layman Looks at the College Character Research Project* (n.p., n.d.).

33. EL to Ernest M. Ligon, 28 Feb. 1939, Ligon Folder, ELP.

34. Ernest M. Ligon, "My Autobiographical Adventure in Research Design with Which to Explore Human Potential," typescript, 1970, Ligon Folder, ELP; Eward, *Exploring Christian Potential.*

35. Ernest M. Ligon, *The Psychology of Christian Personality* (New York: Macmillan, 1935), 1.

36. Amos B. Hulen, review, *Christian Century* 52 (1935): 1560. See also Clarence Bauman, *The Sermon on the Mount: The Modern Quest for Its Meaning* (Macon, Ga.: Mercer University Press, 1985), 323-25.

37. *Adventure in Character Education* 8 (12 Dec. 1954): 3. See also Eward, *Exploring Christian Potential.*

38. Lilly Endowment, Inc., *The First Twenty Years, 1937-1957* (n.p., n.d.), 16. Pages 32-37 of this special annual report contain a list of grants made in these twenty years.

39. Ernest M. Ligon, *A Greater Generation* (New York: Macmillan, 1948), 8, 139, 77.

40. Helen Spaulding, "Character Research Project," 19 Sept. 1952, copy in author's possession. I am grateful to C. Ellis Nelson for this memorandum. See also Ernest M. Ligon, *Dimensions of Character* (New York: Macmillan, 1956); Lilly Endowment, Inc., *Report for 1950,* 6; Lilly Endowment, Inc., *First Twenty Years,* 16; C. Ellis Nelson, interview with author, 12 Apr. 1988.

41. Walter Houston Clark, review, *Christian Century* 74 (1957): 268.

42. See EL to Ligon, 12 Jan. 1970, Ligon Folder, ELP, for one of many examples of Lilly's active involvement in Ligon's work. See also EL to Ligon, 15 June 1948, ibid.

43. Wayne R. Rood, *Understanding Christian Education* (Nashville, Tenn.: Abingdon Press, 1970), 149.

44. Clark, review, 268.

45. Harry Thomas Stock, "Christian Education or the Ligon Plan?" 2, in General Board of Education of the Methodist Church, *Evaluation of the Ligon Plan* (Nashville, Tenn.: Methodist Church, n.d.), copy in author's possession. I am grateful to C. Ellis Nelson for this report. See also Nelson, interview with author.

46. No mention of Ligon or citation to his publications is made in the following: Susan M. Hoagland, comp., *Review of Religious Research: 20th Anniversary Index* (New York: Religious Research Association, 1979); Merton P. Strommen, ed., *Research on Religious Development: A Comprehensive Handbook* (New York: Hawthorn Books, Inc., 1971); and Stuart W. Cook, ed., *Review of Recent Research Bearing on Religious and Character Formation* (New Haven, Conn.: Religious Education Association, 1962). The last item, containing papers from a Cornell University conference, was published with assistance of a grant from Lilly Endowment. Ligon's work is noted in Hendrika Vande Kemp, comp., *Psychology and Theology in Western Thought 1672-1965: A Historical and Annotated Bibliography* (Millwood, N.Y.: Kraus International Publications, 1984), 289-90. For a very negative evaluation of Ligon's *Dimensions of Character,* see Gwynne Nettler's review in *American Sociological Review* 22 (1957): 486-87.

47. Nelson, interview with author; B. Edward McClellan, "Public Schooling and the Shaping of Character: American Traditions," forthcoming. I am grateful to Professor McClellan for sharing a prepublication draft of this essay.

48. Duling to EL, 5 Dec. 1958, Ligon Folder, ELP; EL to Duling, 21 Nov. 1958, ibid.; EL to Ligon, 3, 28 Dec. 1958, ibid.; Manning M. Pattillo, interview with author, 6 June 1988. Ligon did not retire until 1977. He died 17 June 1984. Ellen H. Fladger to author.

49. EL to Richard D. McGinnis, 12 Oct. 1960, ibid.

50. EL to Ligon, 2 March 1962, ibid. See also Duling to EL, 29 Nov. 1960, 31 Oct. 1961, ibid.

51. C. Ellis Nelson to Duling, 10 May 1962, ibid.

52. EL to Ligon, 22 May 1962, ibid.

53. EL to Ligon, 10 July, 11 Aug. 1962, ibid.; EL to Duling, n.d., ibid.

54. EL to Board and Staff of Endowment, 28 Sept. 1962, ibid.; EL to Ligon, 17 Oct. 1962, ibid.

55. Duling to EL, 20 Nov. 1963, Lilly Endowment Folder, ELP.

56. Ernest Mayfield Ligon and Leona Jones Smith, *The Marriage Climate: A Book of Home Dynamics* (St. Louis: Bethany Press, 1963). Copy in Eli Lilly Room, Lilly Center.

57. EL to Eugene N. Beesley, 12 Jan. 1967, Ligon Folder, ELP.

58. Leona J. Smith, *Guiding the Character Development of the Preschool Child* (New York: Association Press, 1968). Copy in Eli Lilly Room, Lilly Center. See also Smith to EL, 12 Apr. 1968, Ligon Folder, ELP.

59. EL to Ligon, 14 Apr. 1971, Ligon Folder, ELP. See also John H. Peatling and Lucie W. Barber, interviews with author, 19 Apr. 1988.

60. Contributions Folder, ELP.

61. EL to Beesley, 22 Sept. 1965, Lilly Endowment Folder, ELP; EL to Paul W. Cook, Jr., 27 Feb. 1967, EL Folder, Cook Papers, Wabash College Archives; EL to Landrum R. Bolling,

20 Mar. 1967, EL Folder, President's Correspondence, Earlham College Archives; Bolling to EL, 24 Mar. 1967, EL Folder, President's Correspondence, Earlham College Archives; Bolling to EL, 6 Sept. 1971, Conner Prairie/ Earlham College Folder, ELP.

62. EL to Beesley, 16 Aug. 1971, American Institute for Character Education Folder, ELP. See also EL to Ligon, 3 Dec. 1971, Ligon Folder, ELP.

63. Tiryakian, *Sociological Theory, Values, and Sociocultural Change,* xi-xii. Perhaps more enduring was the Prairie City research of the Committee on Human Development of the University of Chicago, which was supported by the Lilly Endowment in the late 1940s. Little evidence of the nature of Eli Lilly's personal involvement has been located, however. See Robert J. Havighurst and Hilda Taba, *Adolescent Character and Personality* (New York: John Wiley & Sons, 1949), viii.

64. McClellan, "Public Schooling and the Shaping of Character"; Robert S. Wicks, *Morality and the Schools* (Washington, D.C.: Council for Basic Education, 1981).

65. EL, "Confidential: First Marriage, a Confession of Failure" [1968], p. 2, Memoirs, Miscellaneous Cabinet 1. See, for example, Lilly's copy of Pitirim A. Sorokin, *The Ways and Power of Love* (Chicago: Henry Regnery Co., 1964), where on page 195 he underlined the assertion that families without love "tend to produce morally erratic persons, little capable of self-control, selfishly irresponsible, careless of the interests and well-being of others, and frequently criminal or delinquent." Lilly's nephew believed that there was a close connection between his interest in character education and Evie. J. K. Lilly III, interview with author, 4 Sept. 1986.

66. Lilly Endowment, Inc., *Report for 1976* (Indianapolis: Lilly Endowment, Inc., n.d.), 1.

67. Lilly added to this letter: "I should like to have this made clear in our archives." EL to Beesley, 1 Feb. 1967, Beesley Folder, ELP. Just what caused this unusually strong personal claim is not known, though there was some difference within the Lilly family over whose idea the Endowment was. J. K. Lilly III, "Comments on Chitty manuscript," 14 Dec. 1978, Episcopal Church Folder, ELP.

68. Mark H. Leff, *The Limits of Symbolic Reform: The New Deal and Taxation, 1933-1939* (Cambridge, England: Cambridge University Press, 1984), 6, 292; Robert H. Bremner, *American Philanthropy,* 2d ed. (Chicago: University of Chicago Press, 1988), 151-53, 163-65; Francis X. Sutton, "The Ford Foundation: The Early Years," *Daedalus* 116 (Winter 1987): 42-43. When Lilly learned the amount he owed on his 1936 taxes, his brother reported, "The ensuing noise was a cross between a stampede of American bison and a gray-day eruption of Vesuvius, Etna, and Popocateptl, all in one." JKL, Jr., to JKL, Sr., 11 Mar. 1937, JKL, Sr., Papers, Vault.

69. Albert E. Bailey to EL, 27 June 1935, J. D. Pusey Folder, XBLl. See also EL to Bailey, 16 July 1934, ibid.; Bailey to EL, 16 July 1934, ibid.; JKL, Jr., to EL, 20 Mar. 1939, Lilly Endowment Folder, Drawer 3, Cabinet 1, Company History Files. Bailey was working at this time with Lilly on planning the murals for the third floor of his Sunset Lane home.

70. EL, undated notes for talk, ca. 1957, Speeches Folder, ELP.

71. Nielsen, *Golden Donors,* 16.

72. Quotations from Robert F. Arnove, ed., *Philanthropy and Cultural Imperialism: The Foundations at Home and Abroad* (Boston: G. K. Hall & Company, 1980), 1. There is considerable debate about foundations. A good introduction to the subject is Martin Blumer's

and Donald Fisher's comments in "Debate," *Sociology* 18 (1984): 572-87. A strong defense of foundations is Warren Weaver, *U.S. Philanthropic Foundations: Their History, Structure, Management, and Record* (New York: Harper & Row, 1967). More moderate and sophisticated analyses are contained in Nielsen, *Golden Donors;* Ben Whitaker, *The Foundations: An Anatomy of Philanthropy and Society* (London: Eyre Methuen, 1974); Barry D. Karl and Stanley N. Katz, "Foundations and Ruling Class Elites," *Daedalus* 116 (Winter 1987): 1-40; Barry D. Karl and Stanley N. Katz, "The American Private Philanthropic Foundation and the Public Sphere, 1890-1930," *Minerva* 19 (1981): 236-70; and *U.S. Treasury Department Report on Private Foundations* (Washington, D.C.: Government Printing Office, 1965).

73. EL to Bailey, 16 July 1934, Pusey Folder, XBLl; EL to Beesley, 26 Aug. 1957, Beesley Folder, ELP.

74. Susan O. Conner, "Lilly Endowment Inc.: A Family Legacy for a Half-Century," unpublished manuscript, Lilly Endowment, Inc., 1987. The manuscript is unpaged. Eli Lilly gave more shares (4.8 million) than his brother (4.1 million), but his brother made some of his gifts at times when the value of the stock was higher.

75. EL to Lynn, 24 Apr. 1968, Lilly Endowment Folder, ELP. A ranked list of the largest foundations is contained in Nielsen, *Big Foundations,* 22.

76. JKL, Jr., to Homer Capehart, 29 June 1950, Lilly Endowment, XBLl; Lilly Endowment, Inc., *First Twenty Years,* 4-5.

77. A list of annual assets and grants is included in the appendix of Conner, "Lilly Endowment Inc."

78. EL to Nicholas H. Noyes, 1 Apr. 1949, Board and Staff Folder, Drawer 3, Cabinet 1, Company History Files.

79. J. K. Lilly III, interview with author; Lilly Endowment, Inc., *First Twenty Years,* 5-6.

80. J. K. Lilly III to EL and JKL, Jr., 30 Apr. 1954, J. K. Lilly III, Folder, ELP.

81. J. K. Lilly III, interview with author.

82. Lilly Endowment, Inc., *Report for 1952,* 5.

83. EL to Beesley, 29 Jan. 1973, Indiana University Folder, ELP. See also EL to Herman B Wells, 8 Sept. 1972, Lilly Endowment Folder, ELP; Lilly Endowment, Inc., *Report for 1962,* 30-31; David A. Randall, *Dukedom Large Enough* (New York: Random House, 1969), 349-52.

84. Eva Rice Goble to Francis R. Walton, 23 May 1962, Schliemann Folder, ELP.

85. John R. Seeley et al., *Community Chest: A Case Study in Philanthropy* (Toronto: University of Toronto Press, 1957); EL, undated notes for talk, 3; Lilly Endowment, Inc., *First Twenty Years,* 22-24; Pattillo, interview with author.

86. Lilly Endowment, Inc., *First Twenty Years,* 16-20; Paul Bergevin and John McKinley, *Design for Adult Education in the Church* (Greenwich, Conn.: Seabury Press, 1958); G. Paul Musselman, *The Church on the Urban Frontier* (Greenwich, Conn.: Seabury Press, 1960), 27; Nielsen, *Golden Donors,* 286, 419.

87. Donald J. Cowling and Carter Davidson, *Colleges for Freedom: A Study of Purposes, Practices and Needs* (New York: Harper & Brothers, 1947); Gordon Keith Chalmers, *The Republic and the Person: A Discussion of Necessities in Modern American Education* (Chicago: Henry Regnery Co., 1952); Robert Maynard Hutchins, *No Friendly Voice* (Chicago: University of Chicago, 1936); Wallace Brett Donham, *Education for Responsible Living: The Oppor-*

tunity for Liberal-Arts Colleges (Cambridge, Mass.: Harvard University Press, 1944). Marked copies in Eli Lilly Room, Lilly Center.

88. EL to Ivor Griffith, 2 Mar. 1953, Philadelphia College of Pharmacy Folder, ELP; Arthur Osol et al., eds., *A Sesquicentennial of Service: The Philadelphia College of Pharmacy and Science* (Philadelphia College of Pharmacy and Science, 1971), 136, 137.

89. EL to Sparks, 4 Nov. 1943, EL Folder, Sparks Papers.

90. *SuperVision* 2 (Aug. 1947): 10.

91. Eli Lilly and Company, *The First One Hundred Years* (n.p., n.d.), 11.

92. EL to Sparks, 4 Nov. 1943, EL Folder, Sparks Papers. See also EL to Cook, 27 Feb. 1967, EL Folder, Cook Papers; EL to Bolling, 20 Mar. 1967, EL Folder, President's Correspondence, Earlham College Archives.

93. Unsigned Memorandum, 18 Feb. 1963, Wabash College Folder, ELP; Contributions Folder, ELP; *Crawfordsville Journal and Review,* 27 Jan. 1977; Byron K. Trippet, *Wabash on My Mind* (Crawfordsville, Ind.: Wabash College, 1982), 57, 221-23.

94. EL to Sparks, 27 Dec. 1944, EL Folder, Sparks Papers; Sparks, memorandum, 31 July 1952, ibid; EL to Thaddeus Seymour, 14 Aug. 1969, Seymour Papers, Wabash College Archives; Richard O. Ristine, interview with author, 27 Apr. 1988; Byron P. Hollett, interview with author, 24 Sept. 1985; EL, interview with McCormick, 9 Apr. 1973, Wabash Folder, EL Drawer, Cabinet 4, Company History Files. Sparks was a very successful Indiana businessman who decided to leave business, get a Ph.D. in economics, and become a college president, which he did, serving as president of Wabash from 1941 to 1956. He could and did draw on his business experience in attracting Lilly's interest in Wabash. See Sparks to EL, 28 Oct. 1944, EL Folder, Sparks Papers.

95. Lilly Endowment, Inc., *First Twenty Years,* 5.

96. Duling to Manning M. Pattillo, 30 Apr. 1956, Lilly Endowment Folder, Drawer 3, Cabinet 1, Company History Files.

97. Pattillo to Bolling, 18 Mar. 1959, Lilly Endowment Folder, President's Correspondence, Earlham College Archives; Bolling to Pattillo, 30 Mar. 1959, ibid.; Bolling to Lynn, 23 June, 6 July 1962, ibid. See also Lilly Endowment, Inc., *Report for 1958,* 13-18, 22; Lilly Endowment, Inc., *Report for 1960,* 10, 14; Lilly Endowment, Inc., *Report for 1962,* 27-28.

98. Associated Colleges of Indiana, *A Report of Progress, 1948-1952* (n.p., n.d.).

99. Trippit, *Wabash on My Mind,* 73-75; Lilly Endowment, Inc., *Report for 1960,* 28, 58; Sparks to Duling, 2 Feb. 1953, Associated Colleges of Indiana Folder, Sparks Papers; Opal Thornburg, *Earlham: The Story of the College, 1847-1962* (Richmond, Ind.: Earlham College Press, 1963), 375-76.

100. See correspondence in Transylvania College Folder, ELP; Berea College Folder, ibid.

101. Lilly Endowment, Inc., *First Twenty Years,* 14; EL to W. R. Sinclair, 12 Apr. 1951, United Negro College Fund Folder, ELP; Merle H. Miller to EL, 17 Apr. 1959, United Negro College Fund Folder, ELP.

102. EL to Frederick L. Hovde, 11 Nov. 1968, P Miscellaneous Folder, ELP; Lilly Endowment, Inc., *Report for 1960,* 6.

103. Lilly Endowment, Inc., *Report for 1961,* 28; Lilly Endowment, Inc., *Report for 1962,* 36.

104. EL to Beesley, 29 Mar. 1972, Education Folder, Drawer 3, Cabinet 1, Company History Files.

105. Pattillo, interview with author.

106. Lynn to EL, 14 Jan. 1965, Lilly Endowment Folder, ELP.

107. Lilly Endowment, Inc., *Report for 1964,* 33-42.

108. Lilly Endowment, Inc., *Report for 1963,* 9. For a general overview of right-wing movements in post-World War II America see David H. Bennett, *The Party of Fear: From Nativist Movements to the New Right in American History* (Chapel Hill, N.C.: University of North Carolina Press, 1988), 286-331.

109. Lynn to JKL, Jr., 18 July 1962, Lilly Endowment Folder, ELP.

110. Lynn to Bolling, 19 Nov. 1964, Lilly Endowment Folder, President's Correspondence, Earlham College Archives.

111. John P. Craine to Reinhart B. Gutmann, 19 July 1966, Lilly Endowment Folder, Box 404, Records of the Episcopal Diocese of Indianapolis, Indiana Division, Indiana State Library, Indianapolis.

112. Craine to Morton Nace, Jr., 12 Sept. 1966, EL Folder, ibid.

113. McCormick, "A History of Eli Lilly and Company," typescript, 1975, chapter 12, pp. 216-25; Barry Goldwater, *The Conscience of a Conservative* (Shepherdsville, Ky.: Victor Publishing Co., 1960); John S. Lynn, interview with author, 5 May 1988.

114. Lilly Endowment, Inc., *Report for 1966,* 2.

115. Lynn to EL, 19 Jan. 1969, Lilly Endowment Folder, ELP.

116. Contributions Folder, ELP; Lynn to EL, 22 Apr. 1965, Folder 2, Box A, 1, EL Legal Records, Vault, Lilly Center; Howard Peckham, interview with author, 2 Aug. 1985; Peter R. Lawson, interview with author, 19 Sept. 1987.

117. Lynn, interview with author; Pattillo, interview with author. Landrum R. Bolling asserted that Lilly made some of these personal contributions to help Lynn save face after the Endowment board refused larger support to the conservative organizations he favored. Landrum R. Bolling, interview with author, 28 Mar. 1988.

118. Kenneth S. Templeton, Jr., to Lynn, 14 Jan. 1965, Lilly Endowment Folder, ELP.

119. Lilly Endowment, Inc., *Report for 1962,* 33-34. Administrators at the University of Illinois soon advised Kemmerer not to accept a renewal of the Endowment grant. McCormick, "History of Eli Lilly and Company," chapter 12, p. 224.

120. Lynn to EL, 15 Jan. 1965, Lilly Endowment Folder, ELP.

121. EL to Lynn, 18 Jan. 1965, ibid. See also ibid., 15 Feb. 1965.

122. Conner, "Lilly Endowment Inc." A recognition of the growing problems of urban America contributed to the increase in support for community service grants.

123. Lynn to EL, 18 Mar. 1964, Lilly Endowment Folder, ELP.

124. EL to Lynn, 22 Nov. 1965, ibid.

125. Nielsen, *Big Foundations,* 171.

126. Waldemar A. Nielsen, interview with author, 7 Apr. 1988. Nielsen reported part of these conversations with Lilly and Beesley in Nielsen, *Golden Donors,* 287, but he did not idenfify the two men by name.

127. EL to Burton E. Beck et al., 29 July 1971, Lilly Endowment Folder, ELP.

128. Beesley to Bolling, 4 Aug. 1972, Conner Prairie/Earlham College Folder, ibid.; Bolling, interview with author.

129. Bremner, *American Philanthropy,* 180-83, 190; Nielsen, *Big Foundations,* 3-20, 170-71, 290; Nielsen, *Golden Donors,* 25-36; *Forbes* 107 (15 Apr. 1971): 34; Gordon Englehart, "Precarious Purse Strings," *Louisville Courier Journal Magazine,* 23 Oct. 1977, 29-32; Eugene N. Beesley, "Statement of Lilly Endowment, Inc. Regarding 'Treasury Department Report on Private Foundations' to Committee on Ways and Means U.S. House of Representatives," 11 Oct. 1965, Lilly Endowment Folder, ELP; Conner, "Lilly Endowment Inc."; Lynn to EL, 30 July 1962, Lilly Endowment Folder, ELP; Lilly Endowment, Inc., *Report for 1972,* 8.

130. Conner, "Lilly Endowment Inc."; Lilly Endowment, Inc., *Report for 1973,* 7, 10; EL to Bolling, 10 Oct. 1973, Lilly Endowment Folder, ELP; *Indianapolis Star,* 25 Mar. 1973, 27 Mar. 1974; Landrum Bolling, "Some Thoughts for Exploration on Future Lilly Endowment Policies," 18 Aug. 1972, Lilly Endowment Folder, ELP; Bolling, interview with author; Englehart, "Precarious Purse Strings," 29-32; Nielsen, *Golden Donors,* 288-89.

131. *Indianapolis Times,* 17 Feb. 1964; *Indianapolis Star,* 3 Dec. 1976.

132. EL to Beesley, 8 Sept. 1972, Beesley Folder, ELP.

133. *Indianapolis Star,* 3 Dec. 1967, 7 Dec. 1976; Bolling, interview with author.

134. EL to Beesley, 11 Aug. 1972, Philanthropy Folder, Drawer 2, Cabinet 8, Company History Files; EL to Richard Lugar, 14 Aug. 1972, ibid. See also Robert G. Barrows, "Indianapolis: Silver Buckle on the Rust Belt," forthcoming.

135. EL to Richard O. Ristine, 28 July 1975, in Byron Hollett Personal Scrapbook. The issue of fresh food at the market continued long after Lilly's death. Tina Connor, "Study Results in Thumbs Up for Fresh Food in City Market," *The Indiana Preservationist,* 1988, no. 1:2.

136. Thomas H. Lake, interview with author, 27 Aug. 1987; Conner, "Lilly Endowment Inc."; *Indianapolis Star,* 15 Apr. 1973, 24 Sept. 1984.

137. EL to Board of Directors, Lilly Endowment, 12 Oct. 1972, Lilly Endowment Folder, ELP. Beesley succeeded Lilly as president of the Endowment, thus becoming the first nonfamily member at the head of the Endowment as well as the pharmaceutical company.

138. Lake, interview with author. Lake, retired president of Eli Lilly and Company, succeeded Bolling as president of the Endowment in 1977. Bolling became head of the Council on Foundations. Lilly Endowment, Inc., *Report for 1977,* 3. An example of Lilly's continuing involvement in specific Endowment grants was the large grant he approved in 1971 to the Campus Christian Center at Berea College. See Willis D. Weatherford to EL, 20 July 1971, Berea College Folder, ELP; Lynn to EL, 23 May 1972, Berea College Folder, ELP.

139. Peckham, interview with author.

140. Anita Martin, interview with author, 5 May 1988.

Chapter 9

1. Evelyn Fortune Lilly Bartlett, interview with author, 15 Jan. 1986; EL to Carl Voegelin, 14 Apr. 1937, Voegelin Folder, EL Papers, Glenn A. Black Laboratory of Archaeology, Indiana University, Bloomington; Ruth A. Lilly to Miss Koehne, 10 Sept. 1929, Folder 19,

Box B, Records of Christ Church Cathedral, Indiana Division, Indiana State Library, Indianapolis; EL, "Reminiscences," typescript, 1966-69, XBLl.

2. John P. Craine to Irving Rubin, 23 Oct. 1958, EL Folder, Box 404, Records of the Episcopal Diocese of Indianapolis, Indiana Division, Indiana State Library, Indianapolis.

3. Eli Lilly, *History of the Little Church on the Circle: Christ Church Parish Indianapolis 1837-1955* (Indianapolis: Christ Church, 1957).

4. EL to Virginia Lilly, 20 Apr. 1960, Virginia Lilly Nicholas Folder, ELP.

5. Craine to Rubin, 23 Oct. 1958, Records of the Episcopal Diocese of Indianapolis. See also Peter R. Lawson, interview with author, 19 Sept. 1987.

6. Lilly, *History of the Little Church on the Circle,* 321, 322. See also Frederic P. Williams, interview with author, 18 Jan. 1988.

7. EL to Glenn Black, 9 Feb. 1950, Black Papers, Glenn A. Black Laboratory of Archaeology, Indiana University, Bloomington; EL to Craine, 9 Feb. 1950, Christ Church Folder, ELP. See also Lilly, *History of the Little Church on the Circle,* 299-302, 322; Williams, interview with author; Joyce Marks Booth, ed., *A History of the Episcopal Diocese of Indianapolis 1838-1988* (Dallas, Texas: Taylor Publishing Co., [1988]), 100-114.

8. Lilly, *History of the Little Church on the Circle,* 243. The temptation to move Christ Church from the Circle had existed for over a half century. J. K. Lilly, Sr., led a fight at the end of the nineteenth century to keep the church at its downtown location, a fight commemorated on a tablet installed in the church in 1958.

9. Lilly, *History of the Little Church on the Circle,* 312, 325-27. Quotation is on page 325. The Deed of Gift is published in the appendix of Lilly's history, without identifying him as the donor.

10. EL to Craine, 7 May 1958, EL Folder, Box 404, Records of the Episcopal Diocese of Indianapolis; Byron P. Hollett to EL, 13 Sept., 1971, ibid.

11. Lilly, *History of the Little Church on the Circle,* 312-14.

12. Ibid., 243. See also J. D. Forbes, *Victorian Architect: The Life and Work of William Tinsley* (Bloomington: Indiana University Press, 1953), 93. Lilly underwrote publication of the Tinsley biography. John Douglas Forbes to Paula Corpuz, 27 July 1988, copy in the author's possession.

13. EL to James A. Pike, 20 Dec. 1956, Folder 35, Box A, Records of Christ Church Cathedral. See also Pike to EL, 11 Jan. 1957, ibid.

14. EL to Craine, 28 Jan. 1957, ibid.; EL to Richard Lockton, 25 Feb. 1957, ibid.

15. Jervis Anderson, "Profiles: Standing Out There on the Issues," *New Yorker,* 28 Apr. 1986, pp. 41-95; *Indianapolis Times,* 18 Mar. 1957; Paul Moore, Jr., interview with author, 20 Sept. 1987.

16. *Newsweek,* 25 Dec. 1972, p. 57; Moore, interview with author; Williams, interview with author.

17. Paul Moore, Jr., *The Church Reclaims the City* (New York: Seabury Press, 1964), 148.

18. Edwin L. Becker, *From Sovereign to Servant: The Church Federation of Greater Indianapolis, 1912-1987* (Indianapolis: Church Federation of Indianapolis, 1987), 77; Sam Jones, interview with author, 28 Mar. 1988.

19. Anderson, "Profiles: Standing Out There on the Issues," 74-75. See also Moore, interview with author.

20. Moore, interview with author.

21. EL, "Deed of Gift," 1958, Office of Christ Church, Indianapolis. There were other churches still standing in downtown Indianapolis, though none anymore on the Circle.

22. Moore, interview with author; Moore, *The Church Reclaims the City,* 153-57; G. Paul Musselman, *The Church on the Urban Frontier* (Greenwich, Conn.: Seabury Press, 1960), 113-14; Carl R. Stockton, *Christ Church in Indianapolis: A Selected Chronology* (n.p., n.d.), 22.

23. Moore, *The Church Reclaims the City,* 157; Moore, interview with author.

24. Moore, interview with author.

25. Wade Clark Roof and William McKinney, *American Mainline Religion: Its Changing Shape and Future* (New Brunswick, N.J.: Rutgers University Press, 1987), 11-39; James Wood, *Leadership in Voluntary Associations: The Controversy over Social Action in Protestant Churches* (New Brunswick, N.J.: Rutgers University Press, 1981); Charles F. Rehkopf, "Reactions to Events of the '60's and '70's," *Historical Magazine of the Protestant Episcopal Church* 47 (1978): 453-62.

26. Charles A. Reich, *The Greening of America* (New York: Random House, 1970), 4.

27. EL to Hobson Wilson, 14 Apr. 1971, W Folder, ELP.

28. EL to Herman B Wells, 23 Oct. 1968, Black Folder, ibid.

29. Lawson, interview with author; Howard Peckham, interview with author, 2 Aug. 1985.

30. EL to Scott A. Edgell, 26 Feb. 1969, Edgell Folder, ELP.

31. EL to Peter Lawson, 17 Jan. 1964, Christ Church Folder, ELP. See also Williams, interview with author; Virginia Minton, interview with author, 13 Jan. 1988; Fredrick and Margaret Weber, interview with author, 12 Jan. 1988.

32. Lawson, interview with author.

33. John G. Rauch, Sr., to EL, 27 May [1964], John G. Rauch Folder, ELP.

34. Lawson, interview with author; *Indianapolis Star,* 15 Oct. 1964; Rauch to Moore, 27 Jan. 1966, Folder 54, Box A, 2, EL Legal Records, Vault; EL to Craine, 14, 16 Oct. 1964, Episcopal Diocese of Indianapolis Folder, ELP. Paul Moore did sign the petition. *New York Times,* 14 Oct. 1964.

35. EL, "Proposed Talk with Dean Lawson—(but not carried out)," Dec. 1964, Christ Church Folder, ELP. Lilly did meet with Lawson, on 18 Dec., but for some unknown reason did not use the notes he had prepared. EL to Craine, 18 Dec. 1964, EL Folder, Box 404, Records of the Episcopal Diocese of Indianapolis.

36. EL, "Off the Record: Two Subjects That Affect the Diocese and the Cathedral," n.d., Miscellaneous Cabinet 4. From internal evidence Lilly likely made these handwritten notes on 3 x 5 cards sometime in 1964.

37. EL to Lawson, 2 Aug. 1965, Christ Church Folder, ELP; EL to Craine, 21 Jan. 1966, Episcopal Diocese of Indianapolis Folder, ibid.; EL to Donald B. Davidson, 31 Jan. 1966, Davidson Folder, ibid.; Lawson, interview with author.

38. Lawson, interview with author.

39. Lawson to EL, 5 Oct. 1965, Christ Church Folder, ELP. On this letter Lilly wrote "Not Replied to." Lilly was upset with the national Episcopal Church as well and stopped giving to many of its causes. Nonetheless, his and Ruth's contributions to Episcopal causes, totaling over $35 million, made them at their deaths the largest benefactors in the denomination's

history. EL to Arthur Ben Chitty, 20 May 1970, Chitty Folder, ibid.; Arthur Ben Chitty, *Ability, Power, and Humility: Eli and Ruth Lilly and Their Church* (New York: Seabury Professional Services, 1979), 1.

40. *Indianapolis Star,* 23 Feb. 1967; Henry F. DeBoest to EL, 27 Feb. 1967, Christ Church Folder, ELP. DeBoest tried unsuccessfully to affect a reconciliation between Lilly and Lawson.

41. Craine to Moore, 23 Feb. 1966, Rauch to Moore, 27 Jan. 1966, Moore to Rauch, 3 Feb. 1966, all in Rauch Folder, ELP. Craine and Rauch kept Lilly informed of their efforts to remove Lawson.

42. EL to Craine, 8 Nov. 1971, Episcopal Diocese of Indianapolis Folder, ELP. See also EL to Craine, 25 June, 26 July, 11 Aug., ibid.; Craine to EL, 24, 30 June, 9 Aug. 1971, ibid.

43. Report of the Cathedral Select Committee [1973], Folder 71, Box A, Records of Christ Church. Quotations are on pages 3, 5, 9.

44. EL to Eleanor Black, 11 Mar. 1974, Christ Church Folder, ELP. See also EL to Roger S. Gray, 20 July 1973, ibid.; Contributions Folder, ibid.

45. EL to Landrum R. Bolling, 21 Jan. 1974, Lilly Endowment Folder, ELP.

46. Roger S. Gray, interview with author, 18 Jan. 1988.

47. Gray, interview with author; Fredrick and Margaret Weber, interview with author; Merchants National Bank & Trust Company of Indianapolis, "In the Matter of the Estate of Eli Lilly, Deceased," Estate Docket E77-139, copy in EL Folder, Historic Landmarks Foundation Office, Indianapolis; *Indianapolis Star,* 12 Sept. 1986; *Annual Report of Endowment Activities at Christ Church Cathedral* (Indianapolis: Christ Church, 1986).

Chapter 10

1. EL to Frank H. Sparks, 17 Oct. 1950, EL Folder, Sparks Papers, Wabash College Archives.

2. EL to John P. Craine, 8 Nov. 1971, EL Folder, Box 404, Records of the Episcopal Diocese of Indianapolis, Indiana Division, Indiana State Library, Indianapolis.

3. EL to Harry T. Ice, 18 Jan. 1965, Clowes Memorial Hall Folder, ELP. See also Allen Clowes, interview with author, 11 Nov. 1988.

4. EL to Glenn A. Black, 7 Oct. 1957, Black Papers, Glenn A. Black Laboratory of Archaeology, Indiana University, Bloomington.

5. EL to Black, undated postcard, Black Papers.

6. EL, diary of trip to England, 1954, Miscellaneous Cabinet 4; EL, diary of trip, 1957, ibid. See also EL, "Reminiscences," typescript, 1966-69, XBLl.

7. Gene E. McCormick, interview with author, 2 May 1988; Richard O. Ristine, interview with author, 27 Apr. 1988; Howard Peckham, interview with author, 2 Aug. 1985; Frederic P. Williams, interview with author, 18 Jan. 1988.

8. EL, "Shining Phrase Book," XBLl.

9. EL to JKL, Jr., 20 Mar. 1963, JKL, Jr., Folder, ELP.

10. For this and other examples, see Poems Folder, ibid.

11. EL, Diary, 26 Nov. 1955, XBLl; EL to Black, 27 Jan. 1960, Black Papers.

12. EL to Black, 1 Nov. 1951, Black Papers. See also ibid., 4 Aug. 1950; McCormick, interview with author.

13. Service Invoice, 28 Feb. 1971, R Miscellaneous Folder, ELP. Lilly's bill for this service was $3,009.84.

14. EL to Black [16 Sept. 1957], Black Papers. See also ibid., 26 Feb., 3 June 1958; EL to Craine, 1 Feb. 1963, Kemper House Folder, ELP.

15. *Indianapolis News,* 7 Dec. 1940.

16. EL to Maxfield Parrish, 18 June 1962, XBLl. Lilly bought the Parrish paintings two years before the artist's "revival" by New York critics. *New York Times,* 3 June 1964.

17. George H. A. Clowes to EL, 12 Dec. 1945, Chinese Art Folder, ELP; Invoices, C. T. Loo & Co., 18 Mar., 23 May 1947, ibid.; EL to Loo, 5, 23 May 1947, Loo to EL, 9 May, 15 Oct. 1947, 8 Oct. 1948, ibid.; EL, "Reminiscences."

18. Yutaka Mino and James Robinson, *Beauty and Tranquility: The Eli Lilly Collection of Chinese Art* (Indianapolis: Indianapolis Museum of Art, 1983), 7. See also Gene E. McCormick, "Origins of the Lilly Collection of Chinese Art," ibid., 9-12; and Yutaka Mino, "The Indianapolis Museum of Art: The Oriental Collection," *Arts of Asia* 11 (Mar.-Apr. 1981): 73-137.

19. K. K. Chen to EL, 21 Mar. 1949, Chinese Art Folder, ELP; *Indianapolis Times,* 9 July 1949; *Indianapolis Star Magazine,* 9 Oct. 1983, p. 29; EL, "Reminiscences."

20. EL to Loo, 23 Feb. 1948, Chinese Art Folder, ELP. See also EL, "Reminiscences"; EL, "Items at Home," n.d., Chinese Art Folder, ELP.

21. EL to Wilbur Peat, 29 Jan. 1960, Indianapolis Museum of Art Folder, ELP. The total price Lilly paid for the objects donated was $274,823.50. Peat to EL, 5 Feb. 1960, ibid.

22. EL, "Reminiscences"; Chen to EL, 13 June 1950, Shen Ho Shi Folder, ELP; Benjamin L. Jessup, "Eli Lilly and Conner Prairie" (M.A. thesis, Ball State University, 1987), 72-75; *Indianapolis News,* 24 Nov. 1962; *Indianapolis Star,* 15 May 1983. I am grateful to Esther Linenberger for showing me through the Chinese house. The house was given to Earlham College along with the Conner Prairie gift and was later used for meetings and small conferences.

23. EL to Loo, 8 Mar. 1948, Chinese Art Folder, ELP.

24. EL, "Reminiscences." See also F. S. C. Northrop, *The Meeting of East and West: An Inquiry Concerning World Understanding* (New York: Macmillan, 1946). Lilly's marked copy remains in the Sunset Lane library. See also McCormick, "Origins of the Lilly Collection of Chinese Art," 9-10; Lilly's notes in Miscellaneous Cabinet 1 from his reading of Laurence Binyon, *Painting in the Far East: An Introduction to the History of Pictorial Art in Asia Especially China and Japan* (London: Edward Arnold, 1908).

25. EL to Peat, 15 Sept. 1947, Indianapolis Museum of Art Folder, ELP. See also Lilly's notecards on Chinese art, Miscellaneous Cabinet 1.

26. *SuperVision* (Apr. 1947).

27. EL to Herman C. Krannert, 29 July 1970, Indianapolis Museum of Art Folder, ELP. See also, in this folder, EL to Krannert and Robert S. Ashby, 17 Apr. 1961, EL to Art Association of Indianapolis, 16 Jan. 1967, Kurt F. Pantzer to EL, 20, 31 July, 2, 9, 17 Aug. 1967, EL to Pantzer, 27 Aug. 1967, John Rauch, Sr., to Pantzer, 12 Aug. 1967, Krannert to

EL, 25 Oct. 1967; John Rauch, Jr., interview with author, 4 May 1988; Robert A. Yassin, "The Indianapolis Museum of Art Celebrates the Extraordinary in Its Centennial Year," 1983, typescript in author's possession; Carl J. Weinhardt, Jr., interview with author, 16 Jan. 1986.

28. Carl J. Weinhardt, Jr., "Memories of Eli Lilly," 8 Feb. 1977, p. 3, typescript in author's possession.

29. EL to Pantzer, 13 Sept. 1968, Indianapolis Museum of Art Folder, ELP.

30. EL to Eugene N. Beesley, Burton E. Beck, and Henry F. DeBoest, 10 Mar. 1971, Indianapolis Museum of Art Folder, ELP. In 1970 Lilly also contributed $675,250 so that six French impressionist paintings could be transferred to the museum and, more important, so that he could quietly help a friend in difficult financial circumstance. EL to Richard C. Lockton, n.d., ibid.; Weinhardt, interview with author.

31. EL to Beelsey, Beck, and DeBoest, 10 Mar. 1971, Indianapolis Museum of Art Folder, ibid.

32. EL to Weinhardt, 24 Apr. 1972, ibid. See also *Indianapolis Collects: Contemporary Art* (Indianapolis: Indianapolis Museum of Art, 1972); Weinhardt, "Memories of Eli Lilly," 6-7.

33. Weinhardt, "Memories of Eli Lilly," 2, 5; Weinhardt, interview with author; Joseph T. Butler, "Watches from Five Centuries: The Ruth Allison Lilly Collection," *Connoisseur* 184 (Dec. 1973): 279-83. In 1973 Eli and Ruth Lilly contributed $43,200 to the museum to purchase an Indianapolis street scene, painted in the 1890s by Theodore Groll and titled "West Washington Street." Lilly asked that the label for the painting read "Given by a couple of old Hoosiers."

34. EL to Byron K. Trippet, 25 Feb. 1957, EL Folder, Trippet Papers, Wabash College Archives; *Lilly Review,* 25 Jan. 1977, p. 4; Anita Martin, interview with author, 5 May 1988.

35. Beesley, memorandum, 12 Nov. 1952, Organizational Changes, 1952, XCAo; JKL, Jr., memorandum, 14 Nov. 1952, ibid.; Gene E. McCormick, "A History of Eli Lilly and Company," typescript, 1975, chapter 12, pp. 131-32.

36. William R. Spurlock, interview with McCormick, 9 Aug. 1968, pp. 81-82, Drawer 1, Cabinet 3, Company History Files; EL to Beesley, 22 Sept. 1961, 2 Nov. 1960, 29 Jan. 1965, Beesley Folder, ELP; Beesley to JKL, Jr., 13 July 1960, Beesley Folder, ELP; EL, "Notes on Research," 23 Jan. 1969, Research Folder, Drawer 1, Cabinet 8, Company History Files; EL to Richard D. Wood et al., 14 June 1974, C Miscellaneous Folder, ELP; Richard D. Wood, interview with author, 5 May 1988.

37. EL to McCormick, 26 Feb. 1969, 31 Aug. 1972, Lilly Company History Folder, ELP; McCormick to EL, 30 June 1966, ibid.; McCormick, interview with author.

38. J. C. Fisher, "Basic Research in Industry," *Science* 129 (19 June 1959): 1653-54. The survey was based on publications abstracted in *Chemical Abstracts* in 1955. Only one pharmaceutical company, Merck, was ahead of Eli Lilly and Company on the list.

39. Leonard Gerald Schifrin, "The Ethical Drug Industry: Practices and Performance" (Ph.D. diss., University of Michigan, 1964), 112, 138; W. Duncan Reekie, *The Economics of the Pharmaceutical Industry* (London: Macmillan, 1975), 33-34; Nicholas N. Noyes to EL, 22 June 1960, Noyes Folder, ELP.

40. *Indianapolis News,* 17 July 1967.

41. See Remington Medalist Scrapbook, XBLl, especially EL, "Remington Honor Medal Acceptance Address," 10 Dec. 1958, EL to L. V. Clemente, 12 Sept. 1958, and Beesley to EL, 19 Dec. 1958.

42. EL, "Remington Honor Medal Acceptance Address."

43. EL to Black, 20 May 1955, Black Papers, Black Laboratory; Kenneth Hartman, interview with McCormick, 10 Dec. 1971, Drawer 2, Cabinet 3, Company History Files; E. J. Kahn, Jr., *All in a Century: The First 100 Years of Eli Lilly and Company* ([Indianapolis: Eli Lilly and Co., 1976]), 160-65.

44. EL to Allen L. McGill, 13 May 1958, McGill Folder, ELP.

45. Thomas E. Dewey to EL, 8 Dec. 1959, D Miscellaneous Folder, ELP; *New York Times,* 1 Dec. 1959.

46. Louis Lasagna, "1938-1968: The FDA, the Drug Industry, the Medical Profession, and the Public," in *Safeguarding the Public: Historical Aspects of Medicinal Drug Control,* ed. John B. Blake (Baltimore: Johns Hopkins University Press, 1970), 171-73; Peter Temin, *Taking Your Medicine: Drug Regulation in the United States* (Cambridge, Mass.: Harvard University Press, 1980), 81-82, 120-26; Glenn Sonnedecker, *Kremers and Urdang's History of Pharmacy,* 4th ed. rev. (Philadelphia: J. B. Lippincott Co., 1976), 222; *Indianapolis Star,* 15 Sept. 1960; Beesley to EL, 3 Aug. 1960, Wholesale System Folder, ELP.

47. EL to Sloane Graff, 16 Oct. 1961, Graff Folder, ELP.

48. EL to Sloane Graff, 3 June 1963, ibid. See also Beesley to EL, 3 Aug. 1960, Wholesale System Folder, ibid.; Kahn, *All in a Century,* 166-67; Eva Rice Goble to EL, 8 July 1963, I Miscellaneous Folder, ELP.

49. Pantzer to EL, 12 Sept. 1959, Pantzer Folder, ELP; EL to Thomas C. Hasbrook, 10 Sept. 1973, Political Contributions Folder, ELP; EL to Ristine, 12 June 1964, Political Contributions Folder, ELP.

50. EL to Sloane Graff, 9 Sept. 1949, Graff Folder, ELP. See also McCormick, "History of Eli Lilly and Company," chapter 12, pp. 216-17. Lilly assumed that Great Britain's new health care system was funded in part by American postwar aid.

51. EL to Sloane Graff, 11 Apr. 1952, Graff Folder, ELP.

52. EL, diary of trip, 22 June 1957, Miscellaneous Cabinet 4.

53. Sloane Graff to EL, [?] May 1952, Graff Folder, ELP, with Lilly's marginal comments.

54. J. J. Wuerthner, Jr., *The Businessman's Guide to Practical Politics* (Chicago: Regnery Co., 1959). Lilly's heavily underlined copy is in the Eli Lilly Room, Lilly Center.

55. Barry Goldwater, *The Conscience of a Conservative* (Shepherdsville, Ky.: Victor Publishing Co., 1960); McCormick, "History of Eli Lilly and Company," chapter 12, pp. 219-20.

56. EL to McCormick, 21 Aug. 1967, Facilities Improvement Folder, Drawer 4, Cabinet 5, Company History Files.

57. EL to Sloane Graff, 4 Nov. 1964, Graff Folder, ELP.

58. EL to Gerald R. Ford, 30 Aug. 1967, Political Contributions Folder, ibid.

59. EL to Sloane Graff, 23 Nov. 1966, Graff Folder, ibid.; EL to Roger D. Branigin, 17 Mar. 1965, Branigin Folder, ibid.

60. Branigin to EL, 21 May 1968, 16 Jan. 1971; EL to Branigin, [May 1968], 20 Jan. 1971,

Branigin Folder, ibid.; Roger D. Branigin, Journal, 8 Apr. 1968, Branigin Papers, Franklin College Library, Franklin, Indiana. I am grateful to James E. Farmer for this last reference.

61. EL, untitled poem, 1 Apr. 1975, Anita Martin Personal Papers, copy in author's possession; Martin, interview with author; Byron P. Hollett, interview with author, 24 Sept. 1985.

62. EL to Allen W. Clowes, 5 Mar. 1973, Clowes Memorial Hall Folder, ELP. There had long been a good deal of squabbling among the city's leading citizens over Clowes Hall. See EL, "Notes on Meeting with Harry Ice," 28 Mar. 1966; Ice to EL, [?] Jan. 1965; Krannert to Allen W. Clowes, 5 Jan. 1965, all in ibid.

63. EL to McGill, 5 Oct. 1973, McGill Folder, ELP.

64. EL to Peckham, 3 Sept. 1971, Peckham Folder, ibid. See also EL to Frederick Appel, 20 Feb. 1973, A Miscellaneous Folder, ibid.

65. Weinhardt, "Memories of Eli Lilly," 1.

66. *Syracuse* (Ind.) *Mail-Journal,* 26 Jan. 1977; Peter R. Lawson, interview with author, 19 Sept. 1987; Landrum R. Bolling, interview with author, 28 Mar. 1988.

67. Byron K. Trippet, *Wabash on My Mind* (Crawfordsville, Ind.: Wabash College, 1982), 222.

68. J. K. Lilly III, interview with author, 4 Sept. 1986; Evelyn Fortune Lilly Bartlett, interview with author, 15, 16 Jan. 1986; Rauch, Jr., interview with author; Rauch, Jr., to author, 10 May 1988; EL, Deed of Gift, 6 Nov. 1958, Miscellaneous Legal Records, Vault; *Indianapolis News,* 8 Apr. 1982; Evie Lilly Lutz to EL, 11 Mar. 1970, Lutz Folder, ELP; EL, diary, 6 Jan. 1956, XBL1. The pottery plates Evie made are in the Lilly Archives.

69. Rauch, Jr., interview with author; EL to Rauch, Sr., 8 July 1970, Rauch Folder, ELP; Rauch, Sr., to EL, 11 July 1970, ibid.; Hollett, interview with author.

70. EL to Rauch, Sr., 8 July 1970, Rauch Folder, ELP. Lilly sent a copy of this letter to Herbert Lutz, along with a warm invitation to visit at Sunset Lane. EL to Lutz, 8 July 1970, ibid.

71. Declaration of Family Accord, 6 May 1970, Miscellaneous Legal Records, Vault; In the Matter of the Trust Treated U/A Josiah K. Lilly: Final Settlement Documents, 23 Apr. 1973, ibid.; Memoranda, n.d., ibid.; Hollett, interview with author; C. H. Bradley, Jr., to EL, 12 Nov. 1973, Lutz Folder, ELP; Beesley to EL, 9 Mar. 1971, Lutz Folder, ELP; Contributions, 1973, Contributions Folder, ELP. These trusts involved a tangle of complications, including Ruth and Eli Lilly, Evie, and her issue.

72. Hollett, interview with author. The friendship between Lilly and the senior Rauch never resumed after this split. Rauch wrote a memoir that apparently includes his side of the story. He deposited copies in several libraries, including the Indiana State Library, but the memoir is not available until 2000. Presumably Rauch did not tell Lilly of the adoption because of his son's obligation to respect Evie's wishes.

73. EL to H. Roll McLaughlin, 13 Dec. 1972, Historic Landmarks Foundation Folder, ELP. See also EL to Charles Best, 28 Sept. 1971, Best Folder, ELP; J. K. Lilly III, interview with author; Bolling, interview with author; Peckham, interview with author; Martin, interview with author; *Indianapolis News,* 14 Mar. 1973. Typical was Hollett's assessment of the marriage: "I never saw a couple more devoted to each other." Hollett, interview with author.

74. Martin, interview with author; Black to EL, 23 Sept. 1935, Black Folder, EL Papers,

Black Laboratory; Goble to Black, 19 June 1947, Black Folder, ELP; EL to Donald B. Davidson, 31 Jan. 1966, Davidson Folder, ELP; EL to Rowdy Revelers, 15 Mar. 1956, XBLl; EL to Florence B. Kirby, 28 Sept. 1959, Kirby Folder, ELP.

75. EL to Mary Louise Graff, 14 July 1975, Graff Folder, ELP.

76. *Indianapolis Star,* 13 Mar. 1966.

77. Ibid., 30 May 1978.

78. EL to Appel, 2 Jan. 1974, A Miscellaneous Folder, ELP; Martin, interview with author.

79. EL to Best, 3 Feb. 1975, Best Folder, ELP. See also Herman B Wells, interview with author, 30 Oct. 1984; Charles Webb, interview with author, 21 June 1988; Bolling, interview with author; Peckham, interview with author; Ristine, interview with author; *Indianapolis News,* 28 Sept. 1976. Madeline Fortune Elder, sister of Evelyn Fortune Lilly Bartlett and a good friend of Lilly's, stopped at Sunset Lane to extend good wishes on Christmas day after Ruth's death and found Lilly spending the holiday alone. She made sure that the next several Christmases he spent with her family. Madeline Fortune Elder, interview with author, 11 Dec. 1985.

80. EL to McGill, 10 Mar. 1967, McGill Folder, ELP. See also Martin, interview with author.

81. EL to Frank E. Stevens, 30 May 1973, Stevens Folder, ELP.

82. EL to Mary Louise Graff, 14 July 1975, Graff Folder, ibid.

83. EL to Ruth Lilly Van Riper, 3 May 1968, Van Riper Folder, ibid. The coins of J. K. Lilly, Jr., were given to the Smithsonian Institution, in return for which Congress passed a special bill reducing some of the taxes on the estate. See also EL to Wright Patman, 30 Oct. 1967, JKL, Jr., Estate Folder, ibid. The combined value of the net assets of the estate of J. K. Lilly, Jr., and his wife was $69,636,841, on which state and federal taxes totaled $48,978,316.

84. Warranty Deed, 14 Apr. 1965, Apple Farm Folder, ibid. The Lilly brothers had lost money on the orchard but held it for sentimental reasons, since it was their father's special joy. EL to JKL, Jr., 2 Oct. 1952, ibid.

85. EL to Eli Lilly III et al., 25 Jan. 1968, Hollett Folder, ibid.

86. EL to Mrs. George L. Denny, 8 Oct. 1973, Miscellaneous Folder, ELP. In 1976 Lilly added a codicil to his will to set up a trust of $1 million to pay taxes and maintenance costs on the Wawasee property. Seventh Codicil to the Last Will and Testament of Eli Lilly, 4 June 1976, EL Folder, ELP.

87. Herman B Wells to EL, 9 Dec. 1971, Indiana University Folder, ELP; Wells, interview with author.

88. EL to Rauch, Sr., 30 Dec. 1959, Rauch Folder, ELP; C. H. Bradley, Jr., to EL, 14 Feb. 1968, Stock Notebook, Vault.

89. EL to Bolling, 8 Mar. 1968, Conner Prairie/Earlham College Folder, ELP.

90. EL to Rauch, Sr., 14 Feb. 1966, 22 Jan. 1968, Folder 3, Box A, 1, EL Legal Records, Vault; EL, undated handwritten notes, ibid.; EL to Rauch, Sr., 12 Jan. 1967, Rauch Folder, ELP; EL to Rauch, Sr., Van Riper Folder, ELP.

91. EL to Best, 28 Sept. 1971, Best Folder, ELP.

92. EL to Harry T. Ice, 20 Nov. 1974, Butler University Folder, ibid.

93. EL to Alexander E. Jones, 13 Nov. 1967, Butler University Folder, ibid.

94. Bolling, interview with author; H. Roll McLaughlin, interview with author, 18 June 1987; Weinhardt, interview with author.

95. EL to Craine, 29 Sept. 1975, Craine Folder, ELP. He made exceptions, continuing large gifts to favorite institutions such as the Indiana Historical Society in 1973, and giving $1 million to the Society for the Preservation of Maryland Antiquities to restore and maintain the old Ridgely family home in Towson, Maryland. EL to George T. Harrison, 13 Oct. 1973, Hampton, Old Ridgely Home Folder, ELP.

96. Last Will and Testament of Eli Lilly, 29 May 1973, EL Folder, ELP; Merchants National Bank & Trust Company of Indianapolis, "In the Matter of the Estate of Eli Lilly, Deceased," Estate Docket E77-139, copy in EL Folder, Historic Landmarks Foundation Office, Indianapolis.

97. Ibid.

98. Ibid.

99. *Indianapolis Star,* 25 Jan. 1977; *Indianapolis News,* 2 Feb. 1977.

100. Bolling, interview with author; Ristine, interview with author; McLaughlin, interview with author.

101. EL to Wood, 29 May 1974, Wood Folder, ELP.

102. EL to Mary Louise Graff, 7 Apr. 1975, Graff Folder, ELP.

103. James M. Cornelius, interview with author, 13 Apr. 1988; Wood, interview with author.

104. Martin, interview with author; Eugene L. Step to EL, 13 Dec. 1976, Wholesalers Folder, ELP.

105. EL to Hollett, 8 Mar. 1974, Anita Martin Personal Papers, copy in author's possession; Hollett, interview with author; Martin, interview with author; Roger S. Gray, interview with author, 18 Jan. 1988. By the mid-1970s the Episcopal Church was using a new prayer book. In specifying that the 1928 prayer book be used at his funeral, Lilly indicated his preference for the traditional theology and Elizabethan English ritual that he had known for most of his adult life.

Note on Sources

The major sources for this book are located at the Lilly Archives, Lilly Center, Eli Lilly and Company, Indianapolis. The Eli Lilly Papers, abbreviated here as ELP, constitute the most important collection. They are especially rich for the last three decades of his life. Essential also are papers of other family members and the records of the business itself. At the Lilly Archives also are the Company History Files, consisting of original and photocopied material gathered by R. C. Buley and Gene E. McCormick in the 1960s and 1970s. Also in these files are dozens of oral history transcripts, most with retired company employees. Buley and McCormick drafted a manuscript history of the company up to 1932, which also includes biographical chapters on Colonel Eli Lilly, his son, and grandsons. The pioneering but unfinished work of these two scholars has been very helpful. There is no good published history of Eli Lilly and Company. Both E. J. Kahn, Jr., *All in a Century: The First 100 Years of Eli Lilly and Company* (1976) and Roscoe Collins Clark, *Threescore Years and Ten: A Narrative of the First Seventy Years of Eli Lilly and Company 1876-1946* (1946) were published by the company as public relations efforts. They have slight substance.

Other important archival materials are found at Wabash College, Earlham College, Conner Prairie, and the Indiana Historical Society. Especially useful are the papers at the Glenn A. Black Laboratory of Archaeology at Indiana University, Bloomington, which include Black's files and Eli Lilly's archaeological correspondence. At the Indiana Division, Indiana State Library, are the Records of Christ Church Cathedral and the Episcopal Diocese of Indianapolis.

Oral interviews provided information and understanding not available in the written record. Listed below are the interviews done by the author. Those marked with * were conducted by telephone. All others were in-person interviews.

Lucy W. Barber, 19 Apr. 1988*
Evelyn Fortune Lilly Bartlett, 15, 16 Jan. 1986
Landrum R. Bolling, 28 Mar. 1988
Theodore Bowie, 19 June 1987*
Allen Clowes, 11 Nov. 1988
Mildred Compton, 31 Oct. 1988*
James B. Cope, 24 June 1987
James M. Cornelius, 13 Apr. 1988
Madeline Fortune Elder, 11 Dec. 1985
Roger S. Gray, 18 Jan. 1988
James B. Griffin, 26 Dec. 1986
Hubert H. Hawkins, 13 Feb. 1987
Byron P. Hollett, 24 Sept. 1985
John C. Householder, 5 Dec. 1986
Sam Jones, 28 Mar. 1988
James H. Kellar, 27 Aug. 1986
Thomas H. Lake, 27 Aug. 1987
Peter R. Lawson, 19 Sept. 1987
J. K. Lilly III, 4 Sept. 1986
Esther Linenberger, 16 June 1987
John S. Lynn, 5 May 1988
Gene E. McCormick, 2 May 1988
H. Roll McLaughlin, 18 June 1987
Anita Martin, 5 May 1988
Frances Martin, 7 June 1986
Virginia Minton, 13 Jan. 1988*
Paul Moore, Jr., 20 Sept. 1987
C. Ellis Nelson, 12 Apr. 1988*
Waldemar A. Nielsen, 7 Apr. 1988*
Manning M. Pattillo, 6 June 1988*
John H. Peatling, 19 Apr. 1988*

Howard and Dorothy Peckham, 2 Aug. 1985
John G. Rauch, Jr., 4 May 1988
Robert H. Rhodehamel, 18 July, 8 Dec. 1986
Richard O. Ristine, 27 Apr. 1988
Gayle Thornbrough, 16 Dec. 1986
Earl D. Wallace, 4 Oct. 1985
Charles Webb, 21 June 1988*
Fredrick and Margaret Weber, 12 Jan. 1988
Carl J. Weinhardt, Jr., 16 Jan. 1986
Herman B Wells, 30 Oct. 1984
Frederic P. Williams, 18 Jan. 1988
Richard D. Wood, 5 May 1988

Index

Designer: David Stahl
Typeface: Berkeley Oldstyle
Typographer: Weimer Typesetting Co., Inc., Indianapolis, Indiana
Paper: 70-pound Glatfelter B-16
Printer: Malloy Lithographing, Inc., Ann Arbor, Michigan

DATE DUE

APR 3 0 1990			

HIGHSMITH   # 45220